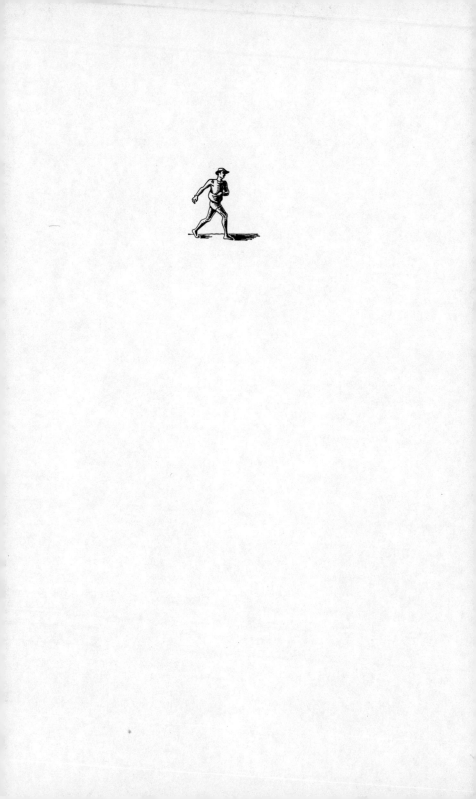

THE BIRTH OF
NEUROSIS

Myth, Malady, and the Victorians

by
George Frederick Drinka, M.D.

SIMON AND SCHUSTER   NEW YORK

Copyright © 1984 by George Frederick Drinka
All rights reserved
including the right of reproduction
in whole or in part in any form
Published by Simon and Schuster
A Division of Gulf & Western Corporation
Simon & Schuster Building
Rockefeller Center
1230 Avenue of the Americas
New York, New York 10020
SIMON AND SCHUSTER and colophon
are registered trademarks of Simon & Schuster.
Designed by Eve Kirch
Manufactured in the United States of America

1 3 5 7 9 10 8 6 4 2

Library of Congress Cataloging in Publication Data
Drinka, George Frederick.
The birth of neurosis.
Bibliography: p.
Includes index.
1. Psychiatry—Europe—History—19th century.
2. Neuroses—Europe—History—19th century. 3. Medi-
cine—Europe—History—19th century. 4. Authors,
European—Psychology. I. Title.
RC339.E85D75   1984   616.85′2′0094   84-10563
ISBN 0-671-44999-0

(Continued after Index)

ACKNOWLEDGMENTS

Straightway, let me thank both A. C. Crombie of Trinity College and G. J. Warnock of Hertford College for granting me a place at Oxford University and giving me supervision as a graduate student from 1973–76. Without those years in England away from the bustle of medical training and practice in America, I would never have had an opportunity to read widely in modern history and literature and try my hand at writing in an organized manner. I would also like to acknowledge Dr. Robert Arnstein and especially Dr. Rosemary Balsam at the Yale University Health Plan for encouraging me to take up again my interest in writing a historical work. It was Dr. Balsam who, upon hearing a paper I delivered on medical history in 1980, put me in touch with the people at Simon and Schuster. Also, I would like to thank Dr. Julia Frank of Yale who did a masterful editing job on a very early version of my book.

The historical librarian at Yale, Susan Alon, and her counterpart at Harvard, Déla Zitkus, deserve many thanks for their work in arranging for me to read the wares of the respective libraries. Ms. Zitkus was of great service in helping me to develop ideas regarding illustrations. I want to express my gratitude to Drs. Bill Beardslee, Dave DeMaso and Jim Herzog of Boston Children's Hospital and the Harvard Medical School, who shaped my schedule in the years 1982 and '83 so that my clinical responsibilities did not inundate me. Special thanks go to Drs. Ken Levin and Gordon Harper for reading progressively later versions of the manuscript. Dr. Levin's remarks were both thought-provoking and encouraging, and those of Dr. Harper were edifying and elucidating on many levels.

Let me communicate my thanks to Fred Miller and his crew of assistants who, with great dispatch and precision, typed and retyped the manuscript.

Finally, and most importantly, let me thank my dear wife, Barbara (enigmatically known as Lady Throckmorton), for her untiring love and care of me, and wise counsel to me, while I was poring single-mindedly over the pages that follow.

For Lady Throckmorton

CONTENTS

PREFACE

We of the late twentieth century commonly look back with some envy on our forebears the Victorians. In the times before Einstein, before Picasso, before Freud, the world must have seemed more whole, more knitted together in an orderly fabric. Absolutes held sway in a manner we can barely imagine today. Heroism, will power, patriotism, womanhood were ideals to which every honest human aspired.

This book sets out to reconstruct an unexpected piece of that lost world of nineteenth-century Europe and America. Using the illness category of neurosis as the template and the doctors, patients, and theories as the material, the pages that follow will refurbish an unexplored aspect of the sensibility of that age. Because of some striking similarities in moral attitudes among the rising middle classes throughout the West, as well as the forms of their neuroses, the word "Victorian" seems apropos to describe not just the sensibility and the neuroses of Britain under Victoria but also those of America and the rest of Europe. To be sure, the sufferings of Victorian neurotics were all too human, timeless, but the forms of the illnesses—the passionate hysterical fits, the God-forsaken sexual perversions, the languishing nervous exhaustions —are bound to their era. They expose to the reader a compelling dark side of the sensibility of the age. The neurotic anguish of many private citizens in the Victorian West was probably the price paid for adhering to such stringent ideas regarding manhood and womanhood, will power and spineless sinfulness.

In perusing this work one quickly discovers the musty language of the Victorian doctors and patients. Like scents from an old wardrobe, the old medical terms themselves—"frayed nerves," "delicate women," "languid tuberculars," "inspired epileptics"— have a deep, almost wistful odor. It is possible to linger over this language, savoring the wish that one could suffer with this or that romantic illness oneself.

What we discover from a closer study of the Victorian language, however, is surprising: that the Victorians called neurotic many, many illnesses that today are understood to have physical, not psychological, underpinnings. Most "neuroses" were thought to stem from weak and delicate nerves, literally stretched or lax, overworked or overexcited. It was only as the Victorian period waned that the question of psychological causation became more central to medical thinking, precisely during the years when genuine physical illnesses were being delineated as discrete medical disorders.

In penetrating behind the language one discovers a collection of forgotten myths residing in the theories about how a neurosis is born. These myths embody many Victorian fears, prejudices, and fantasies. Once brought to light, the myths cannot fail to intrigue and even amuse. The Onan myth, for instance, preached the enervating evils of masturbation; the Noble Savage myth emphasized the nerve-corroding glamour of the burgeoning modern city; and the Degenerate myth posited the notion of a nervous taint, a kind of original sin in the nerves, passed from debauched father to opium-loving son to weak-brained grandson, the last descendant inevitably expiring as a driveling idiot in an asylum. These and all the other myths illustrate the near-literary feel of Victorian medical attitudes toward nervous illnesses. The Victorians, of course, never named these myths, rarely even saw their curious notions of causation as anything but facts of nature. Yet the outlines of these myths are now clearly visible, and they can be lifted whole from the vast store of Victorian treatises on neuroses.

Certainly each myth contains a misguided fantasy but also a fragment of truth. Out of the patchwork of these myths one can reconstruct a Victorian vision of mental illness and human potential. This vision proves compelling, perhaps even believable, in its own right. Though we moderns would like to deny the inevitability of heredity and imagine the individual and his environment as infinitely malleable, the Victorians could never forget the organic absolutes of human nature. Much knowledge involving heredity, the nervous system, and nearly every organ of the human body still lies wrapped in mind-tickling riddles that man may forever try vainly to decipher.

The Birth of Neurosis

ONE

The Age of Nerves:
A Victorian Fantasy

ONE summer day in 1872, when the distant siege of Paris—Prussian monarchists fighting French Communards—was still an agitating memory, a young American was resting in Switzerland. Staying at a country inn nestled on a mountain ledge, the man opened the shutters of his window to discover a rolling valley spreading out before him. Elated by this vision, he wandered to a nearby cliff and there let his eyes run wild over the crests of greens and auburns, the crops and trees, the sheds and cottages below. Contemplating the distant beauty of Mont Blanc, he lost himself in lovely reveries on art. He imagined himself a painter, living in the revolutionary hubbub of Paris, starving in a garret, joyous in his bohemianism.

He sighed to himself, thinking of Jean-Jacques Rousseau, who was drawn to the French culture beyond the Alps, yet worshiped nature. Rousseau, who idealized the Noble Savage embodied in the American Indian, yet never left old Europe. Rousseau, the darling of the French nobility but, in his rarefied ideas, a precursor of the communists. Culture, nature; Europe, America; monarchists, Communards. The tossing back and forth, to and fro, of these thoughts and worries and confusions soon spilled into a maddening stab of fear. A single urge nagged at the young American time and again: to jump to his death, to leap from the precipice and dash the brains out of his skull. Soon his head was aching miserably, his chest becoming tense. He was overcome with one of his vertiginous fits. The mountains reeled and the valley was bled of its colors. He nearly fainted on that cliff, nearly was pulled downward to his death.

Then he heard voices, or simply the edges of words. He wondered if these disembodied voices meant he was a victim of madness, another recurring worry of his. Still the voices recurred, grew more powerful, too real to be figments of his twisted thinking. He turned to see a young couple walking toward him, speaking softly. He recognized his own Boston accent in their tones and listened with astonished attention. Surely they were newlyweds, our unhappy man surmised. The man's deferential treatment of the woman, the way she leaned so clingingly on him, all suggested this attachment of sympathies. They drew closer and looked in his direction. He started with a spark of recognition: it was Alice James and her doting brother Henry, here in Switzerland.

He was acquainted with them through their parents. Their mother was friendly with his sister; both were members of a sewing society from the American Civil War days. His father and theirs were quite closely connected. Both were Princeton men who had spent hour upon hour in their college days, chambered together, discussing philosophy and the great beyond. Though the connection was solid enough, the young sufferer, whom we shall call K., trembled an instant, afraid to approach the sauntering pair. His old fear of appearing awkward in public paralyzed him. Yet Henry recognized him and drew closer, offering his hand with a slight bow. As Alice, wearing milk-white gloves and a halolike bonnet, stood aloof, barely facing him, then turning away, K. had a brief but vivid fantasy of adoring this cool-mannered woman for as long as he lived. His image of her as his obedient wife and the mother of their pack of children, put on a pedestal and worshiped, was a painful, twisted sensation that tore through his brain like fire, like electrical sparks.

K. composed himself, however, smoothing his woolen trousers, pulling at his striped suspenders. The three soon walked to the inn, exchanging news and awkward conversation. K. knew through his mother's letters that Henry had had headaches of his own, that Alice had suffered nervous prostration and had come to

Switzerland for the travel cure with Brother Harry. Of course K. was polite enough not to mention these problems. If his years at Harvard had instilled anything in him, it was good breeding. Nonetheless he felt a great deal of sympathy for both of them, since he sensed that he had fallen in with two other pain-ridden victims of nerves.

Henry spoke warmly of his love of European culture, of the joys of visiting London, Paris, and Venice, with their sumptuous galleries. K. grew sure that Henry's months in London and on the Continent had done wonders for his nervous system. As the three sat eating ratatouille in the old Swiss inn, K. envied Henry's pink cheeks, and he wished that his own doctor's prescriptions for long draughts of Europe had cured him as well as such dosage seemed to have cured Henry James.

K. was an educated man, but his doctors said he had probably read the wrong books. He was also told he lacked will power. His father had destined him at an early age for the ministry, but even as a youth he had preferred reading, underneath his bedclothes, biographies of the great masters of art. Though he never would like the writings of Henry James, finding his novels too verbose, K. admired him for throwing over his law studies and setting off for Europe with a purpose. Coming for a rest, Henry had lingered to write. Poor K. himself was in Europe to recuperate and return to the Divinity School at Harvard to complete his course to become a minister. But every day he rested, he found himself wanting never to go home, wishing to set off for Paris, forswear the ministry, and become a follower of Corot, of Courbet, of anyone French. But he lacked the will.

Though Alice retired early that night, pleading an indisposition, K. spoke with Henry James well into the wee hours. The two men discussed their mutual love of the great masters of Europe, and K.'s eyes widened like those of a man seeing the divinity as he imagined the richness of the Titians in Venice, the vibrant Raphaels in Florence, paintings that James brought alive with his words.

Yet K. always paid for the delight of such conversations. The next morning proved distressful; his head and body had descended into a sea of despondency and self-disgust. He felt like a man recovering from an alcoholic debauch, in ecstasy the night before, in anguish over his ecstasy the morning after. He shunned the company of the Jameses thereafter and soon departed from the inn and returned to America.

The next few years were painful for the debilitated K. Though he returned to the Divinity School in Cambridge and plodded through the courses one by one on his way to a degree, each summer found him on the verge of a nervous collapse. He would then journey to Europe in the dog days of summer and make the rounds of the spas, Marienbad and Teplitz in Bohemia, Vichy in the south of France, Bath in England. Sometimes, partially rejuvenated, he would return to Cambridge in the fall. Other years he would linger in Europe until the spring. So life tottered along for the next few years.

In fall 1879, shortly after acquiring his degree and taking his orders, the Reverend K. suffered a new breakdown, an attack of palpitations, flushing, and blushing beyond compare. This was a serious case of nervous prostration, and he lay in his bed in Cambridge pampered by his mother and his sister, moaning and trying to be idle. Every noise, every creak or jarring in the house filled him with an awful quaking and shaking. Any light would set his head to throbbing. The drop of a pin could send him shuddering. His family walked about on tiptoe. Though his doctors had forbidden him to read—fearing overexcitation—K. coaxed his sister into smuggling popular magazines into his sickroom. So it came to pass that one day he discovered a ray of hope.

This hope appeared in the form of an article in the *Atlantic Monthly* for June 1879. Its author was Dr. George Miller Beard of New York City, the popularizer of thinking about nervous exhaustion, or neurasthenia, its title was "The Physical Future of the American People," and its argument was compelling. Perceiving Americans as an ever evolving and therefore excessively nervous race, Dr. Beard attributed much of American nervosity to the dryness of the climate as well as to the rapid changes in season— painfully hot summers to bitterly cold winters. This climate made the poor northeastern American more prone than the European to great surges of nervous output, which could lead to moments of great inventiveness as easily as horrible bouts of nervous prostration. Beard's cure was an obvious one: to buck up the old nerves. His work with the inventor Thomas Edison at Menlo Park had ignited in his mind an ingenious remedy: the use of electricity. Electricity coursed through the nerves, as every Victorian doctor knew, so if creativity and inventiveness, along with the American climate and civilization, were daily sapping draught upon draught of electricity from the nerves of many noble Americans, then a good shot of electrical current could work wonders. This was only too obvious, even to a layman like K.

K. saw both pent-up inventiveness and drooping nerves as the nidus of his own problem, and so, on the spur of the moment, he decided to set off for New York to see Beard. Unfortunately his symptoms were so severe, his palpitations and blushings so debilitating, that a consultation in New York City had to be put off for months. Though he still felt himself to be a veritable lightning rod for nervosity in the dryness of his sickroom, unable to do anything for more than a year but grow more nervous, K. was finally recovered enough by the early months of 1881 to journey to New York to consult Dr. Beard.

One hopeful spring day K. finally met this chatty doctor in his teeming waiting room on Madison Avenue. After waiting there a long time he was led into the consulting room. The hard-of-hearing Beard told him to sit and asked him questions loudly. The sensitive Reverend K. responded in kind, though he soon found the volume of his own voice nerve-shattering. Yes, he had been a victim of nocturnal emissions. Yes, his last few years he had been susceptible to onanism, an admission that brought on a fit of blushing. Yes, he should marry, that might help. Yes, he intended to take up his profession as soon as possible. Where? That was a difficult decision. It required will power.

After a painstakingly lengthy discussion, Beard shouted, "Let us try a treatment of tonic," and led the impatient K. into his treatment room. He asked K. to take a seat in a hard wooden chair and applied a cold metal cup to the back of his neck, another to a point not far from his umbilicus, his aching abdomen. The Reverend K. panted with admiration and fear. A lever was pressed. The patient sat transfixed, feeling the life-giving force of electricity running through him like life blood, like mother's milk, humming, tingling down his spine. Our young man could feel the fabulous wonders of this cure trembling in his very sinews, the muscles about his spine rising erect.

The Reverend K. returned to Beard's office on Madison Avenue for a total of twelve treatments in six weeks. He felt a renewed vigor. Admitting to Beard that his nocturnal emissions had stopped, he decided to apply for a vicarage in western Massachusetts at a Unitarian church and was even considering seeking a wife. He had two or three young women in mind, and the vision of Alice James shot through his soul. In late 1881 he strode down Madison Avenue clicking his heels, feeling as rich as Vanderbilt, as lively as Chicago. Filled with a newfound optimism and a sense of partaking in the glories of America's manifest destiny, he pounded his chest with delight.

In this exuberant state he made a decision, one that Beard had disparaged but that seemed to make great sense to K. at the time: to enjoy one last tour of Europe as part of a convalescence before taking up his vicarage. K. set sail from New York harbor on the *Hamburg* and cruised across the ocean in an armchair, playing only a little backgammon from time to time. His muscles and nerves had never felt so good! He had never relished the taste of kippers and sausage so much! The ship docked in Liverpool on a brilliant and delightful day. Sunlight splashed and dappled the dock, and he sketched the scene in his mind's eye. He made the trip by slow degrees from Liverpool to London, stopping at many airy wayside inns along the way. The world seemed better and brighter than he had ever known it to be. Then in London came the downfall. He would always think that it was one particular day that proved the turning point of his life.

Our young man was riding the fast train out of Charing Cross Station on his way to the West Country. He was admiring a brilliant sunset that reminded him of paintings by Turner, and a feeling surged through him, a mixture of both delight and regret. The train was proceeding toward Bristol when he suddenly was torn by deep doubts about his vocation. Was he really a minister of God? Even as he saw the depths of his doubts, a terrible and awful shock vibrated through the car, running through his very sinews. The train wobbled on its tracks. Passengers were thrown upon one another. There were screams and screeches. He even heard bones cracking, sinews snarling. The car toppled on its side, and the Reverend K. saw a young woman literally snapped in half by sheets of shattering glass. For an instant he saw his own death. Then he fainted.

He woke up in Guys Hospital, London, surrounded by a cadre of prim and proper gentlemen in long white coats who were taking his pulse and tapping at his knees and ankles with a hammer. A diagnosis of nervous shock was made by the doctors, and K. sank into a despondency beyond belief. The pall of moroseness was only made worse many months later when he heard, via a letter from his aging mother, of Dr. Beard's sudden and tragic death of pneumonia at age forty-two, in New York City.

The next year was perhaps the most desperately melancholic period in the Reverend K.'s life. He learned to walk again, but frequently he had dreams of a train running like a devil through his bedroom. He would wake up in a cold sweat, his clothes soaked through. That year and the following passed, with the young man suffering from a hysteroneurasthenia, prone to loss of feeling in his right arm and shoulder, with funny tingling sensations running up and down his thighs. For six months his field of vision narrowed and he could barely distinguish red from green. His headaches worsened, his backaches and stomach ailments grew unbearable.

Our young man gave up hope for nearly three years. He became a chronic invalid, wintering in Algeria, summering on Cape May, seeming to himself a lost man. His symptoms abated at times, but they could recur if he simply walked down a busy street in New York or London or Paris and heard the clanging of a streetcar. He came to wish that he had died in that train crash, for he was living an empty life.

Back in Boston, he renewed contact with the James family and soon took a passing interest in the work of Henry James's older brother, William. This man, a professor at Harvard, was just then experimenting on the subjects of trance states, séance, and automatic writing. The Reverend K. had long been convinced that he was a victim of self-induced trance states as he lay falling off to sleep. So he was attracted to James's work. After reading a few articles by William James, the Reverend K. became interested in the subject of hypnosis and was soon reading widely in this area.

K. learned that the luminary in the field was Professor Jean-Martin Charcot in Paris, so he eagerly read through his works. He also read the writings of Charcot's contemporaries and admirers, who were studying exhaustively the dual subjects of nervousness and hypnosis.

In 1887 the Reverend K. found himself in Paris. He was not there to paint but to seek a cure for his ailments. His hope mounted when he observed the latest panacea, hypnosis. As he sat in the amphitheater at Charcot's hospital, the Salpêtrière, he grew excited to see himself surrounded by such celebrities as Guy de Maupassant and Emile Zola, Sarah Bernhardt, and many eminent doctors, all hanging on Charcot's every word. The doctor described the illness of hysteria in vivid detail. Then, after using the wonders of projected slides and his own brilliant abilities to mimic his patients, he led his notorious female hysterical patients onto the floor of the amphitheater. Then, touching various areas on their bodies, he sent them into convulsions in front of his astonished audience. The young women were led from the hall to be hypnotized. Returning minutes later, they were reintroduced to the awestruck audience in a trance state, called somnambulism.

The Reverend K. was fascinated by the wonders of hypnosis. Soon he was applying to be examined by Charcot himself. He squandered many months in Paris waiting for the day when he would be led before the great doctor.

Charcot saw many of his patients in his own home, a magnificent structure on the Boulevard St. Germain, cluttered with medieval and Renaissance works. When the Reverend K. first entered Charcot's home, he thought for an instant that he was entering a church. He was filled with a sense of devotion, since many of the windows were stained glass, and the light took on deep tints of reds, blues, and greens as it pierced the glowing panes. The Reverend K.'s spirits lifted.

Charcot stood waiting in his examining room. A short, portly fellow, with a white mane combed back with a flourish, he greeted our hero with a "Bonjour. Asseyez-vous." Ordering the Reverend K. to undress, Charcot began to peer at him from various angles. K. felt that Charcot was looking deep into his very being. As his assistants tapped various reflex points and searched for areas without sensation and zones that would set off hysterical seizures,

Charcot questioned the Reverend K., in English, about the history of his neurosis. K. complained about memory problems and consulted a notebook to get the details straight. Charcot chuckled over this.

Then came the moment of truth. After being told to concentrate his attention on a distant brilliant light, K. passed into a light trance—although it was nothing even close to somnambulism. "Pas grande chose," said Charcot. The light was extinguished and the Reverend K. came to his senses.

Yes, he was a hysteric, said Charcot, but not a grand hysteric. What was he, then? A petit hysteric. Also "un homme de petits papiers," Charcot muttered—a man with little papers—namely, his notebook. Charcot chuckled again. The Reverend K. pleaded with the doctor to hypnotize him again and to make curative suggestions to him, but Charcot refused. When the Reverend K. entreated and nearly threw himself at the feet of the master, Charcot was adamant, stating that a man with petit hysteria could only be made worse by hypnosis, that hypnosis at this stage of his illness might lead to his becoming a grand hysteric. Such a change in the Reverend K.'s nervous condition might be permanently debilitating.

Charcot counseled the Reverend K. to visit spas in the south of France, where he could be given little doses of electricity, receive massages, and be wrapped in hot towels and lie in the sun for long periods of time. Though the Reverend K. still believed that hypnosis could cure his condition, he had so much faith in Charcot's diagnosis and prescriptions that he headed for Pyrmont, where he stayed through 1888.

Soon, however, the Reverend K. doubted that anything there would work. Yet he knew that such self-doubt was precisely his problem. He knew he was suggesting his own symptoms to himself and that somehow he must get himself out of such a state. So he went from one spa to another, one cure to another. Hot springs, cold springs, diets, hypodermic injections of nerve tissue from young animals, the Rest Cure of Doctor Weir Mitchell, even hypnosis: all of these were on the list of panaceas that he tried and that failed. He visited Karlsbad, Marienbad, Bath, Vichy—even Lourdes, he had to confess. But nothing seemed to work; there was always failure, always the recurrence of his contemptible symptoms, his pain, his fears, his urges. Never was he able to launch his career, to become a celebrated minister in the manner of Ralph Waldo Emerson.

Then at Teplitz, in Bohemia, the chronic aches turned into an acute fever of neurosis. It all began when he and a young Russian invalid prince were wading in a hot bath on a fine winter day. The two were exchanging tales of their search for their version of the Holy Grail, the cure, the moment of relief when they, like so many others of this period, would find ultimate health. After K. told the Russian prince of the train crash in 1882 and the lamentable months and years that followed, the Russian prince countered with his most profoundly painful symptom: his sexual perversion.

The Russian explained that he had an all-powerful wish to be tied down and whipped by a woman wearing black boots, a purple brassiere, and little or nothing else. Thrice he had given into this urge and paid prostitutes to gratify it. The tying-down and the whipping had been delicious, and the urge would depart momentarily, leaving a feeling of serene satisfaction. But soon the mad urge would reappear, crashing into the prince's mind, over and over.

The Reverend K. shunned the prince from that day on, finding such urges despicable and sinful. Yet our neurotic hero was intrigued and troubled by the cravings of his acquaintance. Soon he was surrendering to a similar fantasy, though with a personal twist. He wanted very much to watch a shy and pale girl like Alice James go into her bedroom, pleading an indisposition. Then she would reemerge in high boots and milk-white gloves, brandishing a riding crop, uttering unseemly nouns and verbs. Ordering K. to undress and stoop, she would mount him and ride him like a race horse. The poor Reverend K. suffered for months with this fantasy. Then, in 1893, he confessed the thought in fits and starts to a doctor in a sanatorium in the Alps, who recommended that he promptly seek treatment at the hands of one man and one man alone—Freiherr Richard von Krafft-Ebing, Professor of Psychiatry and Nervous Diseases in Vienna.

The result of K.'s meeting with Krafft-Ebing was comparable to a religious conversion. The great Krafft-Ebing—who diagnosed every third patient he saw as a neurasthenic and every fourth as a pervert—was an imposing, serious man who received our neurotic hero with a bow and a greeting in good English. Scanning the leatherbound books and scientific journals lining the consulting room walls, the Reverend K. sat open-mouthed, admiring the Freiherr's knowledge. The professor diagnosed our hero as a hysteroneurasthenic with perverse obsessions and recommended a concurrent treatment of electricity, massage, hydrotherapy, and hypnosis. He sent the reverend to various colleagues for the first three-quarters of the treatment and undertook the hypnosis himself.

Though the reasons were never clear to the Reverend K., he found the trance into which Krafft-Ebing placed him deeper, more soul-consuming than any trance he had ever experienced. With K. frozen in this state, Krafft-Ebing tried long and furiously to convince our young man that women in black boots and high heels were disgusting, that he should scorn the company of men who liked trading stories of their perversions, and that he should go to Viennese prostitutes and perform successful coitus night after night and enjoy it. After he awoke the Reverend K. did as he was told, and the illicit obsessions soon faded, the headaches disappeared. The treatment was repeated on consecutive days, and the day of an ultimate cure seemed at hand. His will power was strengthening by leaps and bounds. He felt a renewed vigor, a wish to live, a hope that he had not felt since first visiting Dr. Beard.

After a night in the brothels of Vienna, K. was breakfasting on a simple fare of fresh fruit and warm milk at the Hotel Maria Theresa. Most strangely, a butler appeared at his side and announced his name. With an impeccable bow the white-gloved butler handed him a telegram on a silver salver. As quickly as he had come, the butler was gone, leaving K. with a heart thumping with apprehension, beads of sweat forming on his upper lip. His hands shook, his ears buzzed, and he panted as he opened the telegram.

Father dead, come home. Mother, the telegram read. His blood jelled with these words; his breathing seemed to halt. K. sat staring at a candelabrum, staring, staring, staring, seemingly self-hypnotized.

Soon he was out the door, running down the street, running

with all his might. Though men in tall hats and women with tight bodices turned and gawked, he put aside all decorum, kept running, and was soon knocking at Krafft-Ebing's door. After a brief explanation of the crisis and a flood of tears, K. was whisked into the doctor's treatment room. Placing K. in a deep trance, Krafft-Ebing repeated the following words time and time again with conviction.

You will be a man. You will do your duty to your family. You will return home, where you will be single-minded, clear-headed, and masterful.

K. awoke gulping, sweating, trembling. But the ringing in the ears had ceased. The urge to jump from high places or to be whipped by cruel mistresses disappeared; his fear of madness vanished. K. shook hands firmly with the doctor and strolled through the streets of Vienna back to his hotel, feeling very much in charge.

That night proved a turning point in K.'s life. He tumbled in his bed clothes. He dreamed he was wrestling with angels, with devils, with himself. He twisted and grappled and sweated manfully.

When he awoke he felt calmer than he had in many years. A strange and amazing peace had come over him. Breathing in and out with great deliberateness, he shaved, pomaded his hair, inserted the studs in his shirt. He felt serene, level-headed, and resolved. After a series of follow-up hypnosis sessions with the doctor, he departed on the fast train for Trieste. There he boarded a huge ocean liner and cruised down the Adriatic, across the Mediterranean, out through the Pillars of Hercules, into the Atlantic. Never once looking back, K. called up images of himself acting with great mastery as executor of his father's will, as family head, as adviser to his mother. The sea air had never tasted so fresh. The salty tang charged his lungs with delight. "My cup is filled to overflowing. The die is cast, the day of judgment is at hand," he said to himself with deep relief.

TWO

Founding Nervous Fathers

K.'S story is fiction, but fiction condensed from and molded by historical reality. In the late nineteenth century, roughly 1870 to 1900, doctors delineated the cluster of specific neurotic illnesses from which K. suffered. In Paris, Charcot popularized hysteria; the term "neurasthenia" was coined by Beard in New York City; sexual perversions were first defined as categories of neurotic illness by Krafft-Ebing in Vienna. In order to tell the history of ideas about neurosis it is best to revert now to the times when the word was first employed.

The word "nervousness" and its Latin counterpart, "neurosis," are of relatively recent vintage. Though many Victorian authors on the subject traced neurotic phenomena back to Demosthenes, the classical Greek stutterer, and Messalina, the decadent Roman nymphomaniac, thereby suggesting that nervousness had always been with us, the words themselves were comparatively new in 1870. They first came into use during the so-called Age of Reason and became central issues in medicine only around the time of the French Revolution.

"Nervousness" as an empirical term simply means "edginess or worrying, sadness or apprehension," all mild emotional disturbances. But the development of this word in the West has implied that these mental states are brought about in human beings through the medium of the nerves: that various unpleasant stimuli enter the body via the five senses, traverse its various parts, and bring about mild symptoms, some emotional, some physical, some behavioral, all mediated through the nerves. But if one looks back through ancient, medieval, and early modern times, one finds body parts other than the nerves as more central in explanations of emotional, physical, and behavioral symptoms that would later be called nervous or neurotic.

Probably the most ancient concept that nervousness and neurosis eventually replaced is melancholia. The word "melancholia" can be traced to the Greeks. Its literal meaning is "black bile," and it is a central notion in the major theory of illness that predominated in the West well into the seventeenth and eighteenth centuries—namely, the humoral theory of disease. Put succinctly, this held that all emotional, physical, and behavioral symptoms were related to an imbalance of the four humors: blood, phlegm, and the yellow and black biles. Blood and phlegm are fluids we can still identify today. By yellow bile ancient physicians meant what we today call bile, a substance that is made in the liver, percolates through the biliary tract and gall bladder, and mixes with other juices in the intestines to aid in digestion. By black bile they meant a black substance that is found in the spleen. We know now that this black bile is really just coagulated blood, but the ancients were impressed by it and related it to melancholy.

Doctors in ancient times perceived the body as seething with these various humors. They complicated matters by describing three spirits—the vital, the natural, and the animal spirits—which mixed in the body with the humors. The four humors were also connected with "qualities": cold, heat, dryness, and moisture. Diseases, then, involved an imbalance of the four humors and qualities and the three spirits. Too much heat and dryness were thought to lead to one symptom, such as fever, just as too much cold and moisture led to another, such as pus formation, and so on. In this imaginative prescientific era, melancholia was a disease of cold and dryness, which makes some sense, since a gloomy pall would fall across the features of a melancholic, and he would lack interest in food, drink, or warmth of any kind.

A second ancient theory of causation for emotional, behavioral, and some physical disorders involved another body organ, the uterus—the *hystera* in Greek. Since the days of Hippocrates, female physical problems were regarded as emanating from the uterus instead of from the nerves. Hippocrates believed that in women's illnesses the uterus literally moved through the body, wandering, like Odysseus, through a highly permeable realm. Rising from the pelvis to pinch and irritate other body parts, the meandering *hystera* could cause a host of symptoms, such as a sensation of strangulation caused by an imagined lump in the throat (globus hystericus), as well as paralyses, seizures, headaches, and fits of crying and flushing. Any and all symptoms in women could therefore be classified as hysterical.

Later a Roman physician, Galen, developed a more subtle theory. The uterus did not literally wander, he posited, rather the symptoms were products of a substance that an unmarried or widowed woman could not dispel from her uterus because of her celibacy, a substance comparable to sperm in males. To Galen this was a liquid or vaporous substance that flowed and ebbed through the body, thickening and accosting its different parts. Smelling salts could drive the uterine vapors back into the pelvis, and so the symptoms would vanish.

Both of these theories of hysteria and the humoral theory persisted into the eighteenth century as explanations for many mild cases of mental distress. And the tracing of women's bodily, emotional, and behavioral anomalies to the uterus, the seat of menstrual flow, survived well into the nineteenth century.

A third and final concept that was later subsumed under the ideas of nervousness and neurosis was hypochondria. Although today we use the term to mean simply a tendency toward interpreting every ache and pain as an augur of severe disease, the ancients used the word more generally to describe many other illnesses, some emotional, others physical, and still others behavioral. The word also implied a site for the breeding of these symptoms. The hypochondrium is the area below the rib cage—the stomach, the liver, and the pancreas, all body organs that partake in digestion—and the essential notion was that much hypochondria is caused by what one ate.

The three ancient terms—"hypochondria," "melancholia," and "hysteria"—that were used to explain the causes of many obscure symptoms of the emotions, behavior, and the body that later would be called nervous and neurotic emphasized vague causative elements. Interestingly enough, the seat of disease in all three theories was localized literally below the waist—in a wandering uterus, disturbed black bile, or an upset stomach. Only gradually did the idea that the nervous system was the primary source of these symptoms become popular.

The story of the modern understanding of nervousness begins in the early eighteenth century when a Briton, Dr. George Cheyne (1671–1743). In *The English Malady*, he described as "nervous . . . low livers" patients who in the past would have been called hypochondriacal. Like so many medical writers about neurosis, Cheyne himself suffered grievously from the affliction he described, namely "nervousness." Born in a rural area of Scotland and originally destined for the ministry, Cheyne instead moved to London, where he mixed with "the young gentry and free livers." Gorging on tavern dinners and growing extremely popular with members of the better classes for some years, he grew despondent. In about 1715 he gave up his "holiday companions." Passing through a moral and physical crisis, during which he suffered from headaches, giddiness, and loss of appetite, Cheyne found happiness only by taking a course of the waters at Bath and placing himself on a meatless diet. Summering in London and wintering in Bath for many years, he subsequently developed a problem with obesity. Often weighing about three hundred pounds and nearly squashing his horse beneath him, Cheyne led a life of great feasting punctuated by long fasts. Time and again he would put himself on meatless diets in an attempt to lose fifty to one hundred pounds; he would succeed, then relapse, then diet again.

Cheyne's understanding of the human body, as laid out in *The English Malady*, is exceedingly imaginative. It combines the humoral theory, Galen's hysterical idea, and Cheyne's own new "nervous" concept of disease. "All nervous distempers whatsoever from Yawning and Stretching, up to a mortal fit of Apoplexy," he wrote, "seem to be but one continued Disorder, or the several steps and degrees of it." The symptoms of nervousness arise from "a Relaxation or Weakness, and the Want of a sufficient force in Elasticity in the Solids in general and the Nerves in particular."

He saw the human body as a mass of solids and nonsolids. The nonsolids, variously called humors or vapors or juices, seem to bubble and seethe through the body among the solids. If the juices are not sweet enough, if they grow caustic, they grate the solids to shreds. So nervousness involves the solid nerves and sinews and muscles literally being frayed by the bitter juices.

Cheyne saw nervousness as a class problem. The genteel classes in England possess more finely tuned nerves, he reasoned. Being wealthy enough to buy tangy food, especially meats, they eat and drink themselves into disease, since strong spirits and spicy foods render the juices of the body caustic and bitter.

Cheyne's cases of nervousness include some individuals hereditarily endowed with delicate nerves and others rendered nervous by low or high living. One young woman of "tender and delicate Constitution" eats "too strong and high Food while at a Boarding School in London." Another young lady, "of an Honorable and Opulent Family of the Finest Parts I ever knew in the Sex," inherited weak nerves from her family, and "for want of due Care and proper Management, brought on at last the most violent, Extreme and Obstinate Nervous Paroxysms I have ever seen." He treated many ladies of distinction, as well as country gentlemen, clergymen, doctors, and even himself.

In this first work on nervousness we find the first and probably oldest myth about neurosis, what can be called the Angelic Invalid myth, which would continue to influence thinkers on neurosis throughout the eighteenth and nineteenth centuries. Whether a young, delicate member of the better classes, frequently a woman, or a sensitive man such as Cheyne himself, the Angelic Invalid inherits delicate nerves from her or his forebears. He or she is a walking raw nerve, waiting for a caustic assault; food and drink often prove the culprits.

To Cheyne spicy foods and strong drinks are not only noxious to the nerves but foreign to England. "Since our wealth has increased," he writes, "and our Navigation has been extended, we have ransacked all the Parts of the *Globe* to bring together its whole Stock of Materials for *Riot, Luxury* and to provoke *Excess*. The Tables of the Great (and indeed of all Ranks who can afford it) are furnished with Provisions of Delicacy, Number and Plenty,

sufficient to . . . gorge the most large and voluptuous Appetite."
The delicate and susceptible English person can become nervous
by gorging himself on foreign foods.

This is an embryonic statement of a second great myth about
neurosis, which we shall call the Noble Savage myth, yet another
neurotic prototype. The Noble Savage is a human being reared in
rustic simplicity who, upon arriving in the city, surrenders to his
appetites and so drowns his nerves in a sea of foreign luxury and
wanton abandon. Later writers would expand upon this myth in
greater detail.

At about the same time Cheyne was popularizing the word
"nervousness," two scholars at the University of Edinburgh took up
the idea. One, William Cullen (1710–90), latinized the word to
"neurosis." The other, Robert Whytt (1714–66), wrote a much
clearer, less fantastic manifesto than Cheyne's on the anatomy of
the nervous system and the way in which a person is rendered
nervous or neurotic. Cullen and Whytt moved further away from
the humoral, spiritual, and vaporous theories of the past, and in so
doing helped transform neurosis into a more palatable academic
subject.

Cullen set out to reorder medical thinking about all diseases.
He divided the study of pathology into four major categories:
achexia, fever, local disorder, and neurosis. He defined neurosis as
"sense and motion injured, without idiopathic pyrexia [fever] and
without local disease." This awkward, latinate definition implied
that scores and scores of medical disorders were neuroses: coma,
apoplexy, paralysis, fainting, shortness of breath, hypochondriasis,
chlorosis or the disease of pale virgins, cholera, epilepsy, palpitations, asthma, diarrhea, diabetes, hysteria, rabies, melancholy, and
mania and imbecility.

Cullen attempted to demolish the humoral theory, but he
offered another almost as fantastic, though certainly better organized. It relied on a contending ancient theory, the so-called
tonus theory of disease. The humoral and the tonus theories
agreed on one point: namely, that all the diseases were caused by
too much of this quality or too little of that—too much heat or
cold in the humors, too much tension or laxness in the tone.
Cullen agreed with the ancients on this point and conceived of
neurosis as a literal tightening or loosening of the nerves.

His nosology is a ponderously complete system that appeared in synopsis in 1769 and was frequently republished and translated throughout the West well into the nineteenth century. Even though later doctors would find other explanations than simply too much or too little tension in the nerves, the vast organizational work undertaken by Cullen established both the use of the word "neurosis" and the clustering together of "neurotic" illnesses in a manner that would be crucial to all thinking about neurosis throughout the nineteenth century.

In the same decades, 1740–70, when Cullen was writing his works on neurosis, his friend Robert Whytt published his book rather long-windedly entitled *Observations on the Nature, Cause and Cure of Those Disorders Which are Commonly Called Nervous, Hypochondriacal or Hysterical* (1764). This work lays out the causes of neurosis in a more satisfying manner than Cheyne's. Whytt posits one simple but powerful organizing idea regarding how a neurosis comes about: a sensation in one part of the body is carried inward through the nerves, back into the spinal cord and even up to the brain, and then outward through another nerve to another body part, thereby causing a symptom. Calling this phenomenon "a sympathy of the nerves," he cites numerous examples. "The smell of grateful food," he writes, "makes the saliva flow when one is hungry," and an "irritation of the windpipe . . . raises coughing, or convulsive motion of the muscles employed in expiration." Thus do palpitations, giddiness, fits, and many related symptoms occur. The various body parts are too much in sympathy via oversensitive nerves.

Likewise, in hysteria and hypochondria, a painful stimulus creeps into the nerves of the susceptible people—in the uterus and the ovaries in the case of hysteria, and in the liver, pancreas, and stomach for hypochondriasis—and shoots an unhappy message to other parts of the body. "A too great delicacy and sensibility," he writes, "of the whole nervous system may be either natural, that is, an original defect in the constitution, or produced by such diseases, or irregularity in living, as weakened the whole body, especially the nerves. Long and repeated fevers, profuse hemorrhages, great fatigue, excessive and long continued grief, luxurious living, and want of exercise, may increase and even bring on such a delicate state of the nervous system." This delicacy then leaves the individual susceptible to an outbreak of nerves, which spreads from one pained body part to the next.

Needless to say, in Whytt's scheme of things, women and children are more sensitive and therefore more nervous, since their nerves are more tender. "We are told of a lady," he writes, "who, upon hearing the sound of a bell . . . used to fall into fits of swooning which were scarce to be distinguished from death. And I have seen the pain of a toothache throw a young lady, of weak nerves, into convulsions and insensibility." He frequently treated these women with laudanum, an opiate that soon became foolishly prescribed by many doctors to many nervous women. Whytt also describes numerous cases of nervous women who grew faint and anxious near cats and various plants. In these cases he is clearly equating nerves with what we now know to be allergies. But he sees all these delicate females as essentially Angelic Invalids.

His approach to neurosis—though less fantastic than Cheyne's— remains a physicalistic one. He endlessly discusses obstructed menses in women and gout and hemorrhoids in men as playing central roles in causing neurosis, and devotes much attention to wind, worms, and obstructions in the viscera.

Whytt does mention that "by sudden terror, delicate women and children have not only been thrown into fainting and convulsions, but rendered subject all their lifetime to epileptic fits." But even here—like Cullen and Cheyne—he stresses physical disturbances in the nerves that underlie neurosis and nervousness. Relying on the notion that a frightening sound or vision speeds through the eye and ear into the nervous system and, in the delicate human, stirs up the whole body and leads to outbreaks of generalized nervous symptoms, he explains away such psychological events as terror and fright. They affect only sensitive women or weak children who are victims of hereditarily delicate nerves.

The Angelic Invalid myth was not confined to medicine; it had much broader cultural ramifications in the eighteenth and nineteenth centuries. Sensitivity, nervousness, and delicateness became fashionable terms. In Jane Austen's *Sense and Sensibility*, published in 1811, we find a typical case of the Angelic Invalid. This popular novel describes in detail two sisters, the one, Elinor, sensible, the other, Marianne, sensitive. Elinor is exceedingly rational, if somewhat drab and not quite as pretty as Marianne.

Elinor falls in love with a bit of a fidget, Edward Ferrars, whom she eventually marries, while Marianne falls madly in love with a rake, Mr. Willoughby, who woos her, wins her, and leaves her.

Marianne is the successor to Cheyne's Young Lady of Delicate and Sensitive Constitution and a sister of Whytt's woman who swooned on hearing a bell. Led on by the dapper Willoughby to expect a proposal, Marianne waits and waits for the good news. She goes to London to be near him, and waits some more. "For her spirits," writes Austen, "still continued very high." She scarcely eats her meals and anxiously listens to the sound of every passing carriage. The days pass with no Willoughby. He takes his time in coming to see her, and when he does, he treats Marianne coldly. Only when the announcement of Willoughby's marriage of convenience to a wealthy heiress becomes the talk of London does Marianne give up hope. "She could say no more; her spirits were quite overcome, and hiding her face in Elinor's shoulder, she burst into tears." She is given smelling salts, and her menfolk grow "desperately enraged against the author of this nervous distress."

Marianne wastes away, losing her beauty and her appetite and eventually her health. When she leaves London and goes to the countryside for solace, it seems that she may recover. Unfortunately "two delightful twilight walks" in the country, "—assisted by the great imprudence of sitting in her wet shoes and stockings —[had] given Marianne a cold so violent" that the poor, gentle girl is soon desperately ill, burning with fever. "Hour after hour passed away, in sleepless pain and delirium on Marianne's side, and the most cruel anxiety on Elinor's." The situation becomes desperate when Marianne passes into a stupor, and even Elinor grows hopeless, "her thoughts wandering from one image of grief, one suffering friend to another."

But Elinor is too sensible to become ill herself, and Austen is not willing to let poor Marianne die of lovesickness. Soon her pulse grows regular. Then the fever wanes and she returns to her senses. Though Marianne had once declared it indecent for women to love more than once, very soon after the feverish illness nearly kills her she comes to her senses and marries a faithful old gent, Colonel Brandon, who had been waiting in the wings. Finally, she comes to live within a short ride by horse and carriage from her likewise sensibly married sister Elinor.

One final pre-Victorian physician of note, Thomas Trotter (1760–1832), a former Royal Navy physician, developed the thinking of Cheyne and Whytt and also reintroduced the Noble Savage myth in *A View of the Nervous Temperment*, a fascinating, surprisingly readable work, written in 1807. This book commences with a vivid description of a prototypical nervous sufferer, a walking list of symptoms: gout, anemia, Saint Vitus's Dance, dyspepsia, and hysteria.

Like Cheyne, Trotter traces nervousness to the gastrointestinal tract, to various foods that irritate the bowels and the digestion. Trotter, however, indicates a very specific anatomical connection between the bowel and the nerves, one not well-known in Cheyne's time, namely, the sympathetic nervous system. "Anatomists have discovered," we read in *A View*, "an unusual share of nerves about the upper orifice of the stomach . . . These nerves of the stomach are derived from the *par vagum* or eighth pair, which communicates with the *great intercostal or sympathetic*." This rather subtle group of nerves (now called the sympathetic and parasympathetic nerves) linking the gastrointestinal tract and other body parts, such as the heart, to the brain had been delineated anatomically in the seventeenth century but was not investigated in terms of physiological function until the midnineteenth century. Therefore, all of Trotter's thinking was based on clinical experience and extensive speculation.

"The human stomach is an organ imbued by nature with the most complex properties of any in the body; and forming a center of sympathy between our corporeal and mental parts." Trotter does not speak in terms of solids (that is, nerves) or nonsolids (that is, juices or humoral vapors). He does not speak fancifully, as Cheyne had, about caustic juices ripping and tearing the nerves. Nor does he refer to unhappy nerves in sympathy, as Whytt did, or to lax and tense nerves, as Cullen had done. Rather he specified the physical medium of neurotic illness, the sympathetic nerves through which an "unhappy" bowel makes the brain and the mind likewise miserable.

Trotter also identified other causes of nervousness not specified by his predecessors: foul air, lack of exercise, tight-fitting clothing, as well as passions of the mind, intense study, and a sedentary lifestyle. All of these he connected to one sociological factor, namely, the growth of the city. Like Cheyne, Trotter saw luxuries as being at the heart of neurosis. However, he saw the city itself, the hydra-headed monster of corruption that breeds luxuries, as the ultimate agent of nervousness. He wrote at great length about the corrupt nature of urban life, in which alcohol, coffee, tea, laudanum, rich foods, and poor air bombard and devastate the nervous system.

Trotter was essentially a primitivist who cherished the clean air and simple food of the countryside, the British Navy and the primitive kingdoms the Navy visited. He lambasted the fashionable world of 1800, in which it was chic to be pale, delicate, and anemic. He attributed the effeminacy, dandyish ways, and meager physiques of city dwellers to their lack of exercise, clean air, solid food, and sleep.

The Royal Navy doctor loved to compare the savage with civilized man, and in so doing he fleshed out the myth of the Noble Savage. "*The nervous system,*" he writes, "that organ of sensation amidst the unpolluted inhabitants of the forest, could receive none of those fine impressions, which, however they may polish the mind in the largest capacities, never fail to induce a delicacy of feeling, which disposes alike to more acute pain and to more exquisite pleasure." Dividing the society of the city into seven major classes (including literary men, men of business, the idle and dissipated, and the female sex), Trotter tries to show how all were being destroyed by nervousness. Of the literary class he writes, "It is to be supposed that all men who possess genius . . . are indeed by nature imbued with more than usual sensibility of the nervous system." Of the mercantile class: "the man of business, in this commercial age, is not always to be estimated a correct liver. Luxury follows hard on gain." The idle and dissipated: "frequent surfeits from high seasoned food; and frequent intoxication from vinous and spiritous potion, commit dreadful ravages on the human body and mind."

He lingers on the female sex. Despising the chic paleness of women, he admonishes them against reading novels that might implant in their brains fantasies of loving passionately and romantically dying of broken hearts. He also decries the fashion of lacing straps too tight: "I have known instances where young girls have nearly expired in a crowded room of straight lacing." He argues that young girls should not be treated like dolls but rather should be allowed to run about with their brothers. He finally cries out: "amidst the great effeminacy of manners, that is rapidly consuming the very spiritual and physical strength of this age, what may ultimately annihilate all that is great in the character of the Britons, it is somewhat consoling to observe that the seamen of the navy, that bulwark of our liberties, will be the last of the community to feel the effect of those enervating customs."

Herein we can see the influence of his naval service and also of Lord Nelson, who was very much in the public's eye. Nelson stood forth as the manliest of men, not allowing the loss of an eye or an arm to shake his nerves or his bravery in the face of the Napoleonic onslaught. Trotter cites Napoleon himself as an example of a debilitating nervousness—probably because he was French and an opponent of the old, seemingly natural order of things—and contrasts him with Washington, a true Anglo-Saxon, whose revolution was led by gentlemen of the upper classes.

Trotter, like Cheyne and so many other early authors on nervousness, wrote in a rambling anecdotal style, which made him at once readable and unscientific. A View is riddled with nationalism, conservatism, and Francophobia, which mingle with medical diagnosis. All the writings on neurosis before the final decades of the nineteenth century were anecdotal and descriptive. Appearing before the time when neurosis—in fact, all illnesses—could be studied in a rigorously scientific manner, they do not employ empirically refutable analyses. Lacking a thoroughgoing scientific method, they gave to a neurosis a general, all-embracing meaning. Such vagueness in the use of this diagnosis lingered throughout the nineteenth century; the term "neurosis" applied not only to those illnesses we moderns would call neuroses but also to diseases such as epilepsy and chorea, which now are tied conclusively to brain pathology. Even disorders such as goiter, resulting from an iodine deficiency, and tetanus, an infectious illness, were called neuroses throughout the nineteenth century.

In the opening decades of the nineteenth century, ideas about neurosis found their expression in two continental schools of thinking—one in France, one in Germany. Both schools gradually became more scientific than the early British approaches. The older of these two schools, formed in France, was based on the work of Philippe Pinel (1745–1826), who was remembered by

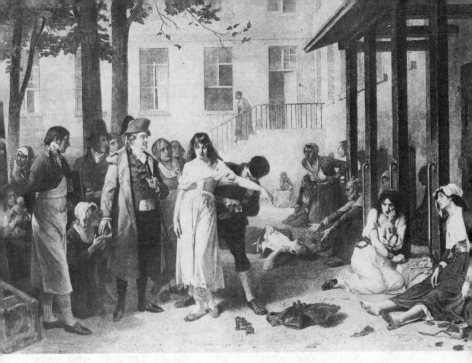

The French school of Philippe Pinel. Antoine Fleury, *Pinel Freeing the Madwomen at the Salpêtrière.* (Rare Book Room, Countway Library of Medicine, Harvard University, Boston)

subsequent generations of French doctors for having unchained the madwomen held captive in the Salpêtrière in Paris during the Revolution. The Salpêtrière is an old mental hospital that, as we will see, played a central role in the history of neurosis. It was in this hospital that the disciples of the French school were trained and went forth to spread the new ideas. The act of unchaining the madwomen in the Salpêtrière was captured in a painting by Antoine Fleury in 1878, which symbolized a major trend in Pinel's medical thinking, namely, the freeing of the study of mental illness from the fetters of ancient and medieval thinking and, within the context of the Revolution, the liberating of the study of humankind in general from old habits of thought. The French school set out to systematize neurosis and link every symptom to brain pathology. Unlike Cheyne's notion of frayed nerves, Whytt's sensitive nerves and Cullen's tense or lax nerves, the French school searched for an actual anatomical lesion, a diseased locus in the brain or elsewhere that could—through the nerves—trigger a neurotic symptom. Pinel wrote, "Let us hope that, as we advance, the material will become gradually clearer and more and more neuroses still of an uncertain etiology will be shown to have lesions in their tissue."

Very bold rhetoric, to be sure. In reality Pinel often fell back on the ideas of his predecessors and invoked, unwittingly, the old myths. He essentially paraphrased Cullen, adding the new French notion of a lesion. Furthermore, he stressed cases in which a general nerve weakness seemed at fault rather than a specific lesion. He describes one young woman, married at fifteen, who suffered "violent chagrin" during her husband's long absence in the Napoleonic Wars. After his return to Paris she gave birth to two infants, had a nervous collapse, and came to Pinel's attention. Resorting to the old ideas of Trotter and Whytt, Pinel attributed her convulsions and eventual premature death to frayed and shocked nerves. The Frenchman followed this case with a description of the weaknesses and delicacies of women in general. He alluded to the seventeenth-century nuns of Loudon, who were supposedly taken over by the devil, as examples of "a great organic delicateness and an extremely nervous susceptibility." For all of his claims of medical progress, Pinel was reduced to the old Angelic Invalid myth. Citing opium, alcohol, and "violent chagrin," as well as too early and too demanding education as causes of neuroses, he called for a return to the natural way of life, the Noble Savage existence of exercise, pure air and water, and simple food. He also called for a return to classical forms of education for young men and women. He perceived these methods as a "strong means of nourishing in the hearts [of the young] a love of their country and a heroic devotion while developing a robust constitution and flourishing health."

He was one with Trotter, his English contemporary, in describing the evils of the city. "So many causes, in the large cities, are present to produce and foment the nervous illnesses! The spread of enervating luxury, of an inactive and sedentary life style . . . continued use of carriages, the use of fermented liquors . . . the torments of ambition, dissipation, pleasure." He agreed with Cheyne's and Trotter's assessment that the malady of civilization, neurosis, had been increasing since the beginning of the 1700s.

In describing the case of "a celebrated actress of the best theatre" who was overcome with "spasms and loss of appetite and a somber mood," he was really touching on both myths. Her cure came only when she "abandoned her drugs, left Paris, the theatre and her admirers; she went on a voyage to Provence where she took sea baths and returned at the end of a number of months, perfectly cured." The movement from city to country, evoked in the same year as the publication of Pinel's essay, by John Keats in his "Ode to Melancholy," is truly Pinel's theme. Molded during the French Revolution, he cites the old regime, with its effete nobility, wallowing in sensuality, as the prototypical era of nervous decay. The Revolution, he surmised, could revitalize man by reconnecting him to a more primitive, healthier life-style.

The Noble Savage myth of neurosis draws heavily on the French thinker whose ideas played a significant role in the coming of the Revolution: Jean-Jacques Rousseau. His arguments about the nobility of man in a savage state and the corruption of body and soul by civilization greatly influenced many thinkers throughout the eighteenth and nineteenth centuries.

The archetypal *philosophe*, Rousseau presents himself in his *Confessions* as a shy and awkward man who found Parisian society more than a little intimidating, the etiquette and pleasures of the French upper classes at once alluring and dangerous. In his essay on the inequality of the human species, Rousseau describes the Noble Savage, who resembles Rousseau, in detail. Somewhere in the mythical past, man lived for eons in a savage state that was pure and healthy. He was honest and virtuous, a veritable Adam in the Garden of Eden. His temptation was not Eve offering him an apple but a wicked human being whose grasping for power convinced him that if he would band together with his fellow beings and give up some of his freedom, he might be not only happier but more noble. This is the tragedy of Rousseau's Noble Savage. He does not find greater happiness and nobility, only the despoiling of his simple rustic joys. All the luxuries of the world and their attendant vices are laid before him, and he is politically enslaved. He seeks greater and greater sensuous delights but surrenders more and more freedom. A simple rustic at heart, he can only suffer. Soon he is burdened with moral and emotional turmoil—with lust, greed, and concupiscence—and they lead to disease, physical decline, and painful death.

Regardless of Pinel's continuing to employ the Noble Savage

and the Angelic Invalid myths, the conception of neurosis adopted
by French medicine and the rest of Europe and America during
the first half of the century stressed the pathological process of an
irritation communicated through the nerves from a lesion. In all
neuroses the brain, the spinal cord, or the nerves were imagined as
being irritated by acute, chronic, or subacute inflammation, softening of the nerves, or apoplexy. The movement of French medical sciences was away from the vague metaphysics of the eighteenth
century, toward the gathering together of symptoms into syndromes, and ultimately the linking of these syndromes to specific
anatomic lesions in the nervous system.

This French emphasis on static lesions as the causes of all
neuroses continued into the last few decades of the nineteenth century. A product of this way of thinking can be found in the article
on neurosis written by Dr. Alfred Luton in the forty-two-volume
French dictionary of medical and surgical practice (1872–79).
Luton cites Cheyne, Cullen, Whytt, and Pinel as the forefathers of
the idea of neurosis, then launches into an argument that the
group of neuroses for which no cause was known was shrinking as
medical knowledge of specific lesions advanced. He set out to show
that hitherto unexplained illnesses were caused by discrete lesions
in the nervous system. To be sure, vague generalizations abound
in this article. Generally mixing sociological and neurological
causes, he argues that somnambulism, bed-wetting, and convulsions in childhood could all be seen as resulting from nervous weakness and delicacy in children. Nonetheless, he noted some genuine
medical advances since Pinel: the connection of chorea to rheumatism, of tetanus to puncture wounds, and of alcohol to delirium
tremens. In these and at least seven other "neuroses" (as Cullen
and Pinel defined them) the anatomical lesion had been located by
the 1870s. Luton also noted that various infectious illnesses, such as
cholera, typhoid fever, and diphtheria, could lead to changes in
the nervous system and therefore to mild or severe mental symptoms. In short, the French notion of lesion seemed triumphant in
explaining many illnesses hitherto called "neurotic." The limita-
tions of this approach became apparent only as the century waned
and the second great school of continental medicine gained
momentum.

In the latter half of the nineteenth century this second great

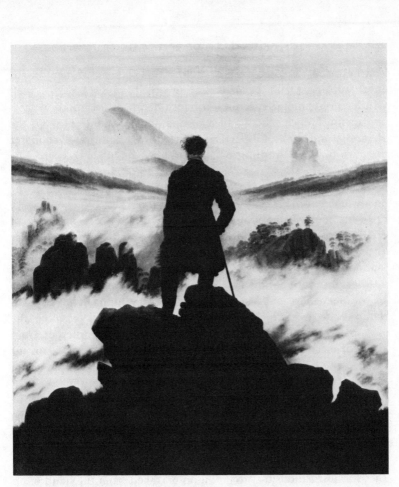

The German school of Johannes Peter Müller. Caspar David Friedrich, *Wanderer in a Sea of Mist.* (Hamburger Kunsthalle, Hamburg)

school of medical thinking developed in Germany. Its inspirer was Johannes Peter Müller (1801–58), a pioneer physiologist and naturalist of the University of Berlin, and its orientation was more physiological and less anatomical than that of the French school. A romantic and a believer in vitalism, Müller held that the life-giving substance within the nervous system was "imponderable"—meaning both immeasurable and profound.

His widely read textbook on physiology (1840) was riddled with fascinating speculations, some physical, some metaphysical. By concentrating on the concept of "nervous spirits" Müller sought more ultimate, and perhaps less practical answers than Pinel; Müller's physiologic speculation had a depth of imagination lacking in the French school's idea of anatomical lesion. Though the dreamy wanderer in Caspar David Friedrich's painting "Wanderer in a Sea of Mist" was not in fact Müller, it might have been. The figure shown gazing over the edge of a mountain pinnacle into a sea of mist represented his spirit as well as the 1878 painting of the madwomen at the Salpêtrière did that of Pinel.

In his book Müller admits that "many physiologists and men of science have not ceased to regard electricity, a force discovered in the 1790s, and nervous power as principles in a certain degree similar." Yet he disagrees; after a close inspection of all the data Müller draws the following conclusions: (1) That the vital actions of the nerves are not attended with the development of any galvanic occurrence which our instruments can detect. (2) That the laws of action of the nervous principle are totally different from those of electricity. (3) To speak, therefore, of an electric current in the nerves is to use a symbolic expression as if we compared the action of the nervous principle with light and magnetism."

Müller sees the evanescing soul or vital principle at work in living matter. "Life," he writes, "is not simply the result of the harmony and reciprocal action of the parts; but it is first manifested in a principle, or imponderable matter which is in action in the substance of the germ." This germ, the sperm or egg, explains the near-miraculous fact that "an onion taken from the hand of an Egyptian mummy, perhaps 2000 years old, was made to grow." It can also explain the more mundane but equally wondrous fact that "branches of plants separate from the trunk, being planted, to form new individuals." To Müller this life force might be beyond science's powers of discovery.

It is almost disappointing to note that Müller's star pupil, Hermann von Helmholtz (1822–94), succeeded in advancing science into precisely the area Müller thought would never be conquered. In 1847 Helmholtz measured the speed of nerve conduction and equated it with electricity. This discovery made in a physiology laboratory seemed to shed light on clinical thinking. It seemed that the laxness or tension of which Cullen had spoken could now be measured.

Another follower of Müller's, Moritz Heinrich Romberg (1795–1873), composed an early German neurological tract, *A Manual of the Nervous Diseases of Man*, between the years 1848 and 1852. Building on Helmholtz's ideas regarding the motion of electricity in the nerves, he regarded imbalanced motion as the central concept in an understanding of neurotic illness. This was a new medical idea—faulty physiology, rather than anatomical lesion, as a cause of disease. Romberg tried in a Herculean manner to explain neurosis using Helmholtz's measurement of the speed of nervous energy. He characterized neuroses of sensory function as being due to either excessive sensation (hyperesthesia) or absent sensation (anesthesia), motor neuroses as being caused by either depressed or exalted movement.

Though Romberg's emphasis on motion in the birth of neuroses stands forth as a second brilliant medical notion, physiological analysis per se bore meager fruit when compared with anatomical studies. This failure on the part of physiological study is not surprising if one realizes the primitive nature of physiological tools of measurement as compared to the more sophisticated techniques of gross autopsy and histological sectioning available to anatomists during Victorian times.

Ironically, certain medical thinkers who embraced the anatomical paradigm of lesion-causing neuroses pushed the idea too far. Even though autopsy examinations of persons who died while suffering from such severe "neuroses" as mania, dementia, and imbecility did not always show brain lesions, the theory of lesion gave rise to two highly imaginative new myths about neurosis. The great Degenerate myth owes its development to Benedictin Augustin Morel (1809–73), and the Genius myth is found in the works of his near contemporary Jacques Joseph Moreau (de Tours) (1804–84). Both men were trained at the Salpêtrière of Pinel and spent their lives toiling with severely disturbed mentally ill patients, whom we would now call psychotic. Yet in their theoretical works both argue backward from the severely mentally ill, the psychotic, to discuss the mildly mentally ill, those we now call neurotic.

In the formation of their myths these two Frenchmen relied on the thinking of Franz Josef Gall (1758–1828), an Austrian, who was the founder of phrenology. Today phrenology seems only a

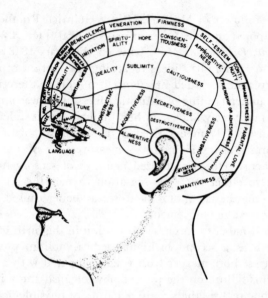

F. J. Gall's brain of phrenology. (From A. A. Roback and T. Kiernan, *Pictorial History of Psychology and Psychiatry*)

fanciful system of assessing an individual's personality by feeling bumps and indentations on his head. But in the 1850s it was a forward-looking system, since Gall argued that the brain was divided into discernible portions. He and his followers made up maps of the brain, which connected its various parts to specific human attributes, such as will, memory, or emotion. If one portion of an individual's brain—the emotion part, for instance—was relatively large, he was necessarily very emotional. If the part corresponding to memory was small, he had a poor memory. Though neither Moreau nor Morel was a phrenologist, each man applied this idea to neuroses. They imagined that some part of the brain of a neurotic was over- or underexcited. This was the site of lesion.

Morel, who practiced at an asylum in Rouen, clearly delineated his intellectual roots in the preface of his great work *Treatise on the Degeneration of the Human Species* (1857). He paid tribute to the Baron Cuvier and the Comte de Buffon, two early nineteenth-century naturalists whose work with animals and prehistoric human bone specimens spurred thinking about the vastness of life on earth and the interconnectedness of man and animals.

Morel's panoramic view of human history, involving hundreds of thousands of years, led him to make large claims about the races of man and the breeding of mental illnesses. He believed that the various races were members of the same species but that some were degenerate forms of a perfect race of Adams and Eves. And to Morel, degeneration literally meant a degenerating lesion in the brain.

It was his belief that he could trace the essential character of epilepsy, hysteria, hypochondriasis, as well as mania, general paralysis, and mental retardation back to a fundamental trouble in the organism, back to "an essential lesion of the central nervous system." The specific neurosis depended on which brain portion was degenerating.

He argued, for instance, that the American Indians were really degenerates who "join in themselves the pugnaciousness and vapidness of the child and the mental slowness and brittleness of the old man." They were not the ideal primitive man of whom Trotter had spoken. Likewise Morel believed that the Hottentots of Africa were brutish and stupid, and the South Sea Islanders indolent and dull. All of these primitives he imagined as afflicted with brain lesions that caused their vapidity, indolence, or brutishness.

Like all of his contemporaries, Morel did not have available to him the fairly well delineated categories of mental illness established today. He also lacked our anthropological perspective, which is rooted in relativism. So he saw the apparent ignorance and savagery of the races of Africa and America as comparable to the defects of mentally retarded and mentally ill people. But between the most savage Bushman of Africa and the healthy and civilized European, Morel believed there was more similarity than between the same healthy European and "the degenerate being whose intellectual arrest" had led "to a diseased state which we designate by the name imbecile, idiot or demented."

Morel believed, like so many of the early writers on neurosis, that "the existence of dangerous and unsafe occupations, life in overly populated and diseased cities, submit the organism to new causes of decline and degeneration." He postulated that various intoxicating agents, such as alcohol and poor diet, lead to the formation of lesions in the central nervous system of the civilized human being, which then cause degeneration. This degeneration, Morel posited, is then passed on through "the germ," that is, the sperm, from father to son. He argued that over a few generations individuals with a "vicious organic disposition"—cretinism (mental retardation resulting from iodine deficiency), rickets (vitamin D deficiency), and scrofula (an infectious illness akin to tuberculosis)—would die off in idiocy and madness. Knowing as we do today that women who suffer from such conditions give birth to children with faulty nervous systems or bone formation of the cranium, we can see how Morel concluded that they were degenerates.

To Morel, cretins and marsh dwellers (who commonly suffered from endemic malaria) were "degenerates par excellence." He also believed that alcoholism could have a similar degenerative effect. Indeed, he thought that the children of alcoholics were precisely the individuals who came to fill the asylums of Western Europe and North America. The morose Swedes were notorious in the nineteenth century for their rampant alcoholism, just as the indolent Chinese were for their consumption of opium. To Morel, this meant that the next generation of Swedes or Chinese would be born both addicted and hysterical or epileptic. The third generation would be suicidal and delusional. The fourth, imbeciles and idiots. The fate of such a family over four generations was expressed in the Degenerate myth of neurosis, to which many later nineteenth-century thinkers returned time and again.

The Morelian Degenerate is a distant relative of the Cheynian high liver and tavern diner, but the effects of his drinking absinthe and carousing in red-light districts are not snuffed out by his death in some Parisian brothel or London side street. Rather, his sins are handed down to his son and daughter, who inherit—though they may struggle to be good and healthy—his nervous curse, which then passes on to grandchildren and great-grandchildren, who finally die as driveling idiots, the last of a palsied race. Morel searched for many explanations for the passing on of lesions from parent to child: an upbringing in slavery, faulty re-

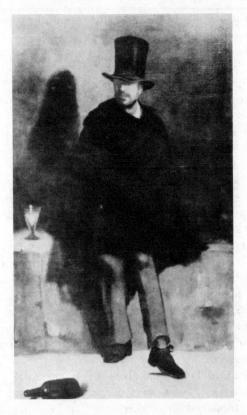

The Absinthe Drinker by Edouard Manet, or B. A. Morel's degenerate forebear par excellence. (Ny Carlsberg Glypotek, Copenhagen)

ligious beliefs, social prejudices, even incest, as well as tobacco, opium, malaria, tuberculosis, and of course vitamin D and iodine deficiency. But this multiplying of causes only increased the scope of his theory.

The influence of the Degenerate myth extended beyond medicine to the broader culture of the nineteenth century. Emile Zola's *Rougon-Macquart*, for example, is, among other things, a twenty-volume description of five generations of a degenerate family along the lines spelled out by Morel. Zola had in fact read Morel and a number of other medical authors in his preparation for the writing of this work, and he apparently kept abreast of new medical ideas about neurosis as he wrote.

Zola begins the story with Adelaide Fouques, who suffers from a "disequilibrium in the blood and the nerves," and so experiences recurrent "nervous crises" and "terrible convulsions." Capricious, passionate, overly emotional, she marries, on the spur of the moment, the near-imbecilic, stuttering Pierre Rougon.

When he suddenly dies of sunstroke, she takes the alcoholic Macquart, a smuggler, as her lover, and has two children as a result of her scandalous affair. Macquart is finally shot dead by the police, and when Adelaide receives the news she has a series of hysterical fits that leave her half demented. She remains in this state for a number of years, till a great-nephew named Silvere, a political fanatic, is shot dead by the police. After this terrible news Adelaide is taken away to an asylum to live out her days.

Meanwhile the multiplying Rougon-Macquart clan is showing signs of the hereditary taint. Some become religious fanatics, others murder with insane glee. Many are simply immoral and opportunistic. Still others go raving mad and commit suicide. All the gory facts of the Rougon-Macquart family are scrupulously recorded by Dr. Pascal, a grandson of Adelaide and Rougon who has gone into medicine.

Though certain family members are momentarily successful—one grandson rises to the level of vice-emperor and another becomes an extremely rich banker—the family is threatened with extinction by the fifth generation. Many of the fourth generation fail to reproduce, and those who do have weak, anemic sons and daughters. One of these sickly great-great-grandsons, Charles Rougon, is sent to live with a debauched uncle near the asylum in which Adelaide resides, and he squanders many an hour sitting with his demented forebear. His death comes in his teens when he suddenly bursts a blood vessel in his nose and slowly bleeds to death while the demented Adelaide watches. The resulting shock sends Adelaide to her grave, while the surviving family members watch their anemic offsprings with trepidation, fearing extinction.

Zola's literary creation follows lines laid out by Morel in his *Degeneration*. In the manner of an epic novelist, Morel composed sweeping panoramic descriptions of the collective health of the nations of Europe. Like the tales of Herodotus, his work is half myth, half history—the Christian notion of original sin embodied in the nervous system. Appealing but unprovable, his sweeping notions hint at a population still plagued with devastating vitamin and mineral deficiencies resulting in pellagra and cretinism, widespread chronic infectious illnesses such as tuberculosis and malaria, and alcoholism and narcotic addiction, which were growing into major social problems. Since he was ignorant about the causes of these and other medical conditions, Morel made some magnificent imaginative leaps that influenced thinking about neurosis for half a century.

Meanwhile another French doctor, Jacques Joseph Moreau (de Tours), who was also trained at the Salpêtrière, took up threads of this argument and moved in a different direction, which ultimately resulted in another myth about the cause of mental illness, the Genius myth. Moreau worked most of his life at the Bicêtre, the counterpart of the Salpêtrière for men.

In 1859 he wrote *Morbid Psychology*, a less anthropologically based, more psychologically minded work than Morel's *Degeneration*. Moreau argued that human inequality was due not to education but to heredity. Contradicting the thinkers of the French Revolution, who stressed the importance of upbringing, Moreau emphatically believed that there was nothing more to the soul or animal spirits, or Johannes Müller's vital fluid, than psychocerebral vitality. He believed that all mental illnesses were caused by "vital modifications, dynamic troubles," in the brain. Influenced by the phrenologist Gall and probably by the German Romberg, Moreau defined these modifications and troubles as overexcitations of brain parts. A convulsion, for example, results when the part of the brain specializing in movement becomes overexcited and thus works too hard; raving madness occurs when the part specializing in thinking becomes overexcited. To Moreau, other illnesses such as idiocy or anesthesia (loss of sensation) can occur when the part of the brain meant for intelligence or feeling grows weak or underexcited.

Moreau believed that nervous energy can become more concentrated and active in certain individuals, usually because of hereditary problems. In this he followed the lead of Morel. But for Moreau, the nervously unstable individual is not only or not always the Morelian degenerate, enervated and feebleminded, expiring as a masturbating moron in an asylum. He can also be one of the very movers of civilization—the prophets, the geniuses! The imbalance of nervous energy heightens the moral force in one or two select ancestors. Like Morel's Degenerate myth, this Genius myth would haunt the thinking of Western doctors throughout the late nineteenth century.

Moreau argued that starvation, a technique constantly used by prophets and religious men as a means of inducing visions and entering into trances, could illuminate the link between madness and genius. Like those who take opium, ether, or hashish, the starving prophet, who is a kind of religious genius, often experiences a "gay delirium." Moreau sees such an exalted state of mind as following from a heightening of nerve force, of vital energy. Through this kind of heightening, genius can spring forth into the world.

Moreau argues that the idiot, the hysteric, the epileptic, the madman, as well as the genius, are all alike in that they are all "born and developed under the same influence, like the effects of the same cause, like branches growing from the same tree." Indeed, his work is accompanied by a drawing of the tree of "idiosyncratic hereditary nervous states." On this tree criminals, eccentrics, prostitutes are all closely connected. Geniuses, such as painters, musicians, and scientists, occupy yet another branch, and the various nervous illnesses are depicted as leaves growing out of still other branches. As for the disappearance and reappearance of genius and madness, hysteria and idiocy in various families, Moreau argues that a close study of the apparently healthy members would show that their ancestors and descendants were scrofulous, tubercular, skittish in temper, or at least eccentric.

Like all the early great thinkers about neurosis, Moreau was searching for an overarching theory at a time when medical men were quite ignorant of the causes of a host of illnesses. So he confused many illness categories. Tuberculosis, malaria, and syphilis, three infectious diseases, are thrown together by Moreau into one category with cretinism, rickets, and pellagra, three diseases resulting from vitamin and mineral deficiencies. Likewise, nearly every term that Moreau used as a diagnostic label was characterized by a vague, almost literary tone. For instance, he described various patients as consumptive and rickety idiots. This might mean someone with tuberculosis and vitamin D deficiency who also was mentally retarded. But the specific meanings of such terms may have little or no correspondence to specific modern categories of illness. "Rickety," for instance, meant not only vitamin D deficient but also run down and creaky. A consumptive could be not only an individual suffering from an infection by the tuberculosis bacillus but also any wasted, pale, and slowly dying patient. Similarly, the word "idiot" could mean mentally retarded but could also refer to those whom we moderns would call psychotic or schizophrenic.

Moreau also described cases in which the idiot-to-be was not an idiot at all as a child but rather a prodigy. "These children," he

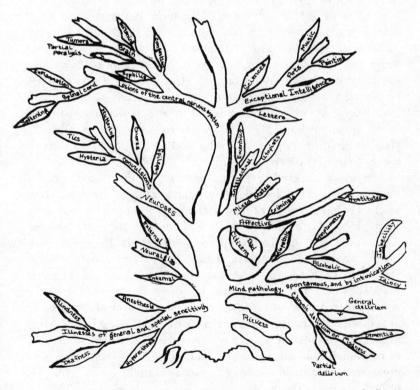

J. J. Moreau's tree of nervosity. (From J. J. Moreau, *La Psychologie Morbide*)

wrote, "are remarkable for the mobility of their thoughts, the instability of desires and wishes, which is only equated by the turbulence, their incoercible urge to come and go, without a purpose, passing rapidly from one thing to another." Arguing from these cases, Moreau stated that "the morbid principle of idiocy tends, primitively and essentially, to augment the intellectual activities, not to diminish it," and the overexcitement of certain brain centers or parts led to a "breaking of the cogs." This image captures Moreau's concept of the mind as a kind of machine that, if overworked, breaks down. Thus a child genius turns into an idiot, a benighted denizen of an asylum. Such a metaphorical way of thinking was at the heart of the Genius myth of neurosis.

In *The Idiot* (1868) Fyodor Dostoevski expresses many elements of this Genius myth. The protagonist, Prince Lev Myshkin, is an idiot in many of Moreau's senses of the term. Reduced to a state of complete mental confusion as a child, he had lived under the care of a doctor in Switzerland for most of his youth. As this novel begins, the prince is on his way back to Russia, apparently in a healthy state of mind. But soon we are introduced to a triumvirate of characters whose workings will drive the prince mad: the half-mad Rogozhin, whose lust for blood is repugnant; Nastassya, the fallen woman whom Myshkin wishes to save; and, finally, the youthful and sheltered Aglaya, who would seem the perfect match for the prince if he were not an idiot.

The prince is a kind of religious mystic, a genius whose uncanny honesty and lack of decorum attract and intrigue the other characters. He has the ability to see to the very core of every person he meets. He looks far deeper into life than other men and women. This vision very quickly complicates his relationship with Nastassya, Rogozhin, and Aglaya. He wishes to marry both women and to make Rogozhin, who has already tried to kill him, his blood brother. The complicated workings of his mind and the equally complicated turn of events lead the poor prince to disaster at a dinner party given by Aglaya's parents. He begins speaking, and at first sounds like a sheer genius, a man whose Christian sense of mission could save the world. But then his thoughts seem to grow overwrought, and in his overexcited state he has an epileptic fit in the midst of the party.

From then on, the prince begins to disintegrate. When Aglaya insists that he accompany her to a confrontation with Nastassya and Rogozhin, the prince cannot tear himself away from Nastassya. He stays behind to comfort and save her. In so doing he ruins his relationship with Aglaya. After Nastassya insists on marrying Myshkin, she runs off with the brutish Rogozhin, marries him instead, and then is murdered by him. The story ends with the unraveled prince back in the Swiss sanatorium, reduced to a state of utter idiocy.

Prince Myshkin is part-genius, part-mystic doomed by neurological destiny. In *Morbid Psychology* Moreau had posited that "the virtue and the vices [of the excessive nervous energy] can come from the same foyer, the virtue being the genius, the vice, idiocy." Although Moreau did give lip service to those who say "the grand social commotion of the French Revolution may have affected the nervous systems" of Frenchmen and Europeans adversely, he was following many of the medical thinkers of the day in stressing that in nine out of ten cases the source of mental illness is heredity, which to the nineteenth-century scientist was an idea quite comparable to earlier notions of destiny or original sin. Genius and madness are not acts of a free will: "Does the writer, the poet, the musician, give himself up freely to inspiration, that sacred fire which consumes them?" No, it is an innate need, an inherited quality.

Like the idiot, the genius receives the germ of nervous overexcitement from a debauched father. The overexcited part of the brain is precisely that which gives rise to great creative work. Of course the genius can easily pass over into idiocy, since he is a monomaniac bent on the one great original idea at the center of his work. Furthermore, he is prone to disturbed states of mind such as reveries, trances, and exalted moments of inspiration.

Moreau's idea is really a tantalizing notion. It binds together many kinds of mental phenomena, some momentarily pathological, such as epilepsy or hysteria, others twistedly and chronically self-annihilating, such as idiocy and dementia, and still others perhaps not pathological at all, such as prophecy and artistic creativity. What unites them for Moreau is overexcitement of the brain, the central nervous system of man, which inevitably leads to a "neurosis," be it an acute seizure, a raving madness, or a split second of creative genius.

By the 1870s there existed in the West a long medical and cultural legacy concerning the complex subjects of neurosis and nervousness. Though the old terms "melancholy," "hypochondria," and "hysteria" had originally implied causative theories that had nothing to do with the nervous system, by the middle of the eighteenth century the concept of nervousness came to subsume them all. Following a period when British medicine developed a number of theories about neuroses, two prominent continental schools of medicine came to flourish. The French school concentrated its theorizing on the idea of a lesion in the nerves, the German school based itself on the concept of unbalanced motion through the nerves.

These two ideas were to have a dialectic relationship throughout the nineteenth century, particularly after the Franco-Prussian War of 1870. The competition between French and German medicine paralleled the growing chauvinism of the century. However, neither the physiological nor the anatomic approaches could remain the property of one nation. Through the international community of science these seemingly contradictory ideas influenced many scientists throughout the Western world. Eventually the dialectic produced a synthesis of the static and the dynamic, which, with the emerging clinical picture of the individual patient, invigorated the theories of the great medical thinkers of the late Victorian period.

Alongside these theories of causation and the scores of inchoate clinical disorders and symptoms called nervous and neurotic, there arose four clearly defined myths about how a neurosis was bred. The Angelic Invalid possesses refined nerves that are susceptible to being frayed and strained. The Noble Savage is destroyed by the evils of the modern city—by alcohol, opium, coffee and tobacco, as well as the city's other luxuries and vices. The Degenerate has inherited his nervous taint from some debauched or overly emotional forebear. The Genius, the son of the Degenerate, may be destined for suicide or idiocy, yet his inspiration bestows on the world priceless pieces of literature, philosophy, statecraft, or science.

In all of these myths environment interacts with heredity. In its purest form the Noble Savage myth seems like an environmental theory, the Degenerate myth a hereditary theory. Yet in each myth resides an element of confusion of heredity with environment, as well as a hint of free will. The would-be Degenerate just might push aside the beaker of absinthe. The Noble Savage might break free of the temptation to surrender to licentiousness. In such a poignant moment of moral decision, when a neurotic patient comes looking for medical help, a nerve doctor could offer some enlightening counsel to drive away the darkening storm of nervosity.

None of these myths, of course, was provable; all relied on personal observations, anecdotes, case descriptions, anthropological and historical interpretations and prejudices. Still, they greatly affected late-nineteenth-century thinkers who were trying to creep forward to make the study of neurosis a genuine science. It was into this confusing and exhilarating milieu that Charcot, Beard, Krafft-Ebing, and indeed the young Freud were born.

THREE

Medical Imagination in an Age of Empire

HE Victorian epoch was a vast scientific exposition, cluttered with such shimmering wonders as the telegraph, the telephone, and the railway, all promising to tie the globe together in one great metropolis. The era seemed a vaulting steel cathedral scraping skyward, upon which the citizenry gazed in awe: the Crystal Palace in Kensington Gardens, jewel of the world exposition presided over by Prince Albert in 1851, or the Eiffel Tower, relic of that magnificent world exposition of 1887 in Paris. These expositions and others displayed the latest technological marvels to an enraptured public—gadgets and buzzers sounding, lights flashing, voices bouncing everywhere.

This world of science captured the imagination of many Victorians, particularly the doctors. Recalling the broad and optimistic horizon that seemed to spread before the late Victorians, the historian Arnold Toynbee later wrote that were he able to decide in which age to live, he would surely choose the nineteenth century. Europe and America were expanding forcefully into many corners of the earth by the 1870s. Inventive Westerners made major advances in many areas, including technology, ideology, and art, but especially science.

Scientific knowledge was expanding as quickly as the British Empire, and medicine fell more and more within the realm of science. In fact, the two worlds, imperial and medical, frequently paralleled each other in their growth. Dr. David Livingstone, the eminent scientific explorer and medical graduate of the University of Glasgow, played a significant role in staking out a large portion of central Africa for the British, as a result of his passion to discover the source of the Nile. Robert Koch, the microbe hunter of the sixties and seventies, cut off his Prussian roots as he cast off his first wife, and in the company of a second, much younger woman, spent the last decades of his life voyaging through Africa, capturing and exterminating microbes.

Medical historians have looked upon this period nostalgically, referring to the closing years of the nineteenth century as the Heroic Age of Medicine. Many medical illnesses won their names from the scientists who first described them during this period. Through a widening array of medical journals, pamphlets, books, and international congresses, physicians of different nations developed more unified paradigms of general disease.

Three revolutionary ideas in science bore specifically on Victorian thinking about neurosis: the germ theory of disease, the theory of biological evolution, and the complicated new anatomical and physiological models of the human nervous system.

Much of medical science in these times focused on the microscope and infectious disease. Louis Pasteur became a French national hero through his work with yeast and rabies, and his fabled intuitive scientific acumen became a national treasure. Koch likewise won acclaim for his studies of anthrax and tuberculosis. His methodical, uninspired approach was seen as a Prussian attribute. These two titans became locked in a struggle in the 1880s when their two nations, France and Germany, sent competing microscopy teams to Egypt to track down the cause of cholera, which was laying waste to the Egyptian populace. Cholera, like many infectious illnesses such as typhus, typhoid, and diphtheria, had stormed across Europe from time to time over the centuries, killing thousands and then vanishing. It was a horrible mystery. When the microscopy teams set out for Egypt, the land of the Sphinx, they were setting out on a heroic adventure.

From this duel Koch emerged victorious, advancing like Tamerlane, chasing cholera into the heart of India, then taking home with him to Berlin the enemy trapped in a vial, the vibrio bacterium. The vanquished French had their martyr in a young microscopist, Louis Thuillier, who perished in Egypt pursuing medical *gloire*.

In the 1880s and 1890s similar medical breakthroughs were made with typhus and typhoid, yellow fever, diphtheria, and malaria by other medical giants of the epoch. Infectious disease became the model of all diseases. A renowned textbook, *Principles and Practice of Medicine* (first ed., 1892), written by the British subject William Osler (1849–1919), who lived for many years in what he called Greater Britain—Canada and America—illustrates the impact of these epoch-making discoveries. The book begins with a lengthy discussion of the symptoms and clinical course of typhoid, then glides into similar accounts of other infectious diseases, and, finally, after hundreds of pages, describes illnesses for which no causative agent was then known. Infectious disease had become the queen of medical science.

Doctors had once been almost of the servant class, coming to the houses of the rich and mighty, fawning and ingratiating themselves with slick statements. Now physicians and scientists in this age who worked with microbes became prominent oracles, national heroes. Pasteur, Koch, Walter Reed, and Joseph Lister grew in international stature, had their portraits painted, found their pronouncements quoted in the newspapers as the reputation of their profession enlarged. The number of doctors who sat in the French Parliament from 1870 to 1900 amounted to nearly one-third of the members. In England the most prominent doctors were knighted, and in America great doctors often accrued fabulous wealth. Furthermore, the writing of medical history owes its inception as a discipline to a number of medical men of this period who decided to write the history of their profession. They frequently could not help themselves when they sang the praises of the great doctors of their time—usually themselves.

Many elements of this growing sense of medical optimism and self-importance can be found in a group portrait of four medical heroes by John Singer Sargent, the portraitist of many prominent Europeans and Americans in the Gilded Age. Sargent depicts the founders of the Johns Hopkins School of Medicine: Osler, the internist and textbook author; Howard Kelly, a gynecologist and evangelical Christian; William Stewart Halsted, a surgeon and cocaine addict; and William Welch, a pathologist interested in

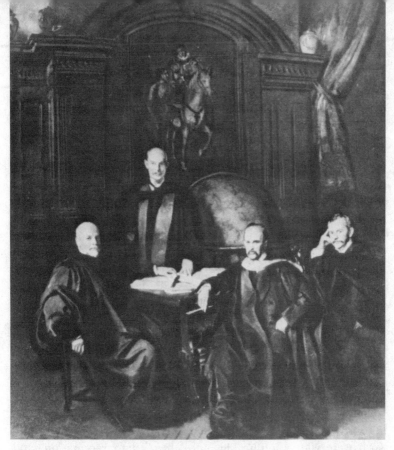

The Four Doctors by John Singer Sargent. (The Alan Chesney Medical Archives, The Johns Hopkins Medical Institutions, Baltimore)

public health and medical history. Each of these four men had an illness, a bacterium, or a surgical instrument named after him.

In this painting the four doctors wear flowing robes, implying both academic and priestly roles. At this time the public was seemingly turning more and more to the academic doctor for healing, away from the clergyman and medical quack. Science seemed to be everywhere, materialistic and victorious, shoving aside would-be competitors. At the center of the group portrait rests a globe, suggesting that medical men saw themselves as internationalists, working for humanity. Scientific medicine knew no barriers. Medical treatises of great length were rapidly translated, ideas won adherents across the spans of oceans within weeks or months, prominent doctors readily shuttled off to nearby countries for medical conventions or conferences. It was almost *de rigueur* for American physicians to travel to London, Paris, and Vienna to top off their training, wandering down the Rhine like Goethe's Wilhelm Meister.

Finally, a painting within the painting looms behind the four men. This painting, *Saint Martin on Horseback* by El Greco, shows the Roman Christian soldier Saint Martin of Tours tearing his robe and giving half to a beggar. So like the medical men of the age to see themselves this way! They saw themselves as a sainted class, helping the poor, the starving, and the distressed of the world with their knowledge. Like Saint Martin, though, medical men stayed on their chargers, safe in their hospitals and laboratories. A widening chasm began to separate the doctors from the patients, who had never understood medical science but who now became its bedazzled beneficiaries. Indeed, medical men saw this chasm, this ignorant hero worship, as a benefit. The doctor could capture some of the mystique that had once belonged only to the religious prophet. Faith or confidence, now called placebo, could be used to work cures.

Yet doctors also knew that their weapons were based on more than just blind faith. The discoveries of men such as Pasteur and Koch were widely applicable, since they led to vaccinations and other techniques of disease control. Likewise, doctors such as Lister in England and Ignaz Semmelweiss in Austria-Hungary applied the germ theory of disease to surgery and obstetrics and so saved thousands of lives. Quarantines screened out potentially infected individuals and prevented new outbreaks of diseases. It is proper to coin the term "medical imperialism" to describe this period in American history. The American conquests of Cuba, Puerto Rico, and later the Panama Canal stand out not only as military or political expansions, the pushing aside of a decaying Spanish civilization and the rising up of a more vital American one, but also as a conquest of infectious disease.

Medical men applied the germ theory to a number of age-old neuroses, including rabies. In this disease the bite of an infected mad dog caused a human being to become delirious. Rabies, or hydrophobia, had remained a mystery since ancient times. Every possible explanation, including possession by the devil or an im-

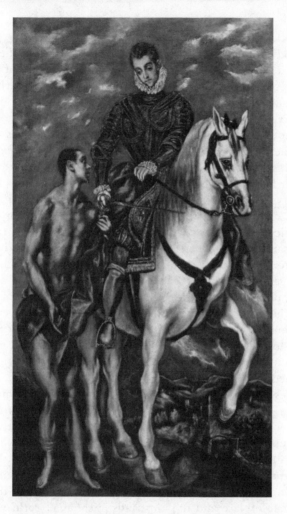

With *Saint Martin and the Beggar*, by El Greco, as backdrop. (Art Museum of Chicago)

balance of the four humors, enjoyed some popularity but offered no cure. The world waited.

Then the great Pasteur arrived on the scene. Fresh from his work with infectious illnesses in silkworms and sheep, the great French scientist posited that a germ, a submicroscopic particle, passed from the dog's teeth into the human flesh and flowed via the blood to the brain. Acting upon this theory, he heroically injected a weakened form of the rabies virus into the brain of a nine-year-old boy named Joseph Meister who days earlier had been bitten by a rabid dog. Following multiple inoculations with progressively stronger forms of the virus, the boy never exhibited any symptoms and returned to his home cured. Rabies was defeated, the world stood astonished and joyful, and the inoculation approach spread.

Similar heroic tales record the defeat of other infectious illnesses such as typhus, typhoid, malaria, and diphtheria, as well as other illnesses, such as cretinism or rickets, caused by vitamin or mineral deficiencies or by toxins such as lead or alcohol. Since these illnesses manifested such mental crises as a feverish delirium and such chronic symptoms as malaise and loss of memory and will, doctors came to believe that many neurotic illnesses—epilepsy, hysteria, phobias and anxiety, even sexual perversion—might also have at their roots various germs, toxins, or deficiencies. As incredible as some of the applications of the germ, toxin, and deficiency theories to nervous illness may appear now, they seemed not only logical but imperative to doctors at the time.

The second popular scientific idea that appeared in myriad, sometimes distorted forms in the medical literature was biological evolution. Usually attributed to Charles Darwin and Alfred Wallace, biological evolution was soon generalized to society. After Darwin published *Origin of Species* in 1859, Thomas Huxley, who, incidentally, had been trained as a surgeon, took up the Darwinian cudgel in science's debate with religion. Huxley and Herbert Spencer popularized the sociological concept that the capitalistic marketplace and the imperialistic colonial world were the arenas within which evolution occurred, and many doctors in the next two decades embraced this thinking. Soon the nineteenth-century Western world was pictured in the popular imagination as the high point of the evolutionary spiral.

Spencer is one of those great figures of the nineteenth century, nearly forgotten today, since his thinking is so riddled with technical errors. However, as Richard Hofstadter writes in his book *Social Darwinism in American Thought,* Spencer enjoyed a vogue across America in the seventies and eighties. He appealed precisely to the American ethos of self-betterment. Though a good Darwinian could pick holes in Spencer's application of evolution to society, many Americans and Europeans liked seeing themselves and their society as highly evolved. Even Alfred Wallace, Darwin's confrere, had argued that the seat of most evolution in man was the human brain. That is, the massive frontal lobes, not the muscles or the limbs or any other part of man, were the biological site where evolution was on the move. Humans, it seemed to many evolutionists, could stretch their brains and grow smarter. This distorted notion of the Darwinian idea of evolution proliferated and captured the imagination of medical men during this period. It was common for scientific figures in the nineteenth century to refer to Darwin when they really meant Huxley, Spencer, Wallace, or especially the Frenchman Jean Baptiste Lamarck, who had posited that an acquired trait in a parent could be inherited by an offspring. This Lamarckian theory was not Darwinian natural selection at all.

As with the germ theory, medical men also applied the evolutionary concept to neurosis. The Western world saw itself as greater than the yellow or the black races, which were in turn greater than the apes and the orangutans, which in turn rose from a long string of species that ultimately rose out of the primordial slime. Since the so-called French school of medicine had for decades conceived neurosis to be caused by anatomical lesions and irritations of the nerves, many doctors came to see neurosis as a product of an irritating struggle of Western man against his ever more complicated, ever more civilized environment. This imagined struggle in the nerves might lead man upward to greater heights of civilization or might lead him downward, through a strain on his brain, to neurosis.

The third cluster of ruling medical ideas during this epoch concerned the nervous system proper. In the 1830s the reflex-arc theory of the nervous system was promulgated by Marshall Hall of Great Britain. This theory stated that a sensory input traveling along a nerve struck against another nerve, whose output led to the movement of a muscle. In the middle of the century a group of European anatomists and physiologists set to work with new techniques for staining, fixing, and viewing the nervous system through microscopes. This work gave birth to a heated argument over the structure of the nervous system. Ultimately, in 1891, a

German named Heinrich Wilhelm Waldeyer posited the neuron theory, according to which the nervous system was not a homogeneous substance but rather a network of separate cells that communicated with one another via long, near-touching tentacles. This too was a major breakthrough.

The concept that the nervous system of man was divisible into discrete centers had grown popular through the impetus of Joseph Gall's phrenology. By the 1850s and 1860s Paul Broca of France and Carl Wernicke in Germany had mapped out areas of brain tissue that specialized in the formation of words. Shortly thereafter the Briton David Ferrier (1843–1928) published his work showing that one very discrete part of the brain of monkeys was specifically connected with sensory input, another with motor output. Arguing by analogy to humans, doctors believed they could literally see into the nervous system of man and see many brain centers that performed discrete tasks. The story goes that in 1881 one of the great systematizers of thinking about neurosis, Jean-Martin Charcot, was present at one of Ferrier's demonstrations on monkeys in London. In the middle of the presentation, as Ferrier attached electrodes to various parts of the brain tissue of his monkeys and made different muscles twitch and vibrate, Charcot leaped up and shouted in English, "It is a patient!" Charcot could see in his mind's eye discrete brain centers in healthy human beings and hence discrete lesions in human patients that would do precisely what the electrodes had done to the monkeys.

This stupendous idea, that the nervous system—the seat of words and understanding—was in fact a delicate conglomerate of single cells divided into various nerve centers, upon which reflex arcs operated, came to intrigue many doctors during this age. The realization that this nervous system was alive with electricity occurred almost concurrently with Hermann von Helmholtz's measurement of the speed of this electricity, and Moritz Heinrich Romberg based his textbook on the concept that neuroses were diseases in which a physiological fault existed.

In the same decades, the 1850s and 1860s, telegraph lines were strung with great rapidity across Europe and America. Two Englishmen, William Cooke and Charles Wheatstone, and the American, Samuel Morse, had invented their telegraph systems almost concurrently in 1837, followed by Alexander Graham Bell, who invented the telephone in 1875, and Thomas Edison with the light bulb in the 1880s. These inventions did not fail to affect thinking about the human nervous system. By the late nineteenth century the nervous system of the neurotic came to be seen as faulty, lacking nerve strength or being low in electricity. Medical textbooks teemed with ideas of fancied nerve centers and overexcitement or loss of nerve energy. Doctors fought intellectual battles over the question of whether or not particular nerve centers existed and whether the waning of nerve energy in a particular malady was hereditary or acquired. Still, these new debates ensued on what seemed solid ground, namely, the anatomic paradigm of brain organization and the physiological postulate that action occurred from neuron to neuron, nerve center to nerve center, via reflex arcs and electrical current.

Though the germ, toxin, and deficiency theories, the evolutionary theory and its extension into social evolution, and the new brain paradigms were best perceived only as scientific hypotheses, they were applied very quickly to real patients, flesh-and-blood sufferers. After all, doctors are not just scientists but also practitioners, who have tended to absorb scientific theories quickly and sometimes apply them wrongly.

What is so perplexing, though amusing—and herein lies a paradox—is that these wrongheaded applications have sometimes led to cures! For instance, when Richard von Krafft-Ebing's *Psychopathia Sexualis* first appeared in the 1880s, various homosexuals, clandestine fetishists, and transvestites read the book and wrote and came to him in droves. His complex therapeutic approach to sexual disorders drew on the deficiency theory, the brain center idea, and the evolutionary theory in a way that now seems to verge on the ridiculous, yet his treatment seemed helpful to his patients. Likewise, Beard's idea of neurasthenia drew on all three theories, but his electrical therapy seemed to work wonders. Hypnosis too seemed a panacea to many doctors. Though Charcot himself doubted the efficacy of hypnosis in the treatment of hysteria and related neurotic disorders, his interest was spurred on by his belief that he could cast new light on both the illness of hysteria and the technique of hypnotism via the three new overarching theories. So were the doctors encouraged to believe in their mistaken theories, and to theorize further.

We must remember that the rapid application of general scientific principles, not just to neurosis but to other subjects in science, had gone on for centuries, long before Charcot, Krafft-Ebing, and Beard came on the scene, and had frequently yielded dazzling new ideas. The doctors writing about neurosis who carved out huge scientific empires had some very solid intellectual comrades-in-arms. Darwin wrote that he stumbled on his ideas of struggle between species while reading the works of an economist, Thomas Malthus. Another economist, Karl Marx, taking back the idea from Darwin, recast this notion as class struggle. So too Spencer, building upon the thinking of the French mathematician and philosopher Auguste Comte, extended the domain of science from physics through chemistry, biology, and psychology to sociology. Going even further, the German scientist Ernst Haeckel wrote an evolutionary work entitled *The Riddle of the Universe*, in which he proposed his own book as the answer. Using humor, cajolery, and vitriol to refute the tenets of religion, he attempted a total synthesis that overreached even the bounds of science as he applied evolutionary theory to religious beliefs.

To understand the Victorian doctors even better we must remember their greatest weakness, namely, their ignorance. Victorian doctors were blind to whole vistas of medicine that are now understood in vivid detail. They knew little or nothing definite about such areas of medicine as immunology, endocrinology, pharmacology, genetics, and laboratory diagnostics. Not knowing when to plead ignorance, they blurred neuroses together with other illnesses in a manner that betrayed their scientific hubris. It would fall to later, less heroic medical scientists to partition these huge mental expanses into minuscule areas of specialization.

Immunology is now a vast field that is clearly connected to the study of infectious diseases. It also includes the so called autoimmune diseases such as rheumatoid arthritis, in which the immunological system seems to attack its own tissue. Likewise, immunology is a central area in investigating allergies and, it now seems, the resistance and susceptibility to many cancers. To Victorian doctors the existence of an antigen-antibody complex—a phenomenon at the heart of immunology—was not known. The argument that a foreign agent such as the tuberculosis bacillus or syphilis spirochete would enter the body and bring forth an immunological response in the body and therefore an inflammation was not at all clear in the Victorian period. Doctors frequently spoke of nervous constitution in cases in which the modern doctor would speak of a lack of immunological response. When the Victorian physician referred to pale and weak individuals with low nerve force, he was sometimes speaking of patients with a poor immunological system.

Similarly, in endocrinology, hormonal agents such as thyroid hormone, insulin, and testosterone were only isolated between 1914 and 1931. Thus it is not surprising to see that goiter, or hypothyroidism, which has profound nervous manifestations, such as imbecility, was long equated with neurosis. Likewise, Graves' disease, or hyperthyroidism, which causes nervousness and anxiety, was considered a neurosis. So too menses, which can lead to mood changes and hot flashes in women, seemed neurotic events. In their ignorance the great thinkers on neurosis ascribed all these phenomena to nerves.

In regard to pharmacology, the great Canadian-American doctor William Osler believed that there were only a few medicines of any value in 1890, namely, potassium bromide for epilepsy and digitalis for heart disease. Osler was what doctors then called a therapeutic nihilist, a doctor who scorned most traditional cures. In reality he was just a good medical scientist who admitted that the pharmacopeia extant in the 1890s was powerless, except as placebo. Although a vast pharmacopeia existed all the way back to antiquity, Osler and other rational doctors discarded many of these plant extracts as being of no value. Eventually this became the stance of all Western doctors. Hence, many of the diseases the Victorians saw, such as asthma, tuberculosis, or thyroid conditions, simply had to go in the direction of what physicians called the "natural history," which meant death. Doctors were reduced to sitting by the bedside watching, consoling, and theorizing.

Likewise, laboratory medicine has made huge leaps since Victorian times. The late Victorians knew how to take temperatures, how to measure urea and diagnose anemia, if crudely, in the laboratory, but really very little else. They had to rely heavily on their physical examinations, their histories, and intuition. The electrocardiogram was first used in 1903, the electroencephalogram twenty-six years later.

Another underdeveloped area of medicine in the nineteenth century was genetics. The Moravian monk Gregor Mendel had in fact done his original experiments with plants and presented his work before the scientific world in 1855. Yet his ideas, which later would become essential to a truly scientific study of heredity, seem to have won no recognition, and so his work lay gathering dust until the early twentieth century. Therefore all Victorian rhetoric about inheritance, hereditary taint, and neurotic forebears was founded on a highly vague, almost literary notion that at times smacked less of the genes than of original sin. When the French poet Charles Baudelaire wrote, "My ancestors, idiots or maniacs, in solemn apartments, all the victims of dreadful passion," he was as close to an understanding of inheritance as most of his medical contemporaries.

Victorian doctors also had an imprecise notion of what was called constitution or predisposition. The confusion of sperm and germ deepened the misunderstanding of constitution. Indeed, the idea of a germ in Victorian times was almost a kind of misunderstood pun. The word "germ" was used to describe not only an infectious agent, such as the rabies germ or the tuberculosis germ, but also the sperm and the egg. Furthermore, many mothers in the Victorian period did pass on infectious germs, not only sperm and eggs, to their offspring. This could involve not only chronic infectious illnesses such as tuberculosis and syphilis, which went from a mother through her placenta to her child, but also the vitamin-deficiency states such as rickets and pellagra.

The great contributors to the modern understanding of neurosis who thrived during this period breathed the air of this heady intellectual hubbub, and their systems of thought reflect the complicated and confusing medical imagination of the times. Westerners in the late nineteenth century were grand systematizers, not only politically but also scientifically and medically. They not only wished to put the chaos of the world in order but frequently thought they could.

This desire to systematize was much akin to the myth-making described in the previous chapter. Charcot, the great systematizer of thought about hysteria and hypnosis, was deeply immersed in a tradition of French neurology that blindly accepted both the Degenerate and Genius myths. Similarly, George Miller Beard, the coiner of the term "neurasthenia," was really reworking the Angelic Invalid myth of Cheyne and Whytt but with an evolutionary twist. The Angelic Invalid, the delicate person of the better classes, became Beard's "brain-worker," the human at the very top of the evolutionary ladder whose nervous sensitivity was both an asset and an Achilles' heel. Finally, Richard von Krafft-Ebing, in his work with perversions and homosexuality, relied not only on the Degenerate myth but also on many elements of the Noble Savage myth. Although he saw many forms of perversions and homosexuality as hereditary, he also saw some perversions as acquired via the evils of civilization. He believed that he could treat only the acquired, not the hereditary form of perversions and homosexuality, and doomed those hereditarily tainted to eternal misery.

In the next three chapters we shall concentrate on Charcot, probably the greatest Victorian student of neurosis. In still later chapters we shall return to Krafft-Ebing and Beard. Each of these three doctors, along with a number of other Victorian medical figures, pressed the four old myths in brilliant new directions. Stimulated by the germ theory, the evolutionary theory, and the new paradigms of the human nervous system, they looked more deeply into the subject of neurosis and popularized three more myths about how a neurosis came to flourish.

FOUR

A Tale of Two Neuroses

CLEARLY the most prominent neurologist in this age of noble doctors was the great Charcot (1825–93), a short and stout Parisian professor with an eye for the visually dramatic. A close second was J. Hughlings Jackson (1835–1911), a shy Englishman with a meticulous, almost obsessive style of thinking, writing, and public speaking. Each of these men, perhaps following his own idiosyncrasies, chose to circumscribe one specific neurotic illness and tried to sound its depths more deeply than anyone who had come before. The Briton focused on epilepsy, the Frenchman on hysteria.

It is impossible to stress too much the fact that for centuries epilepsy and hysteria were difficult to distinguish from each other. Both the epileptic and the hysteric would fall to the ground, make odd noises, flail about like one possessed. In fact, an amalgamated term, "hystero-epilepsy," had existed for a few centuries before the time of Charcot and Jackson. To many doctors these two diseases of the nerves were really one, or at least bedfellows, the epileptic lying beside the hysteric in the same hospital ward, their names appearing as nearly touching leaves on Moreau's Tree of Nervosity.

Jackson and Charcot admired each other. Charcot even kept a plaque of Jackson in his office. Ultimately, however, their investigations went in very different directions. Each attempted to remain true to the scientific method, yet each reached very different conclusions about an issue as basic as the proper role of a physician.

Charcot rose from very humble roots. The second son of a carriage builder, he was a self-made man, and his plodding determination was the key ingredient in his success. The story goes that

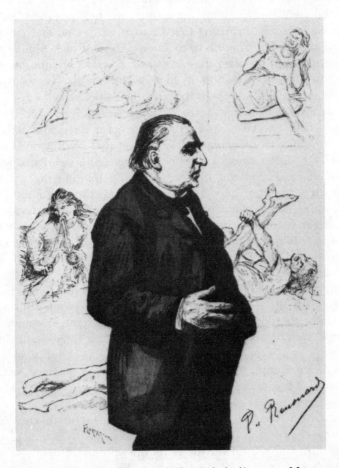

Jean-Martin Charcot, Caesar of the Salpêtrière, world expert on hysteria. Dr. Renouard, *Docteur Charcot*. (Rare Book Room, Countway Library of Medicine, Harvard University, Boston)

his own father, having called his four sons around the family hearth, turned to them and said, "My resources do not afford the possibilities of your all pursuing long and expensive educations. Taking account of your respective abilities, I have made this decision: You, Martin, will be a carriage builder like me; you, Emile, will go into the army; and you, Eugene, into the marines, so that you, Jean-Martin, as you are such a studious worker, will continue in school, and when the time comes you will choose between painting and medicine." Taking into account the heavy burden laid on this son, it is not surprising that Charcot was a cold and taciturn youth, withdrawn from his companions. Prone to sketching at odd moments over the years, he developed a visual orientation that came to play a central role in his slow but steady rise to prominence at Pinel's old hospital in Paris, the Salpêtrière.

By 1870 Charcot had become known as an innovator in the lecture hall. For nearly twenty years he gave a series of well attended, thought-provoking weekly lectures that he illustrated with visual aids such as slides and impersonations of his patients' walks or tremors. He brought disease to life by inviting the patients themselves to enter the lecture hall to reveal their tremors, their deformities, and ultimately their hysterical fits. Charcot developed a flair for the clear, crisp, and succinct presentation, even when lecturing about subjects potentially as tedious as rheumatoid arthritis and multiple sclerosis. His Gallic nose, his aristocratic demeanor, and his literary style won him the nickname of Caesar of the Salpêtrière. Charcot wisely married a wealthy widow, who devoted her life to their two children, Jean and Jeanne, but most especially to facilitating the work of her brilliant husband. Although various anecdotes by his awestruck disciples would have it that he was completely indifferent to thoughts about money, he nonetheless rose to great financial and social prominence, with a salon in the fashionable Faubourg St. Germain, frequented by doctors, wealthy patients, artists, and intellectuals.

Charcot eventually became the famed consultant to kings and princes. His bedside and drawing-room manners were impeccable. His subtle and refined artistic tastes only deepened his appeal to the rich and sophisticated of Europe. Personal friends with M. Gambetta, the French prime minister, he remained for decades the family doctor to both M. Fauld, who had been the French Min-

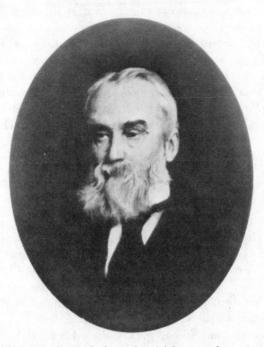

John Hughlings Jackson, father of British neurology, world expert on epilepsy. (From Montreal Neurological Institute, *Neurological Biographies and Addresses*)

ister of Finance under Louis Napoleon, and the Archduke Nicholai of Russia. He is said to have brought Nicholai and Gambetta together one night for dinner at his Neuilly estate and so set in motion the political peregrinations that culminated in the Franco-Russian entente against the Germans.

Despite his social brilliance and artistic sophistication, Charcot's greatest attention was relentlessly fastened on medicine. One day he was on his way to his usual massive lunch at a restaurant near the Salpêtrière when a sick man suffering from multiple sclerosis hailed the carriage, begging for money. Offering to donate his nervous system post-mortem to Charcot, the sick man said he wanted to buy tobacco now. Charcot was said to have smiled and given, for, like his patron St. Martin, Charcot pitied the poor. But unlike Martin, he also had more practical motives: he was after the beggar's nervous system to help him in his dogged search for scientific truth.

Meanwhile, across the English Channel in London, Jackson was developing as a medical thinker. The fourth son of a farmer, Jackson was a shy man with a weak voice and a dislike for long conversations, who also disdained sports, parties, and the theater. When Jackson gave medical lectures from 1860 onward, he seemed to lack stage presence. His lectures at the London Hospital and the National Hospital for the Paralyzed and the Epileptic during half a century were always poorly attended. Though his nickname was "The Sage" and his contemporaries compared him to Sam Johnson, his writing lacks grace and certainly is not good literature.

Jackson was an English eccentric who lacked the refinement of Charcot. He actually bragged in later life about his poor general education. As his colleague Dr. Jonathan Hutchinson writes, "he held that by exemption from overteaching, his mind had retained more freedom and energy than might otherwise have been the case." In his adult years he developed the habit of ripping in half the Victorian thrillers to which he was addicted. This way he could insert one half in one pocket, the other half in another, and read through them at vacant moments while riding in his carriage. At the theater he would lose interest in any performance, good or bad, and leave Covent Garden after the first act with some stuffy medical question filling his mind. He seems never to have remembered the names of his patients and usually referred to them by their diseased body part; the disease rather than the human being was the central issue. This ability to disregard the person and focus on the disease would prove quintessential to his success as a medical thinker.

Back in Paris, Charcot was toiling away in the Salpêtrière, an old saltpeter depot converted into a state haven for women in the seventeenth century. When Charcot first arrived there as a young doctor in the 1850s he found nearly five thousand women lying in massive, ill-lit, and poorly aired rooms in the impersonal Florence Nightingale ward style typical of the times. Many of the women manifested what modern doctors would separate into neurological, psychological, and social illnesses. There were syphilitics, epileptics, alcoholics, and aging prostitutes. They lay like odd

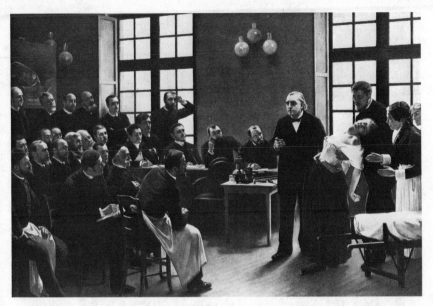

The school of Jean-Martin Charcot. André Pierre Brouillet, *A Clinical Lesson of Dr. Charcot at the Salpêtrière*. (Rare Book Room, Countway Library of Medicine, Harvard University, Boston)

crustaceans or fungi, growing old and dying in the classical-style buildings on the banks of the Seine.

Never losing heart, Charcot, in the 1860s and 1870s, went from room to room, and, just as Adam named the animals in the Garden of Eden, he named various neurological illnesses for the first time. He was the first to describe multiple sclerosis, amyotrophic lateral sclerosis, and syphilitic joints. He also first delineated a muscular disorder now called Charcot-Marie-Tooth disease. His biographers have said that his relentless visual orientation and medical intuition led to his success. They describe Charcot as having been able to sit for hours in the presence of a patient with an unexplained symptom; he would ponder, look, ruminate, breathe heavily. He would examine with his hands, hit a reflex or two, reflect on his ideas, and have his disciples do likewise. Then—in the manner of a scientific genius—the symptoms would suddenly fall into a definable order in his mind.

A famous medical painting by André Pierre Brouillet called "A Clinical Lesson of Doctor Charcot at the Salpêtrière" (1887) shows Charcot supporting a fainting hysterical woman, presumably while describing her symptoms. The audience consists of a host of his prominent followers, all important neurologists of the day. Charcot encouraged the brilliant neurologists he collected around him to be innovative in their own right. They responded favorably, circumscribing various illnesses and implementing procedures for the first time, sometimes naming their discoveries after themselves. For instance, Joseph Babinsky gave his name to an important neurological reflex and Georges Gilles de la Tourette gave his name to a very intriguing neurological disease. Another notable in the painting, Desiré Bourneville, wrote a ponderous book about epilepsy and hysteria. Tourette and Paul Richer composed voluminous tracts on hysteria. Dr. Paul Regnard introduced the camera into the halls of the hospital, to capture the split-second commotion and static symptomatology of the patients on film. Dr. Victor Burg introduced magnets, Dr. Romain Vigouroux electricity, both as therapy for neurotic illnesses. Finally, Pierre Janet was conducting in-depth studies of the mental conditions of his patients.

It was not simply Charcot's personal brilliance that made him famous but the impetus he gave to his men. Because of his sensitive, if sometimes imperious manner, these men acted almost like Charcot's understudies. The enormous output of this group of doctors introduced a vivacity and excitement into medicine that influenced doctors, patients, and the lay public across all of Europe and North America.

The biographical sketches by Charcot's former disciples written after his death would have it that chance brought the hysterics of the Salpêtrière to Charcot. Apparently a part of the ancient buildings housing the hysterics and epileptics was condemned, and its inmates needed to be placed elsewhere. So the epileptics and hysterics were transferred to Charcot's care, giving him the opportunity to study the two groups. Though this story is true, it is also a fact that hystero-epilepsy as a single illness category was a few hundred years old by 1870. With chance and medical custom each playing a role, Charcot and his followers, who often were referred to in historical works simply by Charcot's name alone, turned their attention more and more to patients in the Salpêtrière described as suffering from one illness, hysteria.

As we have already seen, "hysteria" means simply "uterus." Both Hippocrates' theory that hysterical symptoms were products of uterine wanderings and Galen's notion that hysteria was caused by a vaporous substance exuded from the uterus survived into the eighteenth century. Spiritual theories of various mental and bodily illnesses were also intertwined with these medical doctrines. Medical men such as Cullen had tried to follow new lines of development by spinning new theories that stressed the importance of the nerves. But even by the time Charcot took an interest in the subject, hysteria—defined as a neurosis in women marked by fainting, convulsions, loss of sensation, and a host of other symptoms—continued to be described in medical textbooks as a woman's disease related to the ovaries or the uterus through the passing of unhappy sensations via the nerves to the brain. Treatment by surgical removal of the uterus and ovaries remained common.

When Charcot ran up against hysteria, he was unable to locate a lesion in the nervous system. All autopsy studies showed no pathology. Thwarted in his attempt to find a lesion, as he had in cases of multiple sclerosis, Charcot fell back on his visual talent. He undertook a careful study of the clinical phenomena of the disorder and scrupulously classified the symptoms he saw.

His classification divided hysteria into two major clusters of symptoms. The first, the seizure proper, was appropriately called the seizure portion of the disease. The second he called the stigmata, meaning the symptoms present between the seizures.

One stigmatic symptom was anesthesia, the presence of areas on the body where the hysteric felt no sensation. Two more were tremors and paralysis. A fourth was contracture, or the tendency of the hysteric to become paralyzed so long in a particular position that an examining doctor could apply all his physical force without being able to change it. A fifth symptom was astasia-abasia, or difficulty walking and standing. This Latinized-Greek term really meant tottering and near swooning. Next came tunnel vision, a narrowing of visual fields that permitted the hysterical patient to see only objects directly in front, not off to the sides.

The last stigmatic symptom was the presence of hysterogenic points on the body. French neurologists had found that most of their patients subject to hysterical fits possessed a number of points

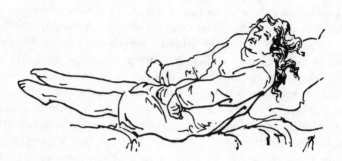

Phases of the grand hysteria: I. Epileptoid. (From Paul Richer, *La Grande Hystérie*)

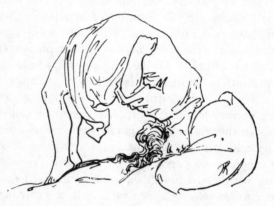

II. Grand movement: *arc-en-cercle*. (From Richer, *La Grande Hystérie*)

on their bodies that, if pressed, either caused a seizure or aborted one. A number of sketches in French publications depicted these so-called hysterogenic points on female patients' bodies. Explanatory theory relied heavily on the reflex-arc idea: pressing the skin must cause an electrical impulse to pass inward through the nerves to a point in the spinal cord or brain where, through reflex action, a second electrical impulse, moving outward, culminated in a fit or the cessation of a fit. In accordance with this simplistic theory, Charcot and his followers, and indeed many great neurologists in distant cities, felt that the hysteric had more weakened and impressionable nerves and therefore was likely to react more calamitously to slight pressure on particular body points than a normal man or woman would. And the reflex thus set off was strong enough to send the whole nervous system into a fit. It would begin with a slight aura, or tingling, around the hysterogenic point and then rise up into the stomach, then to the throat, and finally set off a generalized fit.

Charcot divided the seizures themselves into four parts. First came the epileptoid phase, which seemed to resemble fairly closely the convulsions of epilepsy. The patient would spontaneously drop to the floor and go through tonic and clonic movements (flailing and jerking motions). Then, in the second phase—that of grand movements, or clownism—peculiar twists and turns, bizarre and grotesque feats of dexterity were performed. The ultimate grand movement, the pirouette of hysteria, Charcot called *arc-en-cercle*. Herein the patient arched her back, balancing on her heels and head like an acrobat.

Next came the third period, that of passionate attitudes. This proved to be the most intriguing phase in hysteria. In this phase the patient experienced various false sensory or mental images, reveries, had visions of snakes, brigands, and monsters, and seemed frightened or glad, morose or giggling in turn. The patient would babble and shout, repeat phrases and gestures. Charcot would listen, detecting experiences from the patient's past or her imagination.

Fourth, and last, would come the delirious phase, when the patient entered into noisy weeping and lamentation, or laughing and giggling mixed with stupor.

During the later years of his career critics of Charcot would state that florid phenomena such as arc-en-cercle and passionate attitudes were not seen in hysterics outside of Paris. Charcot countered that the illness category he was describing was grand hysteria, the full-blown, perhaps most degenerated form of the disease. Other less dramatic symptoms—a minor paralysis or only

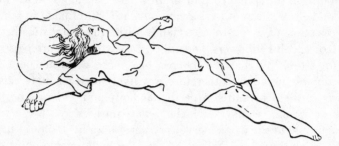

III. Passionate attitude: crucifixion. (From Richer, *La Grande Hystérie*)

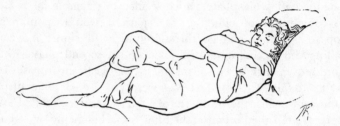

III. Passionate attitude: erotic posturing. (From Richer, *La Grande Hystérie*)

an occasional swooning—occurred in what he called petit hysteria.

While Charcot's curiosity over hysteria grew in Paris, J. Hughlings Jackson had already begun similarly meticulous work on another neurosis, epilepsy. A rather taciturn, thoughtful, and precise man with a sad, bearded face, Jackson had in his youth apparently debated studying the evolutionary philosophy of Herbert Spencer instead of medicine. Then, like most young men in England who decided on medicine as a career, he had trained in London, concentrating on the use of the ophthalmoscope, which he always employed with painstaking precision. Jackson seems to have seen the ophthalmoscope not only as a literal way of looking at the living optic nerve but also as a means of peering into the seat of the soul of man.

Jackson arrived in London in 1859 to seek his fortune and there

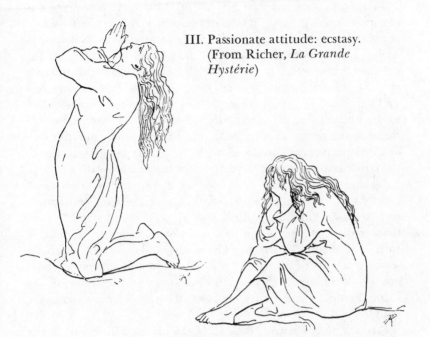

III. Passionate attitude: ecstasy.
(From Richer, *La Grande
Hystérie*)

IV. Delirium: weeping and lamentation.
(From Richer, *La Grande
Hystérie*)

fell in with Dr. Edouard Brown-Séquard, a flamboyant French-American neurologist who had come to work in a new hospital there. This hospital, the National Hospital for the Epileptic and the Paralyzed, had been founded by two maiden ladies, Joanna and Louisa Chandler, whose much beloved grandmother had suffered from an apoplectic paralysis and had died without any good medical facilities available to her.

These two spinsterish women had set to work fired with the determination to rectify the wrong. By making and selling ornaments of shells, beads, and pearls they had soon accumulated two hundred pounds to establish a medical facility in a house in Queens Square, London. In 1860 they invited Brown-Séquard to take command of this incipient hospital for the paralyzed and epileptic. Four years later he talked Jackson into joining his staff.

In 1865 Jackson married his cousin. After only a few years of marital happiness Mrs. Jackson developed cerebral thrombosis. As the years passed she came to suffer from focal seizures. Not surprisingly, Jackson began to center his professional attention on epilepsy. Even before his wife's death, in 1876, he began to study cases of presumed epilepsy that ended in death. In case after case Jackson found that particular parts of the nervous system known to be related to particular normal movements were diseased through tumor or scarring or syphilitic infection, and that the diseased parts were correlated with the abnormal movements or the symptoms seen in the patients when they had been alive.

Jackson was especially fond of cases in which a patient would manifest not a generalized seizure but a very discrete movement such as a twitching in one limb, which would then "march" across the nervous system, causing new areas of the body to tremble in turn from second to second. The study of these cases, which resembled the fits of his wife, was critical to the discoveries of Jackson. He could see the correlation of anatomy and behavior, of the lesion found in some autopsies and the specific movement, the symptom.

Like his hero, Spencer, Jackson began his theorizing with a few basic evolutionary premises, namely, that the human species was at the upper extreme of animal development and that the nervous system of man was the acme of human evolution, the part of man where evolution was occurring. He began by dividing the nervous system into three levels. The lower level included the spinal cord and the brain stem. The middle level included those parts of the brain devoted to movement and sensation. The third level was the frontal lobe of the brain, the "organ of mind."

Jackson next proceeded to use these evolutionary premises to conceptualize how the disease of epilepsy occurred. Arguing that a counterevolutionary process, a "dissolution of the nervous system," was at work, he relied to an extent on Spencer's evolutionary language. Yet he shied away from making any expansive pronouncements that might seduce him from the study of neurology as an organically based discipline that could connect anatomy to physiology and physiology to movement and even to loss of consciousness. He employed evolutionary thinking wisely and fruitfully.

Through the ages, the confusion of epilepsy—which in Greek simply means "seizure"—with either satanic possession or inspiration and prophecy had always muddled medical thinking. The epileptic's falling into a fit of writhing and twisting smacked of possession and mysticism and visitation by God. By concentrating his attention on seizures that might begin in a finger, then extend to the whole hand and arm, and only then to the entire body, Jackson dissolved the religious mystique around the illness. Furthermore, by dividing the brain into the three levels, he could envision in a comprehensible manner how loss of consciousness could occur in a full-blown epileptic fit, namely, by the spreading of the focus of irritation to the frontal lobes, the "organ of mind."

Although he used such old terms as "nervous irritability" and "exhaustion," Jackson meant something precise, namely, that the nervous tissue in certain parts of the epileptic brain was prone to "firing" extravagantly because of an anatomical parasite, a "discharging lesion." When it discharged, it produced a widespread convulsion by impelling healthy nervous tissue to cooperate in its excess. We can easily see at work in Jackson's thinking the Franco-German synthesis connecting a clinical picture with both an anatomical lesion and a physiological imbalance. Whereas normal nerve tissue would fire only in concomitance with a certain movement—say, lifting a glass to the lips—diseased tissue would fire chaotically and so set the hand to shaking and stiffening. Cells nearby would then be affected, and soon the whole arm would be shaking, then the neck, the legs, and the other arm. Soon the epileptic fit would generalize and the patient would become unconscious.

Jackson argued that the pathology of epilepsy was due to arterial blood flow. He suggested that the reason for the alternating firing and easing up was problems in nutrition. Nerve cells require much blood, and Jackson believed that tumors, cysts, and abscesses, the anatomical lesions, upset the blood flow and produced seizures by expanding and squeezing nerve cells. Though Jackson's theory may have oversimplified the situation, the British neurologist had nonetheless taken huge strides toward explaining epilepsy, once and for all, to the medical world.

Back in Paris, Charcot was likewise trying to puzzle his way toward an explanation of his favorite neurosis, hysteria. With its fits and stigmatic symptoms, this disease had, however, begun to grow intriguing to more than just the world of medicine. Therefore, when he delved into the area of causation, and stumbled on hypnosis as a diagnostic tool, the popular appeal of his studies was heightened even further.

At this time, 1870–1900, many intelligent men and women who hitherto had looked to religion for ultimate answers were now turning toward science. Charcot's sedulous study of hysteria offered some novel and interesting ideas about religion. Those who in the past were considered saints were now called hysterics by Charcot, for in their odd reveries and ecstasies saints looked quite a bit like hysterics in the middle of passionate attitudes. Furthermore, Charcot now depicted the miracles that the saints wrought as hysterical cures, since in many cases the sufferers fell down and ranted and raved in the manner of hysterics going through the first two periods of the hysterical fit—namely, the epileptoid phase and the period of grand movements. Also, the myths of the Degenerate and the Genius had a wide appeal, since they offered—through the vehicle of hereditary taint—a scientific-sounding substitute for original sin and God. So when Charcot spoke on hysteria, many ordinary, and some extraordinary, people came flocking to his lecture hall.

Charcot's lectures were packed with physicians and litterateurs, who waited expectantly for his announcements, especially when he spoke of neurosis and hypnosis. One eyewitness, an English doctor, states in the medical journal called the *Lancet* that Charcot invited the prime minister, Léon Gambetta, to hear his talks; another eyewitness, Dr. Axel Munthe, a Swedish doctor trained in Paris, claimed he actually met the writer Guy de Maupassant at one of these talks. In *The Story of San Michele,* Munthe's autobiography, he exclaims, "I seldom failed to attend Professor Charcot's famous Lectures of Tuesday at the Salpêtrière, just then devoted to the grand hysteria and hypnosis. With the great lecture hall filled to the last place with a multi-colored audience drawn from all of Paris, authors, doctors, leading actors and actresses, fashionable demimondaines, all full of morbid curiosity to witness the startling phenomena of hypnosis . . . It was during one of these lectures that I became acquainted with Guy de Maupassant." This famous naturalist author was himself a perfect specimen of both the Degenerate and the Genius. He was one of Emile Zola's adherents and therefore highly interested in nervous illness and hereditary taint. He also was a mental patient himself who eventually went mad and died in an asylum.

This popular appeal of Charcot's works also found its roots in a much larger problem then facing the French nation: the humiliation of the French at the hands of the Germans in the 1870–71 Franco-Prussian War and the growing sense that France was on the decline. Hysteria and hypnosis, which mingled the scientific with the histrionic, played into this growing national concern. The hysteric was seen as both a degenerate and a kind of genius, or at least a great actress, and the French nation saw itself as at once the nation with the greatest science in the world, the finest art, and the greatest nerve weakness. Charcot was obviously aware of the connection between the hysteric and the artistic genius and the degenerate since on a number of occasions he used the catchphrase of the Decadent movement, "art for art's sake," in describing his hysterics.

In his lectures Charcot would make some introductory remarks on hysteria or hypnosis, then present the history of a particular patient, who would enter to be questioned. After Charcot or one of his assistants had pressed on a hysterogenic zone, or after the patient had been removed from the hall to be hypnotized, the patient would suffer a seizure, a fit of great singularity, before the eyes of all those present. All four phases of the hysterical fit would occur. The onlookers would sit in awe. Although he thought he was using the tools of a neurologist, Charcot was also an incipient psychologist and a bit of a showman. While he was certainly aware that his performances were theatrical, he was not altogether sure whether the performance got in the way of the science.

Charcot's female patients won fame in Paris and in the international world of medicine for their performances, from which they stood to gain a great deal—namely, attention and notoriety. It is also clear now that they were unwittingly trained by their doctors. After being examined by physician after physician in the Salpêtrière, they gradually collected ideas of how they should behave when having a fit or when hypnotized. Besides, they watched each other and learned; some even learned from the epileptics who lay in the beds next to them. These hysterical patients had been

gradually collecting in the Salpêtrière, since doctors in other
mental hospitals throughout France respected Charcot and sent
him their most difficult patients. However, the hysteria that Charcot described was not simply a fraud. There is quite a bit more to
the story than vanity, trickery, and imitation.

Some critics of Charcot quickly realized that something more
than just an anatomical lesion or an imbalance in physiology was
at work in the illness. For instance, Munthe, who was proud to
have studied under Charcot, was also acutely aware of the evils of
the social situation in the Salpêtrière. He perceived how a gullible
country girl could arrive in the big city and be seduced into becoming a photographed and carefully studied patient in the
greatest hospital for hysteria in the world. Munthe tells of meeting
the simpleminded country parents of one such inhabitant of the
Salpêtrière. This young girl had come to the hospital to be a
housekeeper but had been wooed into becoming a grand hysteric.
Munthe counseled the unsuspecting parents, who had come to
Paris looking for their daughter, to return to the country and
promised that she would be with them shortly. In the manner of a
Victorian hero, he planned to rescue the woman from the clutches
of the doctors at the Salpêtrière. His rescue was nearly completed
when Charcot and his followers waylaid the girl, aborted the
abduction, and embarrassed Munthe professionally. Charcot apparently blackballed him, and the sophisticated city doctor was
banished from polite Parisian medicine and had to move his genteel practice to Rome.

This story—which must be regarded with some suspicion, since
Munthe liked to romanticize himself—can be seen as one piece in
a large puzzle. To Charcot, the hysterical fits, the hysterogenic
zones, the hypnosis, the audience, the "morbid curiosity" remained mysterious pieces of a vast nervous puzzle called hysteria,
which he hoped to assemble into a picture. However, he was only
dimly aware of the interplay of patient, doctor, and audience, and
he set out to codify complex facts with little understanding of
significant pieces in the puzzle.

Charcot was not, for instance, very aware of the importance of
the relationship between doctor and patient. Though he had an
inkling of the importance of psychology, he was not truly aware
of what we would call the psychodynamics of psychological ill-

nesses, nor was he aware of group dynamics. That the patients of the Salpêtrière were often attractive young women, usually of the poorer classes, while the doctors of the Salpêtrière were often handsome and ambitious men, usually of the upper middle classes, seems not to have influenced his theories. Indeed, in reading Charcot's lectures today one recognizes the attempt to omit all mention of these and other interpersonal and social realities.

Munthe's autobiography and other literary works in which physicians play significant roles, such as Henry James's *The Wings of the Dove* and Theodor Fontane's *Effie Briest*, leave little doubt that the nineteenth-century physician set out to woo his female patients through charm, intuition, and the capacity to instill hope. In *The Wings of the Dove* a young woman, Milly Theale, is suffering from an incurable disease, probably tuberculosis. The last of a wealthy family, Milly sets off for Europe to make the grand tour before she dies. In London she makes the acquaintance of Sir Luke Strett, a prominent English doctor. He peers into her eyes, seems to intuit something inscrutable, and in a mysterious way reinstills in her a wish to live. This wish remains with Milly for a good part of the story. It departs only when she is jilted by a young man. At this point the inconsolate Milly turns her face to the wall, gives up hope, and dies in Venice.

In Fontane's novel Effie Briest is forced to marry a much older man. After being nearly bored to tears by provincial life, she has an affair with a military man. Then, feeling extremely guilty, she feigns paralysis and pain while on a visit to Berlin. She takes to her bed. Soon she and her husband move permanently to Berlin. There a Dr. Rummschuttel attends her and guesses that she is hiding some sin. A bit of a misogynist and a bit of a flirt, Rummschuttel continues with her but never really forces her to talk to him. He keeps her life and her symptoms relatively under control for a number of years. Unfortunately the husband learns about the long-buried affair, kills the ex-lover in a duel, and then disowns poor Effie, with the doctor standing by, compassionate but inactive.

The male doctor-female patient relationship in the late nineteenth century usually smacks of an intuitive, somewhat deferential stance on the part of the doctor and a quiet and helpless prostration on the part of the patient, be she wealthy or poor. Since this inequality was so embedded in his society, Charcot's inability to recognize the character of his relationship with his hysterics is far from surprising.

Nonetheless he forged ahead. A good scientist by the standards of the times, he first codified the symptoms of hysteria and then— in the style of French medicine—began to work toward uncovering the presumed lesion. He believed that hysteria should be no exception to the rule that where there was a neurotic symptom, there had to be a lesion.

Thus he would lecture on a hysterical symptom with the patient in the lecture hall, precisely the way he had with other neurological illness such as multiple sclerosis. He would describe such symptoms as left-sided weakness or tunnel vision. He would demonstrate reflexes and map out areas of anesthesia. Then, with great precision, he would press a so-called hysterogenic spot on the woman's body. Or he might order the patient taken from the room to be mysteriously hypnotized by his assistants, as he continued his untiring search to comprehend the nature of the lesion in his hysterics and their illness.

Charcot had inklings of the startling new notion of studying not only the illness but also the patient, the person in whom the illness flourished. He even invited the young psychologist Pierre Janet to do research at the Salpêtrière in the mid-1880s. Yet Charcot never pushed this idea to its limit. His attention rested for a long time on the description of the symptoms. Meanwhile his disciples and admirers did take the time to record and publish voluminous histories of the lives of the most prominent hysterics. In these novellalike histories we can catch a clearer vision of the hysterics as human beings. We learn much by passing into the lugubrious wards of the Salpêtrière and meeting a few of the patients, the poor hysterics. Whereas we can only imagine the personal pain of Edgar Degas's somber ballerinas, painted in the same epoch, the case histories by Charcot's men spell out the desperate details of the lives of these Frenchwomen.

One of the most interesting and significant of the women in the Salpêtrière was Geneviève. Born in Loudon, where the famous "devils" had been prominent in the time of Richelieu, she was an orphan who went to live on a farm in the country. Fits of anger and a generally temperamental nature led to her early hospitalization. She was soon sent to a second farm. A laborer from an early age, she had no formal education whatsoever. At age twelve, she cut her hand and was left with a slight scar. Then her fits of anger worsened.

At age fifteen, she fell in love with a young man named Camille, to whom she became engaged. Most tragically, Camille died that year of "cerebral fever." When her foster father refused to let her go to the funeral for fear of her nervousness, the young Geneviève escaped from home and ran to the cemetery at night. Trying to dig up the remains of Camille, she was overcome with a crisis and was found unconscious by his grave. She remained in this state for twenty-four hours.

For the next year she was sad, withdrawn, refusing to talk, often angry. When her foster mother died she was sent to the hospital in Poitiers, and it was here that she began her career as a professional hysteric. Hospitals were to become her only home.

She was discharged in about a year and established as a chambermaid in Poitiers, where her master seduced her. She returned to the hospital apparently in a pregnant and hysterical state. Her pregnancy, in fact, was a hysterical (imaginary) one. Shortly thereafter Geneviève attempted suicide, first with pills (belladonna) and then with scissors on the left side of her abdomen. From then on, the left side of her body would remain insensible, or anesthetic.

At seventeen, she escaped from the hospital with a medical student, with whom she became sexually entangled. Spending the next two years in and out of this relationship, in and out of mental hospitals, she eventually went to Paris as a chambermaid in 1863. She would often have fits on the street and on one occasion was saved from leaping to her death from a bridge. She was first admitted to the Salpêtrière in 1865.

Her frequent escapes from the Salpêtrière, her fits, her teasing, vain character were described in detail by Charcot's followers Bourneville and Regnard in their book, *Photographic Iconography of the Salpêtrière* (1877–80). Twice she escaped and became pregnant. First she gave birth to a girl, whom she left in the country, and then a boy, who died of exposure.

Charcot appeared in her life from 1874 onward, mostly in order to press the hysterogenic point in the area of her left ovary, which would alternately cause and stop a fit. Charcot's disciples divided her seizures into three parts: tonic, clonic, and delirious. Described most vividly and in greatest detail is the last part—which coincides with Charcot's period of passionate attitudes—in which Geneviève went back and forth between ecstatic and crucified poses. Both poses resembled the dramatic postures of Louise Lateau, a stigmatized saint living in Belgium, who was a current favorite of the Paris newspapers. Intermingled with these poses were a series of erotic gestures in which she would plead for kisses and sexual intimacy from the doctors and attendants in the hospital, uttering such words as "vagina" and "penis." Back and forth, back and forth she would go, saint to prostitute, saint to prostitute, in minutes.

In 1875 she created a scene of some sort in front of Charcot and was banished from the Salpêtrière. She wandered in the direction of Lille, hoping to see her "sister" Louise Lateau. However, on the way she had a hysteric seizure in a barroom. Originally taken for a drunkard, she was treated cruelly by one doctor. She was then removed to an asylum, where a second doctor, familiar with the work of Charcot and perhaps with Geneviève's case, pressed on a hysterogenic zone, and her seizures diminished. The diagnosis was made. The doctor sent Geneviève back to Salpêtrière with a letter beginning "Monsieur and cher maître" and detailing the events. Back in the Salpêtrière for the next few years, Geneviève was a victim of frequent hysterical attacks.

At this point Regnard and Bourneville began a photographic study of her and also recorded her words in detail. Geneviève seems to have fallen in love with an employee, possibly a doctor, at the Salpêtrière, a M. X, who she thought looked a lot like the long-lost and much loved Camille of her adolescence. She was eventually placed in a cell because of the incredible nature of her passionate attitudes. Using compression on her ovaries and amyl nitrite, the doctors of the Salpêtrière were able to stop, start, and stop again her fits, bringing her from one phase of the fits—tonic, clonic, and delirious—into another. Back and forth, in and out, ecstasy, arc-en-cercle, ecstasy, erotic posturing, laughing, crying, giggling, crying, she spoke into the ears of Regnard, Bourneville, Charcot, and M. X.

"I suffer," she cries, "I have had enough, have pity on me. I am not a sordid woman, like the prostitutes. I do not love a man one day and another the next. To make love with a man that one does not love is filthy."

"I love M. X. When he sees me, he will say, 'Hark, how pale she is.' " She would fall and tumble on the floor as if making love,

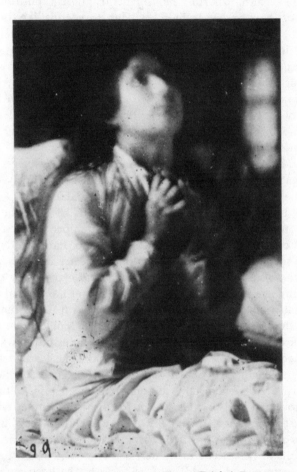

Geneviève in an ecstasy. (From Désiré Bourneville and Paul Regnard, *Iconographie Photographique de la Salpêtrière*)

then in a minute strike the crucifixion pose or be in ecstasy like a saint. She was visited in dreams by Camille and by M. X, who she hoped would save her from the Salpêtrière. Geneviève's story ends with her escaping with another hysteric and returning appre-hended, claiming that M. X had helped her to escape.

In her delirious dreams Geneviève seemed to be crying out to the doctors to save her. The French doctors stood by, recording her symptoms, eternalizing her movements in photographs, but surely they must have wished to help her. Her story reads like the tale of a pitiful heroine in a stock Victorian novel. This tattered and beaten-down woman must have tugged at the heartstrings of these brilliant Parisian doctors. Yet the cold-bloodedness required to do good medical research allowed them to pull back one step. Both the medical student who ran off with Geneviève and Munthe, who tried to abduct another hysteric, may have surrendered to their desire to be saviors. Yet Charcot and his followers resisted this temptation.

Another case illustrates this tension between the roles of com-passionate doctor and cool-minded researcher. It involved prob-ably the most photogenic hysteric at the Salpêtrière, a woman named Louise, who entered the hospital in 1875 at the age of fifteen and a half and remained there for a number of years.

The oldest of the seven children of two Parisian domestics, Louise survived into adolescence along with her brother Antoine, while the other five died in infancy. Like so many other children of the nineteenth century, she lived with a wet nurse until she was six months old and only then went to live with her parents, with whom she stayed until she was about six years old. Then she was sent off to a boarding school run by Catholic nuns, where she remained until she was thirteen and a half. She learned to read, write, and sew in the convent school, where she was also punished liberally. Sent to her cell and sometimes beaten for refusing to read aloud the lives of the saints or for throwing temper tantrums, she must have been a real rebel. On a few occasions she was caught masturbating with two other girls, and the three were tied up in their cells as penance. During her fits of temper, when she would refuse to obey and would hold her breath, the good nuns seem-ingly considered her to be possessed and so threw holy water in her

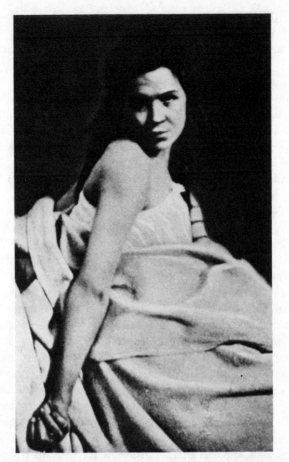

Louise with a hysterical contracture. (From Bourneville and Regnard, *Iconographie Photographique de la Salpêtrière*)

face. On one occasion they had her exorcised, or so Louise told the interested doctors at the Salpêtrière many years later.

During vacations and free days she visited a woman near the school who had befriended her. Here she witnessed the woman's drunken husband beating his wife and dragging her around by her hair. She also visited her brother Antoine, who was then doing an apprenticeship in Paris. In her conversations with him she first learned how babies were born. Finally, during a visit to her parents' home, she met a mysterious M. C., whom her mother forced her to kiss and insisted Louise call "Papa."

Once finished with school, she went to live with M. C., his wife, and children in the capacity—it seemed—of apprentice in sewing at M. C.'s clothing store. But M. C. was sexually estranged from his wife, and after unsuccessfully propositioning Louise on a few occasions, he threatened her with a razor. Though she pleaded for mercy, he made her drunk and then raped her.

The morning after her rape Louise awoke to find her genitals very sore and her legs weak. She told no one her secret, although Mme. C. suspected something and sent the poor girl home. There she began to vomit and complain of abdominal pain. A doctor, without examining her, diagnosed the onset of menses. A few days later, while lying in bed, she awoke to see green cat's eyes staring at her. She screamed and had her first fit. The attacks occurred frequently thereafter.

Treated with bloodletting cups on her back, she seemed to improve and was sent as a maidservant to live with an old spinster in Paris. There she became sexually involved with two adolescent boys. Her parents learned about her sexual activities and called her home. Ensuing family quarrels brought to light that Louise's mother was a long-standing lover of M. C., and Antoine was probably his son. As these revelations unfolded, Louise's hysterical fits worsened markedly, bursting forth many times daily for longer and longer periods, sometimes for hours. Admitted to one hospital for six months, she was then transferred to the Salpêtrière, where her condition remained essentially unchanged for at least the next five years.

Examination revealed partial paralysis and complete anesthesia over the entire right side of the body, as well as a decrease in hearing, smell, taste, and vision on the right side. Also, Louise manifested some of the most violent and dramatic hysterical fits, with all four phases represented, especially the phase of passionate attitudes. In this phase she not only had hallucinations of cats' eyes, snakes, and other reptiles but also slipped back into the past and relived episodes from her life. Her experiences with M. C., her adolescent affairs with her two young men, especially the one named Emile, her conversations with her mother, all came flooding back. She would pass into trancelike phases and seem to see her mother, M. C., or Emile looming before her. She would talk to them and hear them reply. She would plead for mercy from M. C., giggle and shout for joy with Emile, grow upset and angry with her mother. Day in, day out, these fits occurred intermittently for more than five years in the presence of the doctors at the Salpêtrière.

What makes this case so intriguing is at once the similarity and dissimilarity to contemporary cases of sexual molestation. Louise was raped by M. C., and then, not being able to tell anyone her secret, she became sexually promiscuous, thereby setting off a chain of events that led to that great revelation that her mother had herself been the lover of M. C. However, what is so preeminently Victorian about Louise's case is the form of the illness, the chronic and debilitating hysterical illness, with its weakness, its anesthesia, its hysterical fits. What also seems culturally deter-

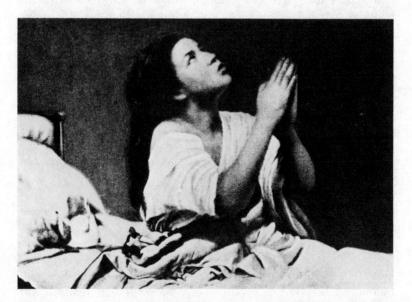

Louise in a passionate attitude: pleading for kisses. (From Bourneville and Regnard, *Iconographie Photographique de la Salpêtrière*)

mined is the doctor's failure to try to empathize with the patient and persuade her to talk about her feelings, her rage, her despair, her sadness.

Charcot, however, sat, viewed, listened, and contemplated. Out of these details he conjured some original theories that caught the eye of many a doctor. Though he never seemed to be in touch with the pathos of these women's lives, he called into question certain age-old ideas that pervaded the study of hysteria. He described a number of cases of male hysteria, quite similar to those of Geneviève and Louise, thereby destroying the ancient notion that hysteria was concerned with the uterus. He let these male patients stay in the Salpêtrière in a separate wing so he could study them carefully.

Though he questioned the connection between the symptoms and the woman's uterus, Charcot did not discard the notion of a physical cause for hysteria, but rather shifted the lesion from the uterus to the nervous system. This was of course not a new idea at all, as Robert Whytt and George Cheyne had already made the same point long ago. But Charcot did something new with his material. He identified the etiological moment as a psychic trauma, like the death of Camille or the rape by M. C., suggesting that hysteria could not be perceived as a purely organic illness, one in which the nerves alone were at fault. Indeed, in many of his lectures he stated that he did not regard hysteria as an organic illness at all.

Nevertheless Charcot was hardly a psychologist in dealing with cases like those of Geneviève and Louise. He and his followers still used the terms "trauma" or "shock" to describe a strain on the central nervous system—a kind of electrical shock—similar to Cheyne's frayed nerve or Whytt's nerves in sympathy but with electricity doing the fraying or sympathizing. Furthermore, Charcot always believed that the major causative agent in every case of hysteria was hereditary taint; in other words, hysteria remained the result of an organic predisposition. His hysterics came from nervous families, as they did for Morel and Moreau. Charcot saw hysterics as victims of moral degeneration or faulty heredity and, therefore, as possessing faulty cerebrums. Their neurological systems lived on the edge of dissolution. To Charcot, in the fight for the survival of the fittest, hysterics were creatures burdened with central nervous systems that could not withstand any variety of stress, psychic or physical. Furthermore, the majority of hysterics were women, creatures more emotional than men, with smaller brains and muscles. Some of the male hysterics were described as effeminate, and Charcot believed that those males who were not effeminate had usually inherited the taint from their fathers or their mothers. Nonetheless he did admit that in some of these cases he could find no real underlying hereditary taint. It is this open-mindedness that made him a good scientist, even when dealing with the slippery subject of hysteria.

In about 1880, still on the track of the presumed hysteria lesion, Charcot made the pronouncement that if a patient was hypnotizable he was potentially hysterical. Charcot defined the hysteric as suffering from hereditary taint that made the nervous system weak and susceptible to domination through hypnosis. A hypnotic trance, which caused symptoms similar to a hysterical fit or could even create stigmatic symptoms, was to Charcot an artificial form of hysterical neurosis.

To illustrate this point, the Caesar of the Salpêtrière created through hypnosis a condition seemingly comparable to a psychic or physical shock and capable of inducing a hysterical symptom. In his lectures he would produce for his followers and admirers a number of convincing, well delineated pairs of patients. The first patient—a man—possessed a hysterical symptom such as a paralysis or an area of anesthesia, resulting from a trauma—a psychic or physical shock. One such man was Porcz, a cabman who had suffered a terrifying fall from the seat of his horse-drawn carriage. Another was Pin, a laborer who had stood transfixed with fear before a rolling barrel that had broken loose from a pulley. (The barrel had not touched him.) The second patient in the pair was always one of the famous female hysterics of the hospital, such as Louise. She would come forth hypnotized. Before her entrance into the amphitheater, one of Charcot's men would suggest to her under hypnosis that she should develop a hysterical symptom to match the man's. To the audience's astonishment she would comply, manifesting onstage a paralysis or area of anesthesia identical to that of Porcz or Pin. Thus Charcot isolated, in an electrifying new way, the moment when hysteria burst forth.

Still, Charcot remained a believer in the Degenerate myth. In

his eyes the emotional outbursts of such hysterics as Louise and
Geneviève, especially in the period of passionate attitudes, only
confirmed his belief in their nerve weakness. Furthermore, Charcot's atheistic prejudices blurred his scientific acumen. The
antireligious legacy of the French Revolution is apparent in his
thinking. When Geneviève compared herself to Louise Lateau,
Charcot drew the same comparison. His attempt to equate saints
with the nervously weak, and miracles with hysterical fits, was
intriguing but also a case of scientific empire building.

At the same time, Charcot was ignorant of many basic elements
of psychology and sociology. He never completely understood the
mass hysteria of the Salpêtrière—how the hysterics affected one
another and how his presentation of them to an audience really
encouraged their symptoms to grow more dramatic. He also never
completely understood psychosexual factors in hysteria (except to
the extent that the nervously weak woman was a potential prostitute). Charcot did not concentrate on talking or listening to his
patients. The words of Geneviève about Camille or of Louise
about M. C. were only a small part of the larger neurological
picture.

Finally, Charcot misdiagnosed some of his patients. A close reading of some of his case histories suggests his patients may have had
organic illnesses for which Charcot lacked the laboratory acumen
to make a solid diagnosis. For example, Porcz had underlying
rheumatic, or autoimmune, illness, which may have explained his
paralysis and areas of anesthesia, while Pin had cardiac illness,
which may have explained his similar symptoms. It is also conceiv-
able that even such famous hysterics as Geneviève and Louise
suffered from some obscure form of epilepsy.

Nonetheless Charcot was brilliant in his presentations, and doctors all over the world sat up and took note. His works on hysteria
were quickly translated into English by two interested doctors in
London, and many English doctors went to visit him in Paris.

Back in London, the less sensational, more meticulous work of
Hughlings Jackson continued. Having already deduced that an
actual anatomical lesion existed in his favorite neurosis, epilepsy,
Jackson offered a very convincing and scientifically viable explanation of how this anatomical lesion worked: through a
physiological upset of the blood flow to parts of the brain, which

set off a "march" of faulty firing of nervous energy and of twitching movements in one body part, then another. This "march" was one kind of seizure. Another kind could culminate in a loss of consciousness and a full-blown fit, or grand mal.

Jackson carried on his very sober scientific scrutiny through the eighties and nineties. Like Charcot, he scrupulously studied individual cases. But unlike Charcot, he did not choose debilitated women as his subjects. Such individuals would have carried the taint of the Degenerate. Rather—and here Jackson made a subtly wise choice—he described in most detail a certain medical man who had epilepsy.

This highly educated medical man, named Quaerens, presented a particularly valuable and timely case. Quaerens began his own case description in college. In 1871, while waiting for a college friend on a stairway, he suddenly seemed to lose all recollection of his surroundings. A few minutes later the friend found him leaning against a wall, looking pale and puzzled. Quaerens had had a staring fit but did not know it. These staring fits continued for a couple of years. He first tried to laugh them off, then sought medical attention, but he failed to get any explanation, so he continued to handle the matter casually. Only in 1874 did he have his first grand mal, in which he lost consciousness and fell down in a state of shaking and quivering. From a London physician he then learned the nature of his disease—epilepsy.

The puzzling little attacks in which he only lost consciousness continued to predominate. Yet no real decrease in his mental powers occurred during these years. He was even able to complete his medical training and to take a job as a physician. In fact, he found that he would often be able to complete his work as a doctor when he was in the midst of some of these puzzling little attacks. His habits seemed so ingrained that he would come to himself after having accomplished a medical task. It almost seemed as though he were acting like an automaton.

For instance, while he was using a stethoscope to examine the lungs of a boy with the symptoms of pneumonia, he apparently lost all memory. The next thing he recollected was sitting at the writing table in the house of the patient. He was curious as to what had happened, and so he returned to the sickroom, where the patient lay in bed. He found a note in his own hand that said "pneumonia in the left base" and learned that he had advised the patient to go to bed immediately. In short, Quaerens had done precisely what was proper while he was in the midst of an epileptic attack.

When Jackson found that the autopsy on Quaerens—the doctor-patient had died of an overdose—revealed a small lesion in the left temporal lobe of the brain, it strengthened his hypothesis that these funny states, in which grand mal or "marches" did not occur, were different forms of epilepsy. In the grand mal the fit was a confused and meaningless thrashing around. In the "march" a twitching began in one extremity and spread in moments to other parts of the body, often stopping short of a loss of consciousness. In Quaerens' case Jackson saw the seeds of two other kinds of epileptic seizures. The first, the staring fit, was a petit mal. Jackson postulated that somehow the "organ of mind," the frontal lobes, were being affected by the anatomical lesion in the temporal lobe and an obscure physiological fault radiating from the temporal lobe. The second kind of seizure, in which the doctor-patient lost consciousness while performing such a meaningful act as an examination, Jackson called "mental automatism." Habitual, or automatic, action was able to continue even while the organ of mind was out of commission because the lower levels of the brain and spinal cord continued to work properly. Precisely how a lesion in the temporal lobe could touch off these seizures was not completely clear to Jackson, but he sensed that he had begun the task of clarification. He had explained, at least partially, the anatomical, physiological, and clinical concomitants of four different kinds of epilepsy, from the simplest of the four, the "marches," to the most complicated and most strange, the "mental automatism."

This delineation of the four basic kinds of epilepsy was an astonishing accomplishment. By way of meticulous argument he had explained fairly convincingly how all four kinds of seizures occurred through an anatomical lesion, which led to a physiological upset of blood flow to various parts of the brain, which then led to a specific part of the brain's firing awry. In certain cases that went to autopsy he had shown lesions matching the specific symptom. He then generalized these findings to other epileptics. The various symptoms—trembling and jerking of an arm in the "marches"; falling to the ground, flailing about, and loss of consciousness in the grand mal, and so on—resulted, he posited, because that part of the brain controlling normal arm or hand movements or conscious thoughts had momentarily gone mad.

Jackson, of course, borrowed from the old, imprecise language of Cheyne and Whytt, of Morel and Moreau. Nervous "instability," "exhaustion," and "dissolution of the nervous system" are all potentially imprecise terms. But Jackson imbued them with a crispness and a precision of meaning in which anatomical lesion, physiological fault, and clinical symptoms are delineated and described.

In dividing the brain tissue into three parts—the brain stem, the brain parts dealing with movement and sensation, and the frontal lobes, which he called "the organ of mind"—Jackson was drawing on the ideas of Morel and therefore touching on the Degenerate myth of neurosis. Yet Jackson culled from the myth a theory that not only was stripped of the vagueness inherent in that myth but also was scientifically useful and eventually provable. Though he was able in autopsies to demonstrate various parts of his theory, his great creative idea of connecting anatomical lesions to physiological faults and clinical symptoms remained largely a hypothesis for decades until it was confirmed by twentieth-century investigations with the electroencephalograph, which can actually measure the physiological imbalance. This instrument shows conclusively that the electricity in the brain of the epileptic discharges in precisely the way Jackson had suggested.

Although Jackson mentioned Charcot in his writings, he rarely treated cases of hysteria and never spoke of Charcot in relation to abnormal mental behavior. However, showing from autopsies that an underlying lesion did exist in many epileptics, he posited that similar lesions, certainly more subtle, would be discovered in such abnormal mental conditions as "insanity"—meaning psychosis—schizophrenia or manic-depressive illness. He believed that the highest level of the brain, the "organ of mind," was malfunctioning in these diseases. "In every insanity," he wrote, "there is a morbid affection, more or less, of the highest cerebral centers, or synonymously, of the highest level of evolution of the cerebral subsystem, or again, synonymously of the anatomical substrate of physical bases of consciousness. There may be discoverable disease destructive of nervous elements, or there may be loss of function from some undiscovered pathological process inferred from symptoms." Jackson had the good sense, however, to limit himself to the more profitable study of his pet neurosis, epilepsy, and in so doing he began to detach this disease from its long interconnection with its much stranger bedfellow, hysteria, an illness in which emotions played such a significant role.

Jackson insisted on a split between those studying neurology and those studying emotional and psychological phenomena and argued that there was a need to separate the two subject matters, the brain and the psyche, by using two different languages. This insistence is comparable to saying that there is a difference between a neurologist and a psychologist. Jackson insisted that such phrases as "the psychology of the nervous system" or "the physiology of the mind" engendered a confusion that could be traced back to Cheyne's frayed nerves and Whytt's nerves in sympathy. This was also true, he felt, of the imprecise use of the terms "nervous" and "neurotic." He believed that physicians should leave the psychological alone and concentrate on the organic. "Our concern as medical men is with the body," he wrote. "If there is such a thing as a disease of the mind, we can do nothing for it."

Charcot certainly agreed with Jackson that hysteria and epilepsy were separable entities, and he and his assistants compiled a list that made this clear simply by observing some of the basic differences between a hysterical fit and an epileptic seizure. Even the nurses in the Salpêtrière seemed to learn to see the two as separate and distinct entities. However, Charcot never ceased believing that hysteria, in many ways an illness of the psyche, should remain a fit subject for the study of doctors. Furthermore, most neurologists of the late Victorian period seemed to agree with Charcot when he posited the existence of a generalized or nonspecific lesion in the hysteric, a "dynamic lesion," as he named it.

This idea of dynamic lesion is tricky. On one hand, the oft-repeated term amalgamates the anatomical lesion of the French and the dynamism, or physiology, of the Germans. In fact, Charcot never gave up the notion that the ultimate cause of hysteria was an unbalanced nervous system. On the other hand, Charcot was flirting with psychological explanation. As we shall see, the Master's emphasis on the possibility that a psychic trauma could precipitate hysterical symptoms opened the vast subject of psychology to Western medicine.

Yet Charcot's term "dynamic lesion" confused the languages of the organic and the psychological, as Jackson warned. Charcot, however, was both a researcher and a practicing physician, and doctors always and everywhere have dealt with patients in whom the emotional and the physical mix. So Jackson's suggestion that medical men forsake the treatment of maladies of the mind could be made only by a researcher such as Jackson, who could not remember the names of real patients and called them by their diseased body parts.

Furthermore, Charcot's own cases were a very confusing and sticky conglomerate of physical and emotional elements. Hysteria always seemed a mixture of emotional and neurological instabilities. Some of his hysterics may have suffered from a then undiscovered epileptic illness such as the bizarre automatism of Quaerens. Many of Charcot's female patients at Salpêtrière manifested fits that looked like epileptic seizures on one day, then on another day like full-blown hysterical fits that went through the four stages of hysteria. So the term "hystero-epilepsy" made sense in describing these patients. Furthermore, epilepsy remained a disease of degeneracy, which implied an emotional and mental component. Many other patients at the Salpêtrière who were frankly epileptic, with no tinge of hysteria, still had the look of degenerates. They had a shriveled limb, for example, and their seizures would break out with a trembling in that limb and then become generalized epileptic attacks. These women were often mentally retarded and seemed as dull and listless as a Morelian idiot.

The "correctness" of Hughlings Jackson's views on epilepsy has only become clear with the passage of time. For many years, despite Jackson's work, the description of epilepsy remained in neurological textbooks in the same section as hysteria. Even to this day psychomotor epilepsy, or "mental automatism," implies an emotional instability.

Yet the confusions that coiled together the studies of epilepsy and hysteria, and the epic research of these two men, fired the enthusiasm of many doctors to peer more deeply at these illnesses. We shall turn now to the work of Charcot and some of his contemporaries in the exciting area of psychic shock.

FIVE

The Railway God

IN the 1890s a little-known Viennese neurologist, Sigmund Freud, wrote a letter to a friend in Berlin. In it he described one of his first childhood memories, an experience on a train. In 1858 the young boy, then called Sigismund, boarded a train in a village in Moravia, a province in the vast Hapsburg empire in Central Europe, and rode with his family toward the imperial capital of Vienna. His family coming from the primitive countryside of Galicia, his imagination fired by stories about the horrors of hell told him by a Catholic servant, Freud later remembered that the gas lanterns in the provincial capital through which the train passed looked to his young eyes like the very lamps of hell.

This train ride is especially noteworthy, since years later Freud believed that he remembered seeing his mother naked during the trip. In the 1890s, while undergoing his self-analysis, Freud wrote to his mentor, Wilhelm Fliess, in Berlin: "between the ages of 2 and 2½, my libido was stirred up towards *matrem*, namely on the occasion of a journey with her from Leipzig to Vienna, during which we must have spent the night together and I must have had an opportunity to see her *nudam*." In short, the young Sigmund saw on that very night the object of his Oedipal wishes and his fear.

By the nineties Freud had developed a train phobia. He felt anxious when he came near trains, and he began to attribute this fear to his childhood experience and to his Oedipus complex. What is so interesting is that a careful reading of the medical literature on neurosis during the 1880s and 1890s reveals that railway neuroses were a common phenomenon. Cesare Lombroso, an Italian doctor, describes such a phobia of the great composer Gioacchino Rossini. The Berlin neurologist Hermann Oppenheim wrote, "I have several times had occasion to treat persons with fear of railways and travelling." The American neurologist Philip Knapp made a similar statement. Charcot and Gilles de la Tourette in France likewise spoke of railway neurosis. In short, train neurosis was a significant medical and social problem in late Victorian times. It is hard to believe, however, that not only Freud but also Rossini, Oppenheim's and Knapp's patients, as well as those of Charcot and Gilles de la Tourette, all saw their mothers naked on trains. Only Freud suggests this etiology. It seems more likely that the railway itself played a crucial role in the birth of these neuroses, as all the other great neurologists of the day contended.

It may be difficult now to picture the fear and wonder that grasped the very soul of the Victorian who experienced the railway train for the first time. But such a recapturing of the past may shed some light not only on Freud's phobia but also on a larger social and medical issue. Though not all of the train neuroses were phobias—many were cases of hysteria, anxiety, or nervous exhaustion—the patients had in common the experience of fear or fright while in the proximity of the railway.

The idea that fright caused nervousness is present in Robert Whytt's description of the delicate woman who hears a bell and literally swoons. We find it in Jane Austen's picture of Marianne, who, on hearing the news that the wicked Willoughby is marrying for money, grows tearful, hysterical, and eventually feverish. In Charcot's Salpêtrière, Louise's hysteria surely grew out of the frightful experience of being raped.

Fright—or anxiety, as we might call it today—has obvious physiological symptoms: the eyes grow saucer-wide, the heart pumps rapidly, the breathing quickens, the hands grow clammy and trembling. These are responses of the sympathetic nervous system, which supplies sensation not only to the stomach, as Trotter had emphasized, but also to the heart, the skin, the muscles, and to many other parts of the body. This response has won the name of the "fight or flight" reaction.

No one had given fright a central position in the explanation of a neurosis until the late nineteenth century, when Charcot looked carefully at the relationship of fright and neurosis. In so doing he stumbled on the tiny thread of an idea that he spun into a new myth about neurosis, one that can be called the Zeus myth.

By the 1870s Charcot was coming across baffling cases in his wards. Men and women were developing quasi-neurological symptoms similar to the hysteria of Geneviève and Louise following some shock, some trauma, either psychological or physical, on train trips. As a result of their often crippling symptoms these individuals wanted to sue the railways for compensation. Such cases had already won the nicknames of the "railway spine" and the "railway brain" because doctors originally believed that the spine and the brain must have been injured in every case. Yet the search for a minuscule lesion caused by the accidents proved fruitless and soon gave way to extensive speculation about psychic causation. There followed one of the most bedeviling yet intriguing chapters in the history of neurosis in Victorian times.

Between 1850 and 1910 the railway systems of America and Europe became webs binding together the landscapes into skeins that could be traversed in hours rather than days. Between 1850 and 1860 the French railway system expanded from 3000 to more than 9000 kilometers of track. By 1880 the French railways had almost tripled in size again, and by 1910 redoubled, so that many of the provincial sections of France could be reached from Paris in hours. Similar statistics and comparable mobility were also the case in Germany, Britain, Italy, especially America, and even Russia. The railway—like the telegraph and later the telephone—stands out as a technological wonder tying the national landscapes together and telescoping time and distance in a manner unimaginable to earlier generations.

Behind much of the excitement of technological advance there usually crouches a tiny bit of fear. Novelty is frightening to many people. One fascinating, if evanescent, bit of documentation of this fear can be found in *The Story of San Michele*, the autobiographical work of Charcot's colleague Munthe, who describes his own fear of the railway. As we have already seen, Munthe had unsuccessfully tried to rescue one of Charcot's hysterics from the Salpêtrière and restore the girl to her simple parents from the countryside. Munthe seemed to fear the Salpêtrière and to an extent the city generally. In his book Munthe relates that he has grown weary of the fast pace of life in Paris and so returns to his home in Lapland to rest and recuperate. There, one night, he has a funny dream in which he and a troll enter into a discussion of the pros and cons of civilization and, most specifically, of the railway.

The little gnome tells the dreaming Munthe, "I have heard strange noises in my ears ever since you big people began that dreadful blasting in the mountains around us," and he shakes his head disconsolately.

> Some Goblins say you want to rob the Trolls of their gold and iron [he continues]. Others say that it is to make a hole for that huge, yellow iron snake with the two black strips on his back who is wriggling his way over fields and forests and across the rivers, his mouth foaming with smoke and fire. We are afraid of him, all the animals in the forests and fields, all the birds in the sky, all the fishes in rivers and lakes, even the Trolls under the mountains are flying north in terror of his approach. . . . I tell you times are hard, there is something wrong with your world, there is no peace anywhere. All of this incessant rattle and noise is getting on my nerves.

Although the gnome never seems to contract a good case of hysteria, phobia, or nervous exhaustion, his fear of the train spewing smoke and churning through the wilds of Lapland in Munthe's half-fictional anxiety dream paralleled the palpable fear of railways that was widespread at that time. Starting in the 1830s, when the first railway line opened between Liverpool and Manchester in England, common folk came to fear that the railway would make barren the fields through which it passed and dry up the rivers and streams. The air would be poisoned, cows would lose their milk, horses would become sterile, and all hunting animals would grow sickly. In 1842 a great railway crash near Paris created such a stir that the citizenry talked of literally destroying the train.

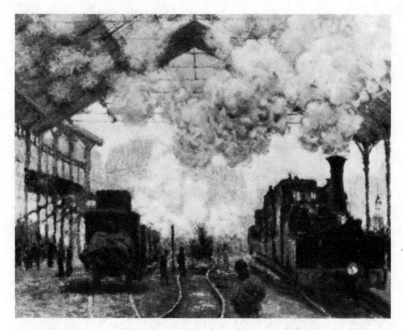

La Gare St-Lazare by Claude Monet, or the railway as an agent of nervous shock. (Fogg Art Museum, Harvard University, Cambridge, Mass.)

Though this widespread fear gradually diminished as trains grew safer and the citizens of Europe and America took to the railway of necessity, much of the fear lingered, resurfacing after a great train wreck. Thus the magic and flair of the railway, mixing together wonderment and fright, smoke and fire, made it an image of impersonal power in an age of mechanized empire and its evil, neurosis.

Along with Charcot, Herbert Page (1845–1926) and Hermann Oppenheim (1858–1918) were pioneers in the study of nervous illness caused by railway accidents. Charcot discussed the phenomenon in his lectures. Page wrote an influential book *Injuries of the Spine and Spinal Cord* (1883). Oppenheim challenged Charcot's equation of the railway spine and brain with hysteria and coined the term "traumatic neurosis." Out of this literature arose the Zeus myth of neurosis, which stressed the importance of both electricity and ideas in the breeding of a neurosis.

Page is an obscure historical figure whose only claim to fame is a medical tract he wrote that eventually fell into the hands of Charcot, spurring the imagination of this great thinker. Neither an asylum doctor nor a neurologist, Page was a surgeon for the London and Northwest Railway in Great Britain. He examined many men and women who had been involved in railway collisions and who had brought suits for damages. He came to treat them in the capacities of both physician and as a medicolegal expert establishing bona fide cases of neurosis caused by psychic jarring. Page had to sort out those with genuine organic nervous injury from the malingerers and the frightened nerve-sufferers.

In his book he cites more than two hundred cases of possible hysteria. Though the majority of these cases remained women, a number of his patients were men who manifested many of the symptoms of hysteria described by Charcot. Furthermore, he intermingled cases of anxiety, phobia, and nervous exhaustion, calling most of them hysterical or nervous.

The usual scenario of these cases involved an unsuspecting passenger—often female—riding to Newcastle upon Tyne or Bristol or Yarrow by the sea. She is looking forward to a reunion with her married daughter, or Christmas dinner with her mama, or perhaps worrying about a sick friend in the distant city. All of a sudden the train jerks on the tracks. A cry goes up. A crash may be heard. Glass shatters and the car reels. The poor innocent passenger is wrenched from her seat and is sent flying into a luggage rack or is left staring, her veins running cold, at a fellow passenger whose brains have been dashed out by a whizzing shard of glass.

The surviving passenger is helped from the train. Though a day or two may pass when the poor innocent feels nothing but a slight agitation, within less than a week the patient is prostrate, suffering a grievous outbreak of hysteria or some related neurosis.

Perhaps the most compelling case found in Page's book is "that of an apparently strong and healthy girl, nineteen years of age, in good position in life, who was in a most serious collision. She received no bodily injury, but the night of the accident she woke screaming that the engine was rushing into her room . . . and she died in five weeks, no structural disease whatever being found after death." In many ways the successor of Whytt's bell-jarred swooner or Austen's Marianne, this lamentable case, if more poignant and disturbing than most cases of the railway brain and spine, nonetheless captures the ultimate Victorian fear, both medical and more general. The railway could dissolve the human nervous system in an instant, a cataclysmic split second of fright.

Charcot remained the final arbiter of neuroses due to fright or shock. In the mid-1880s, within a few years of the publication of Page's book, Charcot delivered a number of lectures in which he described neurosis engendered by fright or shock. In the cases of Porcz and Pin he depicted men who experienced falls and traumas and later developed hysterical symptoms—namely, paralysis and anesthesia. As we have seen, he then brought into the amphitheater at the Salpêtrière famous hysterical female patients. After having them hypnotized he suggested they develop the same symptoms that had appeared in the traumatized males. To his surprise and pleasure the women hysterics did so, and the diagnosis of hysteria in males sparked by "nervous shock," as he put it, seemed clear.

Charcot believed that the fright in his male patients—a fear of imminent death, of crippling injury—was translated into an electrical shock that spread through the nerves and so brought down the nervous organization. The moment of looking death in the eye had jarred the nervous system, toppling it like a house of cards. So hysteria had broken out.

Charcot further believed that within the nervous system of the hysterical women, such "old reliables" of the Salpêtrière as Louise and Geneviève, there already existed a nervous disorganization: a "dynamic lesion." Through hypnosis the doctor could push the nervous system of these female hysterics in any direction he desired. He could reshuffle the cards of the hysteric's nervous system and elicit the same symptoms that the male had suffered via a nervous shock. Charcot was, of course, generalizing from railway jolts to other instances in which human beings could be jarred into hysteria. The connecting link was an unexpected shock, some fright. So many of the traumas from which his patients suffered were caused by civilization and its new machines. Even when the jolts and shocks of civilization were not to blame, when the cause was a natural force, such as gravity or lightning, he felt he could delineate an underlying fear of the forces of civilization.

One of his cases involved a man carried to the Salpêtrière in May of 1889. "Our invalid was walking on foot along a highway from Noisy-le-Sec to Paris," Charcot said to his colleagues. He described the man as a brave soldier in Algeria and Mexico who had recently lost his parents and had grown morose and run down. Charcot then asked the patient to tell the rest of the story.

"It was three or four in the afternoon," the man said. "The sky was black, the thunder was sounding for some time already, but I was not paying any attention to it. But suddenly a clap of thunder sounded . . . I don't know why, I grew frightened. It gave me the idea that I could be hit by lightning . . . and I began to cry . . . then . . . I saw the lightning and heard the thunder. . . . The sound *resembled a cannon which . . . could break me in a thousand pieces.*"

Charcot: "You saw the lightning near you? Please tell us about that in detail."

The patient: "In the same instant that I heard the thunder and saw the lightning [strike the earth], I saw . . . a brilliant spinning fire. . . . *This ball of fire gave forth three clouds of smoke . . . which resembled the smoke coming from the chimney of a locomotive and which gave off a suffocating odor.* . . . I lost consciousness."

The patient then developed weakness on his right side and anesthesia. Comparing his case with others, including trauma caused by the railway, Charcot believed that fear or fright ignited by terrifying ideas could cause hysterical neurosis. All of these anxiety-provoking ideas—cannons, the railway, death—that lightning elicited in a trembling human set off the chain of events ending in a neurosis. Thus it seems proper to call this new myth of neurosis the Zeus myth, for just as Zeus the Thunderer had set many a mythical Greek to trembling, the railway and the machinery of civilization had, Charcot believed, shattered many unsuspecting nervous systems.

What is novel in this and other cases of traumatic hysteria is that Charcot and other doctors were dealing not just with nerves but with ideas. "It gave me the idea that I could be hit by lightning," says the invalid. Somehow the vision of lightning gets connected with the idea of cannons and the railway and the fear of getting killed. With the Zeus myth of neurosis, the virtuoso neurologist of the Salpêtrière truly became an incipient psychologist.

Charcot could not completely escape his organically based intellectual heritage, however, and still continued to see shock as a stimulus in the nerves. Drawing on the experiments of an older colleague, Guillaume Duchenne (1806–85), Charcot attempted to explain scientifically how fright could be turned into an electrical impulse, or, put differently, how the idea of being killed could be transformed, like lightning itself, into electricity.

In the 1870s Duchenne (best remembered today for his work with muscular dystrophy) had done extensive experiments with the phenomenon of fright. He was especially interested in how a slight electrical shock administered to a specific facial muscle could bring about an expression resembling fright. The imaginative and

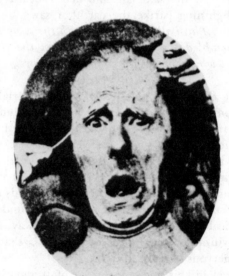

An expression of fright produced by an electrical current. (From Charles Darwin, *Expression of the Emotions in Man and Animals*)

scientifically astute Duchenne had photographed the expressions of his anguished subjects, largely in order to prove that the muscles of the face work in synchrony to express an emotion. Though one muscle is stimulated electrically, a cluster of muscles move together to make an expression of fright.

Charcot connected Duchenne's work to his own research on hysterics. In 1882, quoting Duchenne, Charcot wrote that in a hypnotized hysteric the same muscles could simply be pressed with a stylet through which no electrical current was traveling, and the same expression could be produced. He argued that the hereditarily weakened female hysteric was much more susceptible to weaker stimuli than the constitutionally strong subjects of Duchenne's experiments. Charcot posited that just as in the case of the old soldier frightened by lightning, an idea of dying had been translated into an electrical shock. This psychic shock then imbedded in the individual's body and brain a devastating neurotic symptom.

Charcot was flirting with the relationship between ideas and nerves, a provocative new concept he could only partially explore. Shortly thereafter it was necessary for him to fight a sort of rear-action skirmish with a German neurologist in Berlin who took him to task for his equation of the railway neurosis with hysteria.

Starting in 1888, Hermann Oppenheim published some papers and soon an entire book on cases of trauma he had been treating in Berlin. Out of his work he compiled a list of neurotic symptoms caused by railways and mechanized modern civilization. His patients heard ringing, even singing, in their ears, experienced stabbing pains in their bodies, had terrifying dreams in which they relived traumatic events. Many fainted regularly. Others could barely walk, and when they did, they staggered about like drunkards. Many stuttered or felt their hearts pounding faster, faster. Some broke out in sweats, blushed or flushed in an instant.

Many of the cases involved previously strong men who worked for the railway and had been involved in collisions on the job. One forty-one-year-old conductor developed headaches, chest and back pains, areas of analgesia, and general weakness following a train wreck. His symptoms barely improved during six months of hospitalization, and he died shortly after he was discharged. Another railway employee, also forty-one, was struck on the back during a railway collision and subsequently developed back and extremity pain on the left side of his body, as well as a swimming in the head, narrowing of his left visual field, jitters and tremors, night terrors, and problems with walking. Treated with warm baths, he showed significant improvement after many months and was sent home. A third man, employed as a railway secretary, was struck on the head and back and developed marked anxiety, stuttering and trembling as well as an inability to write. A fourth developed head and back pains, visual problems, urinary frequency, areas of anesthesia, and tremors. And a fifth—who was not struck at all during an accident, but was simply frightened— developed great anxiety, sleeplessness, problems with memory, and supposedly an epileptic disorder.

Oppenheim postulated that a mixed group of neuroses could break out following railway trauma. To be sure, some patients showed signs of hysteria, such as anesthesia or paralysis. But others were best diagnosed as suffering from anxiety, nervous exhaustion, even epilepsy and dementia. Hence he frowned on Charcot's all-encompassing idea of traumatic hysteria and coined the more amorphous term "traumatic neurosis" to describe these cases.

Also, the German doubted the importance of ideas in the breeding of such neuroses and concentrated on the nerves and specifically on electricity coursing through the nerves as the causative agent in these illnesses. He expanded on the physiological aspects of lethal shocks to the nervous system, looking to electrical theory to explain the importance of electriclike stimuli coming from the environment into the sensory organs, passing through the nerves, and causing a neurosis. Though he used the phrase "psychic shock" to describe the experience of many of his patients who were not physically traumatized, he wrote, "We assume that in the functional disorders, [that is, the traumatic neuroses] molecular alternations occur in the central nervous system." Both psychic and physical shock he saw as acting upon the nervous system to "evoke molecular alterations in the same areas which govern the higher psychic and the motor and sensory functions and those of the special senses." He warmed to the comparison of these cases to instances in which persons were actually struck by lightning, and he stated emphatically, "This theory is opposed to that of Charcot who regarded traumatic hysteria to be secondary to auto-suggestion," that is, a frightening idea in the mind of the patient.

Regardless of Charcot and Oppenheim's disagreement, many doctors in the late nineteenth century believed that they had at least the beginnings of a scientific understanding of traumatic neurosis. From the 1880s onward, myriad lawsuits reached the courts, and many doctors felt they had something to say as expert witnesses. Cases of railway spine or traumatic neurosis due to railway accident clutter nineteenth-century legal and neurological textbooks in Europe and America.

The questions with which the court wrestled were, first, when was a railway responsible for an injury, however apparently trivial, to one of its passengers? Second, how were malingerers to be detected? And third, if an expert witness, such as a neurologist or expert in nerves, were called to testify, how was his testimony to be employed?

From 1880 to 1910 the railways were increasingly being judged responsible for mental shocks. Doctors played a significant role in diagnosing litigants' suffering from traumatic neurosis or the railway spine. Doctors felt confident enough to try to distinguish between malingerers and genuine neurotics. Finally, doctors came to pronounce which neurotics were hereditarily weakened, with a train accident only the catalyst for an inevitable process of nervous degeneration, and which neurotics were strong before the accident but propelled by trauma into a downhill neurotic course.

In the case of the Louisville and Southern Railway Company versus Minogue, 1890, a Southern belle named Mary Minogue "was by the jar of the collision thrown from the seat to the floor of the car in which she was riding . . . the appellee sustained external bruises, and her nervous system was greatly shocked. . . . None of her bones were broken, but . . . ever since, she has been troubled with partial paralysis, or an insensibility in one leg from the knee down." The medical testimony was described as unsatisfactory in this case because the doctors disagreed on whether the injuries were permanent or not. The physicians nonetheless agreed that the railway should pay something since this was clearly a case of the railway spine.

An 1891 case involving the Pittsburgh Railway Company and a woman named Eva Ewing was based on the following claim: "The

defendant company ran one train of cars . . . against and upon
another car [in consequence of which cars] were broken, over-
turned, and thrown from the track and fell upon the ground and
premises of the plaintiffs . . . and against and upon the dwelling
house of the plaintiff, and by reason thereof, greatly endangered
the life of Eva Ewing . . . and subjected her to great fright, alarm,
fear and nervous excitement and distress, whereby she then and
there became sick and disabled and continued to be sick and
disabled from attending to her usual work and duties, and continued to suffer great mental and physical pain and anguish, and
is thereby permanently weakened and disabled." It seemed apparent that slight collisions or even fears of collisions could cause
damage: nervous shock was a reality. The nervous system of
humans, and especially of women, seemed delicate and much
prone to being shaken by violent outside forces and impressions,
particularly those related to the railways.

The theory could be stretched even further to encompass not
only patients who had feared railway accidents but also others who
were simply near railways, thereby heightening their nervous susceptibility to any terrifying nervous stimuli. For instance, a Mrs.
Mitchell was about to step from a train when "a horse car of the
defendant came down the street. As the team attached to the car
drew near, it turned to the right and came so close to the plaintiff
that she stood between the horses' heads when they had stopped."
She testified that fright and excitement caused by the approaching
team left her unconscious and also caused a miscarriage and subsequent illness. Medical testimony was given to the effect that the
mental shock she had received was sufficient to produce those results. Similarly, in the 1897 case of Spade v. Lynn and Boston
Railroad, Margaret Spade was frightened when another passenger
was disorderly on the train she was riding. A quarrel ensued between him and the conductor, who acted with "carelessness,
negligence, and with the use of . . . unnecessary force." Mrs. Spade
testified about her terror in the train: "It seemed as though I had
turned to solid ice. My breath was cut right off. I could not have
spoken; I tried to speak, but I was chilled so I kept growing stiffer
and stiffer, until I do not know when they got me off the car." In
both cases the women had fainted, perhaps following a strong
sympathetic nervous system response. But the actual fainting fit

was caused not by a train accident but by some agitating experience simply while near a train.

In yet another case a woman was hit in the temple during an accident and thrown into hysteria. In still another, the confusion and fright of a train wreck left a woman nervous and anxious, unable to perform her duties as a mother. In other cases, in almost every state in the Union, boys, girls, women, and men were frightened by railways and lay hysterical, prostrated, anxious, and terrorized. In most cases American juries awarded the poor traumatized sufferers substantial amounts of money. Though higher courts sometimes reduced the reparations, medical testimony and popular opinion concurred in establishing a firm connection between fright, nerves, and the responsibility of the railways. In the last few years of the nineteenth century there were more and more cases in which doctors were willing to step forward and testify that connecting links existed between the collision, the shock, and the symptoms. Outraged with the idea that a sensitive female, especially a pregnant one, could suffer injury and not have reparation, juries tended to agree with the medical testimony. Once they had names such as "hysteria," "railway spine," and "traumatic neurosis," doctors—armed with the theories of Charcot, Oppenheim, Page, and others—believed that the railways were causing profound injuries to many unsuspecting persons.

The railway spine and more general cases of neurosis concentrated attention on the idea that the stress and strain of civilization—of which the railway was the symbol—caused these illnesses. By the turn of the century the symptom pictures outlined by Charcot and others seemed to be well established by science, and the progressive symbols of society, such as the railways, seemed to be responsible for the breakdown of the human nervous systems. As Sir Clifford Allbutt, Regius Professor of Medicine at Cambridge University, put it in his *Contemporary Review* article of 1895:

> To turn now . . . to nervous disability, to hysteria . . . to
> the frightfulness, the melancholy, the unrest due to living
> at a high pressure, the world of the railway, the pelting
> of telegrams, the strife of business . . . surely, at any rate,
> these maladies or the causes of these maladies are more

rife than they were in the days of our fathers? To this
question . . . there is, I know, but one opinion on the subject in society, in the newspapers, in the books of philoso-
phers, even in the journals and treatises of the medical
profession.

All believed that the hydra-headed monster called nervosity was
growing new heads daily and that the hubbub of civilization embodied in the railway was to blame for the ever-mounting number
of cases of neurosis. Indeed the railway spine and brain stands forth
as the classical Victorian neurosis, that is, a psychocultural illness
in which the human psyche collided with the changing nineteenth-
century environment and gave birth to an epidemiclike neurotic
illness whose form and severity are rooted in the Victorian era.

Returning momentarily to the young Sigismund—peeping out
the window of a railway car, imagining the gas lanterns to be the
very lamps of hell, and then turning to see his naked mother—one
gets hints of an explanation other than the Oedipus complex.
Though Dr. Freud never developed the idea, the little boy of two
or two and a half may have been looking back yearningly to the
maternal warmth of old Galicia and even rural Moravia. There
life was simpler, less brutal, there the nerves were less tightly
drawn, there the trolls of Munthe still protected the infant child
from so many nervous shocks.

The Zeus myth of neurosis, which can be attributed to both
Oppenheim and Charcot, set forth an etiological explanation
emphasizing the moment when a vulnerable human collided with
an increasingly complicated and intimidating environment. The
child, the woman, even the vulnerable man, confronted a fast-
paced whirligig world for which he was not prepared. He stared
into the snarling new meshwork of the Machine. His veins ran
cold with fear. Electricity shot through his nerves. He fainted. He
awakened from his deathlike state transformed into a neurotic
sufferer.

SIX

The Mind in Splinters

ON May 6, 1877, a plump and dimpled blond girl named
Blanche Wittman made her inauspicious entrance into the
Salpêtrière. This girl, destined for great things, had a pedigree
common to French hysterics circa 1870. Her father was a carpenter
who went mad and ended his days in an insane asylum. The eldest
of nine children, she was one of only four siblings who survived
into adulthood; four died of "convulsions" and one possibly of
epilepsy. She seemed a typical Degenerate to the eyes of Victorian
neurology.

Blanche was a sickly child. At two years of age she experienced
episodes of convulsions, paralysis, mutism, and deafness. She was
undoubtedly nervously tainted from birth, Charcot and his followers thought when they collected her history. It was only when
she was seven that these early symptoms abated markedly. Poorly
educated because of her long illness, Blanche remained nearly
illiterate. As an adolescent she was prone to outbursts of hot temper, a tendency that her mother quelled with solid Victorian discipline, namely flinging pails of water in her face.

Sent as an apprentice to a furrier at age twelve, she began to
experience convulsions. As luck would have it, whenever her boss
found her alone he would try to seduce her. She rebuffed his
advances, but her "nervous crises" worsened. She would shake all
over, dropping whatever she had in her hands. For the next two

years she barely held her master and her nervous crises in check. When her patron tried to beat her, Blanche escaped from this unbearable situation and ran home.

From age fourteen until fifteen, while living with her mother and working as a laundress, she carried on a sexual affair with a youth named Louis. Then in 1877, when she was fifteen years old, her mother died suddenly, and the poor girl had no recourse but to return to the wretched furrier. When this lecher renewed his advances and her convulsions recurred, she first fought him off and then fled to an aunt's home. Then, taking a job as a nurse, she moved into a nearby hospital. This arrangement gave her some security. She found, however, that her attacks worsened after she took a lover named Alphonse. They overcame her nearly every night and drove her to seek expert medical help at Charcot's Salpêtrière. Here she was admitted both as a nurse and a patient in 1877.

Blanche's sojourn at the Salpêtrière lengthened into her life work. Her hysterical fits were far from sensational to the doctors in the Parisian hospital; Louise's face and form were more photogenic, and Geneviève's life story was more fascinating and morbid. Still, Blanche found a home in the wards of the Salpêtrière.

By 1877 Charcot's growing fascination with hysteria and traumatic neurosis had heightened to the point of his daring to use any technique to plumb the depths of these disorders. He collected around himself an array of seemingly incurable female hysterics, traumatized male neurotics, and curious and inventive doctors. In this Parisian medley Blanche soon rose to a position of prime importance. It is she who falls hypnotized and fainting into the arms of the Master in the famous painting "A Clinical Lesson of Dr. Charcot at the Salpêtrière." It was her facility as a hypnotic subject that helped to rivet the eyes of the medical world on hysteria and hypnotism through the eighties and nineties. It was she who was central to the French effort to analyze the human mind, to break down the mind-brain of the neurotic into nameable splinters and layers. And it was hypnotism that was the primary tool in this amazing analysis of the human mind.

Like a film producer, Charcot possessed the ability to make breathtaking "finds." Blanche and hypnotism were two of his greatest discoveries. Many other doctors and patients bearing their talents—their techniques and symptoms—took themselves to his hospital to be scrutinized by Charcot. Thus did Charcot import Dr. Lambalt to the Salpêtrière, a great expert in the use of the ophthalmoscope. Since one of the major symptoms of hysteria was the narrowing of visual fields as well as a loss of sensitivity to the color red, ophthalmologic examination—examination of the eye with a light and a magnifying lens—became an important part of the diagnosis of hysteria. Also, Charcot brought in Dr. Burq, a general practitioner who for twenty years prior to his "discovery" had been using bars of metal such as copper, silver, and iron in the cure of nervous diseases. Burq made an application to use metallotherapy on the inhabitants of the Salpêtrière, and Charcot simply assented. Then there was Vigouroux, an aging doctor who used electricity in the cure of patients, and the young Regnard, who was not only a good photographer but also an expert hypnotist. Dr. Richer proved an excellent medical illustrator, Tourette and Babinsky superb neurologists and nosologists in their own right. Even Freud visited, and offered himself to the Master as a German translator. The list of brilliant French and foreign doctors is too lengthy to recount and is in fact much longer than the list of famous hysterical women and traumatized men at the Salpêtrière.

Charcot and his followers were so curious about the causes of hysteria that they hurled every potential diagnostic and therapeutic weapon in their grasp at their disabled hysterics; not just magnets, metals, and electricity but also the anesthesia ether, which hysterics loved because it tended to bring on a voluptuous delirium; amyl nitrate, which the doctors apparently preferred since it gave birth to frightening hallucinations; morphine, which led to the death of at least one famous hysteric, Marceline, who succumbed to withdrawal; chloroform; pressing on hysterogenic points; and so on.

Charcot and his men constantly employed an inductive approach. For instance, they observed that the patients sometimes played vicious tricks on one another by pressing on a rival's ovaries and so causing an attack. Sometimes one hysteric helped a comrade by pressing on the points that quelled a fit before the doctors could arrive. As a result the doctors invented a little compressor to help keep pressure permanently applied to ovarian spots. Isolation was another technique Charcot began to use. He noticed that simply keeping a patient separate from family members and other patients often quelled symptoms. Although hypnosis was the most celebrated technique that Charcot used, it seems to have been just one of many approaches he and his followers tried and found worth while at the Salpêtrière.

The story of hypnosis before Charcot is a lengthy tale that is intriguing in its own right. In the various threads of this story we can see the broad popular appeal of hypnosis in nineteenth-century Europe, which probably played a role in the phenomena Blanche and her colleagues manifested when hypnotized. The

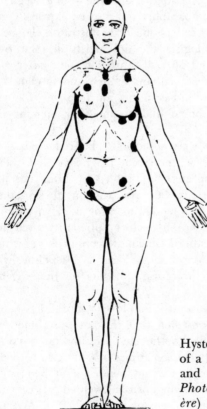

Hysterogenic points on the body of a hysteric. (From Bourneville and Regnard, *Iconographie Photographique de la Salpêtrière*)

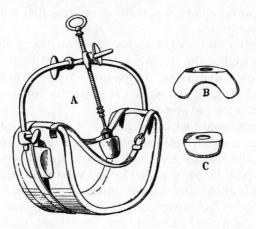

An ovarian compressor to quell hysterical fits. (From Bourneville
and Regnard, *Iconographie Photographique de la Salpêtrière*)

tale begins roughly one hundred years earlier, at about the time
Robert Whytt thrived in Edinburgh and a few decades before
Thomas Trotter was a doctor for the British Navy.

Hypnotic practices began with an eighteenth-century Austrian
doctor named Franz Anton Mesmer (1734–1815). An attractive
man with piercing eyes and impeccable manners, who attended
medical school at the University of Vienna, Mesmer learned an
odd conglomerate of theories in his medical studies which included certain astronomical and astrological notions going back to
Paracelsus, the fifteenth-century German alchemist. Mesmer's own
theory of diseases, combining the Newtonian theory of gravity,
electricity—knowledge of which was much advanced by his contemporary Ben Franklin—and magnetism, drew strength partially
from astrology but also from concepts of curious forces that preoccupied eighteenth-century science.

Mesmer's theory posited the existence in the human body of a
fluid called animal magnetism. He believed there was an axis
passing through men and women from head to foot, something
like the imaginary earth magnet connecting the magnetic poles. In

illness the animal magnetism passing through these poles began to function awry, ebbing and flowing in ways that led to the outbreak of symptoms.

This relatively modern theory drew on the ancient humoral theory as well as the Galenic vapor theory of hysteria. But since Mesmer compared animal magnetism to very real and, in 1780, very novel scientific forces such as electricity and gravity, his theory did not seem too preposterous.

Mesmer posited that the technique of curing involved the doctor's using his own healthy animal magnetism to reorganize the patient's force fields and vital fluids. A physician's therapeutic approach should begin with an elegant entrance into a room, a softness of voice, intense looks into the patient's eyes, firm but gentle touches on distressed body parts. The crux of the cure involved the patient's passing into a trance and then into a crisis. This crisis seemed like a hysterical fit, with the patient striking odd postures, trembling all over, and falling down. Following the crisis, the force fields and the animal magnetism would supposedly slip back into order and the patient would be healed.

Mesmer married an elderly wealthy woman and set up a practice in a splendid mansion in Vienna. He began to apply his theory and technique to sickly individuals and won some acclaim.

In the same period, 1770–80, Father Johann Gassner (1727–79) began a career as an exorcist in the countryside not far from Vienna. Gassner was a bit of a heretic who believed fanatically that he was an agent of God and, further, that many people suffering from all sorts of diseases were simply inhabited by evil spirits. He created quite a stir in Bavaria with his amazing cures. An eyewitness tells how Gassner would make a nervous sufferer, often a peasant, kneel before him. Then he would speak in Latin to the wretch, or rather to the devil inhabiting the poor human. When Gassner ordered the devil to display his power, the patient, whether he knew Latin or not, would often display his symptoms. Once the devil had declared his presence, Gassner resorted to the medieval rituals of exorcism. Ultimately he prayed to God for aid. The wretch would cry out, flail about, utter curses in Latin, and then lie still, as the soul of the evil one sailed into the gaping abyss of hellfire.

Both Gassner, the son of medieval Christianity, and Mesmer,

the son of the Enlightenment, won some acclaim as healers. Inevitably the two collided in a controversy over the question of how their cures worked. Each man applied his own technique, each believed in his own theory.

Both churchmen and scientists descended on Gassner's parish in Bavaria to observe his exorcisms. When the King of Bavaria, a liberal with scientific interests, issued an invitation to Mesmer, the Viennese doctor went forth to meet the priest at work. After close observation of his fellow healer, Mesmer reported to the king that Gassner's exorcisms were based on a superstitious theory, whereas animal magnetism was a reality. He described Gassner as a man of good faith who really was an unsuspecting tool, not of God but of nature. In short, he gave credit to Gassner's practice but maligned his theory.

Gassner was soon banned as a heretic by the Church and banished to a monastery by the Bavarian king. Though no one doubted Gassner's power as a healer, exorcism was suspect as theory. Animal magnetism seemed at the time more enlightened, more scientific. Mesmer emerged from this controversy as a highly influential theoretician and physician. With his personal rise to fame his theory of animal magnetism won more adherents. His friends included Mozart, Gluck, and Haydn as well as the Austrian empress Maria Theresa. His practice grew larger, he cured some seemingly incurable cases. His wealth and social position grew.

Then came his greatest test. A young female pianist, the darling of the Viennese court, whose hysterical blindness seemed only to add to her notoriety, came looking for a cure. Mesmer undertook the treatment of this woman. Unfortunately, as her blindness disappeared, her musical talents also seemed to diminish. Her noble family, acclaimed because of their offspring's musical talents, then abducted the convalescent girl from Mesmer. Claiming sexual seduction by Mesmer, the girl's parents influenced the Austrian emperor to send Mesmer out of town.

Following this scandal and his precipitous flight from Vienna, Mesmer deserted his aging wife and traveled to Paris on the eve of the French Revolution. Once there, he developed a new technique: group magnetism. Collecting crowds of prominent Parisians, usually women, around a wooden tub filled with water, he carried on intriguing séances. Two of Charcot's disciples, Binet and Féré, described this tub, called a *baquet*, and the séance in their 1896 work called simply *Animal Magnetism*.

> A circular oaken case, about a foot high, was placed in the middle of a long hall, hung with thick curtains, through which only a soft and subdued light was allowed to penetrate. . . . At the bottom of the case on a layer of powdered glass and iron filings, there lay full bottles, symmetrically arranged, so that the necks of all converged towards the center; other bottles were arranged in the opposite direction, with their necks towards the circumference. All these objects were immersed in water . . . The lid [of the case] was pierced with a certain number of holes, whence there issued jointed and movable rods or iron branches, which were to be held by the patients. Absolute silence was maintained. The patients were arranged in several rows round the baquet, connected with each other by cords passed round their bodies, and by a second chain formed by joining hands. As they waited, a melodious air was heard proceeding from a pianoforte or harmonicon . . . and to this the human voice was sometimes added. Then, influenced by the magnetic effluvia issuing from the baquet, curious phenomena were produced [namely, convulsive episodes, crying, twitching, hiccoughing, and immoderate laughter].

One eyewitness of many séances wrote, "When the agitation exceeded certain limits, the patients were transported into a padded room; the women's corsets were unlaced, and they may then strike their heads against the padded walls without doing themselves any injury."

Mesmer himself often made an appearance to the accompaniment of soft, mournful music. He would pass among his patients draped in a lavender silk robe. Fixing his eyes on each patient in turn and touching the patients with his hands or a long magnetized iron wand, he would send one patient after another into a trance.

Society women suffering from the then popular vapors or fainting fits were drawn to him. Soon a furor developed in Paris. At first the darling of Marie Antoinette and her courtiers, Mesmer was soon suspected again of sexual misconduct and also of charlatanism. Though medical men first came to study with Mesmer in droves, he seems to have had a way of alienating them. Also, he insisted on earning large sums of money. Secret societies—"societies of harmony" as they were called—were formed by him and his followers, from whom he extracted large amounts of money for the sale of his secrets. French scientific commissions came to study animal magnetism in detail, and finally the Academy of Sciences ruled that Mesmer's theories had no scientific basis. The cures themselves seemed real enough. No one doubted them. But it was the theory of animal magnetism that seemed questionable.

Despite the ousting of Mesmer from polite medicine, his popularity was so widespread that he remained the rage of Paris for another decade. His old friend Mozart, who also had migrated to the City of Light, wrote a few lines about Mesmer in one of his operas. Paintings of Mesmer became numerous, some complimentary, some not so complimentary. Marie Antoinette remained his patronne. The societies of harmony grew strong and prosperous.

Yet his practice of extracting large sums of money from his disciples, his sponsoring of showy group mesmeric events, went too far. Gradually the Parisian citizenry turned against him, seeing him as a quack, a mountebank, a moneygrubber. Caricatures and cartoons of Mesmer proliferated. Theatrical spoofs appeared. Humiliated, Mesmer packed his bags and took flight again.

Where he went is unclear. Probably to England and Italy, perhaps to the smaller cities in France. The revolution was under way, and he may have been better off out of harm's way as his unpopularity with the French mob may have made him a likely candidate for the guillotine. Following years of wandering, Mesmer finally settled on Lake Constance in Switzerland, where he lived out his days in idyllic retirement.

The medical community in France, which was then the most mechanistically oriented in the world, banned the practice of animal magnetism, or Mesmerism, for almost a hundred years. Officially, at least, to practice Mesmerism was a medical sin. It was comparable to Leonardo da Vinci's cutting up of human bodies in Florence during the Renaissance. However, it was often done secretly by a doctor here or there. And Mesmer's societies of harmony continued without him.

It was in one of these societies that a new phenomenon was soon born, namely somnambulism. A nobleman named M. de Puységur (1751–1825), who lived in retirement in Soissons, "employed his leisure in magnetising peasants, after the manner of his master," wrote Binet and Féré. To his surprise, one young peasant named Victor was thrown by such mesmerism into a peaceful sleep. He hallucinated and "imagined that he was firing at a mark or dancing at a village fête." In this state Victor showed much more intelligence than he normally did. He seemed to possess a second personality. M. de Puységur could produce these same phenomena en masse by "magnetising an elm tree which grew on the village green [via a series of touches and passes]. The patients were seated on stone benches round this tree, with cords connecting its branches with the affected parts of their bodies, and they formed a chain by linking their thumbs together . . . [certain patients] then fell into ordinary crises, and this soon passed into a sleep in which all physical capacities appeared suspended while the mental faculties were enlarged."

In somnambulism we see a second form of hypnotism, one that complemented the older form, the writhing and wriggling phenomena of Mesmer and Gassner. Though we can only hypothesize about why the writhing fit and the walking sleep were so widespread in late revolutionary and postrevolutionary France, they were indeed quite common. Later, Charcot and his men were just categorizing what they really saw in their patients.

Even though a mechanistic world view dominated nineteenth-century French medicine, in which hypnosis had no official place, trance states truly intrigued the nineteenth-century French. Mesmerism thrived outside French medical circles. Particularly in the form of somnambulism, magicians and stage performers used the wonders of trance induction widely. For a long time the artificially induced trance was not considered an appropriate diagnostic or therapeutic tool by most medical men west of the Rhine. Yet the subject continued to be studied surreptitiously by medical men and was twice brought to the attention of the Academy of Science during the middle years of the nineteenth century.

Meanwhile, in Germany, where a more organic world view held sway, hypnosis lived on as a more respectable medical discipline. Many medical worthies made pilgrimages to Mesmer in Switzerland until his death in 1815. An intimate connection between hypnosis and romanticism, mysticism, and vitalism developed in Germany between 1780 and 1850. The German physiologist Johannes Müller's ideas about nervous energy complemented thinking about animal magnetism.

In 1841, in Manchester, England, the third key figure in the development of hypnotism began his work. One night a surgeon named James Braid (1795–1860) was attending a demonstration of magicians. Featured in the show was a Swiss itinerant mesmerist named Lafontaine. Braid became intrigued, though perplexed, with Lafontaine's tricks on the stage.

Originally Braid was convinced that Lafontaine was an adroit imposter. Yet he was interested enough to attend a second séance. More and more curious, Braid then began his own experiments with trance states, using his family and friends as subjects. First he requested "his friend Walker" to sit down and look fixedly at the neck of a wine bottle, which was placed at such a height as to cause considerable fatigue to his eyes and eyelids when he looked at it attentively, according to Braid's biographer Milne Bramwell. "In three minutes his eyelids closed, tears flowed down his cheeks, and his head drooped, his countenance was slightly contracted, and a sigh escaped from him, and at the same moment he fell into a deep sleep . . . [then] Braid made his wife sit down and fix her eyes on the ornaments of a porcelain sugar basin . . . in two minutes . . . the patient sighed deeply, the chest heaved, she fell back. It was evident that she had passed through a paroxysm of hysteria, and Braid woke her."

In the course of his mesmeric endeavors Braid put forward a new theory to explain the trance phenomenon. The surgeon believed that the cause of the trance lay not within a strange fluidic substance called animal magnetism but within the mind or the nervous system of the hypnotized patient. Somehow the maneuvering of the hypnotist affected the patient's mind or brain in a way that induced the trance state.

Though Braid's theory was never accepted by conservative medical men in his own lifetime, he did leave behind the word "hypnosis," as well as a series of surprisingly modern case descriptions, which were soon to be rediscovered by polite medicine.

Two decades later, in the 1870s, Charcot stumbled on hypnosis.

Precisely how his interest developed is not altogether certain. However, he was much influenced by a colleague, Charles Richet, who had begun investigations with this technique a few years earlier. Despite the official position, it is fair to say that French medicine had never really given up hypnosis as a subject for research. As Charcot wrote in his famous paper "Provoked Hysterical Somnambulism and Catalepsy," he could find as predecessors Braid and a number of significant French doctors whose works dated from around 1860. The problem remained to find an explanation for the efficacy of hypnosis, and so Charcot's interest seems far from extraordinary.

In any event, the wonders of hypnotism seemed incredible to Charcot and his followers in the early years at the Salpêtrière. Some of the hysterical women, such as Louise and Geneviève, had been lying in their paralyzed and anesthetic and seizure-ridden states for decades. Hysteria seemed irrevocable and incurable. Then the patient would be hypnotized. And in this trance the paralyzed limbs would move, sensation would return to the long-anesthetized body part. The chronic hysterical patient seemed momentarily cured. Though such improvements usually vanished after the hypnotic trance ended, the transient improvement seemed inspiring to the doctors. Furthermore, by telling the patients while in a trance that they would remain unparalyzed or would not be blind any more, doctors could sometimes cause the symptoms to remit for long periods of time, though they might recur after some physical or psychic trauma such as a fall down a staircase or a renewed induction of hypnotism by a curious French doctor.

It was not the therapeutic properties of hypnosis, however, that most intrigued Charcot. Rather it was the weird mental and physical phenomena that he and his followers were able to produce in the hysterics. He analyzed these particles and splinters of behavior, and they ultimately led him to pronounce that hypnosis was an artificial form of a neurosis. We have already seen how he could, through hypnosis, elicit in his "old reliables" hysterical symptoms comparable to those seen in traumatized men. Charcot essentially placed alongside one another the various types of hypnotism, the stages of hysteria, and the symptoms induced in patients through trauma, and he drew some interesting, if fleeting parallels. For instance, the hysterical period of grand movements, when the patient did acrobatics, resembled the fits induced by Mesmer. The period of passionate attitudes, when the patient re-lived events from the past, looked much like the somnambulism of de Puységur. From these parallels and those between men who had been traumatized and hysterical women who had been hypnotized he came to equate not only traumatic neurosis with hysteria but hysteria with hypnotism.

Just as he had done with hysteria, Charcot set out to describe and classify the phenomena he and his colleagues were witnessing in hypnotized hysterics, and by way of this classification he assem-bled a sensational new thesis. In his 1882 paper before the French Academy of Science he outlined the three stages of hypnosis: catalepsy, lethargy, and somnambulism. He described the three stages in neurological and medical terms. Reportedly employing a rigorous scientific method, he spoke of tendon reflexes, neuromus-cular excitability, and cardiac and respiratory rates. The Acad-emy, which had damned Mesmer, listened attentively to the prominent French neurologist. Through Charcot hypnotism be-came an acceptable diagnostic and therapeutic technique in France and the rest of the West, and Charcot's thesis defining hypnosis as an artificial or laboratory neurosis became a fashionable medical doctrine.

The first paper written by Charcot, and many later papers pub-lished by his followers, delineated the hypnotic techniques, the various maneuvers and discoveries used in the laboratory of the Salpêtrière. Charcot and his associates had their patients stare into bright lights for long periods of time. The hysterics, notably Blanche, Marceline, and Louise, would then fall into catalepsy, a condition marked by a loss of consciousness. The experimenter would move the limbs of the patient in different directions, and the patient would then hold the pose for long periods of time. Also, when the hypnotist shaped the hysteric's hand into a fist, suggesting anger, or opened and placed her hand above her head, suggesting surprise and fright, this would cause the rest of the body to assume a pose of anger or fright. The teeth would grit, the hands would clench, the eyelids would narrow in anger; or the eyes would grow saucer-wide, the mouth would open as in fright.

The second stage, lethargy, would be brought on by first placing

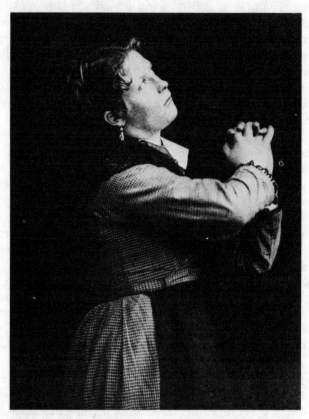

Blanche in a catalepsy manifesting muscular suggestibility. (From Bourneville and Regnard, *Iconographie Photographique de la Salpêtrière*)

the patient in a cataleptic or frozen state and then turning off the light or closing the eyes of the staring hysteric. The patient would then fall down limp. In this state of limpness an exciting new phenomenon was discernible. This phenomenon, called neuromuscular excitability, intrigued Charcot for years. If a muscle was touched it would contract. Once contracted, the muscle would seem paralyzed. No force applied by the doctors seemed to break the paralysis, and in this state the patients sometimes manifested superhuman strength.

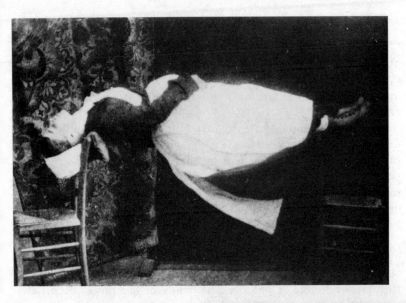

Louise in a lethargy manifesting neuromuscular hyperexcitability. (From Bourneville and Regnard, *Iconographie Photographique de la Salpêtrière*)

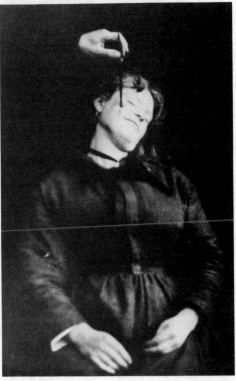

Blanche in a lethargy, limp but hypersensitive to the touch of a stylet. (From Bourneville and Regnard, *Iconographie Photographique de la Salpêtrière*)

A combination of these two stages, catalepsy and lethargy, could also be created by keeping one eye of a hysteric open and the other eye closed. One side of the body would be cataleptic, or frozen, and the other lethargic, or limp, but prone to neuromuscular excitability.

The third hypnotic phase, somnambulism, would be induced by different techniques, such as simply scratching the head of the cataleptic patient. Rather than growing limp, as in lethargy, the patient awakened in a twilight state, walking and talking like a robot. This last state was not investigated in detail by Charcot until later years, and in fact he left most of this investigation up to his more psychologically minded followers.

Blanche Wittman proved the most hypnotizable hysteric. Her induced paralyses, her expressions of fright or anger, her somnambulistic trances proved the most astonishing in the Salpêtrière. Regnard undertook a photographic study of her poses. Brouillet painted her on canvas. Though she had a few fierce competitors, such as Louise and Marceline, by the late eighties she was dubbed the Queen of Hysterics. Her astonishing cataleptic, lethargic, and somnambulistic feats were reported in detail throughout the Western medical world.

Almost concurrently, a renewed interest in the subject of hypnosis was growing elsewhere in Europe. Various stage performers, such as Hanson and Donato, had turned the heads of a number of doctors in Germany, Austria, and France, including Freud's mentor Josef Breuer. In America, William James studied séances with a medium named Mrs. Leanora Piper; and in the same year as Charcot's speech before the Academy of Science, the medical society in the French city of Nancy had turned its attention to the hypnotic cures of a doctor named Auguste Ambroise Liébeault (1823–1904).

Liébeault was one of those general practitioners around whom a great deal of reverence has accrued. Two years the senior of Charcot, he had studied medicine at Strasbourg. The official histories of the early days of his work establish that his interest in hypnosis went back to about 1848, in medical school, when, against the advice of a teacher, he first read two works on hypnotism, after which he laid his reading aside for a while. In about 1850 he moved

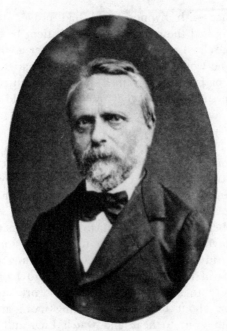

Auguste Ambroise Liébeault, country doctor and
mind healer. (Medizinhistorisches Institut, Zurich)

to a small village outside of Nancy, where he established a successful and lucrative private practice.

In about 1860, working primarily with peasants as patients, he
returned to the study of hypnosis. The story goes that he had a few
early setbacks in his hypnotic practice. One woman, for example,
fell into a violent seizure, like that of Braid's wife, and the ferocity
of the attack led Liébeault to renounce "a process which exposed
me to such an accident." But Liébeault soon returned to the subject and the practice. Eventually he seemed to have gotten the
hang of the technique, and soon he was willing to make a proposi-
tion to his French peasant patients. "If you want me to cure you
by using drugs, you must pay me as before. But if you allow me to
treat you by sleep, it will cost you nothing, and you will be cured
as well." Scores of French peasants, renowned for parsimony, were
soon lining up to be put into trances. Soon Liébeault had gained a

vast experience with hypnosis and had proved to himself its efficacy. He applied the practice to every patient he saw—hysteric, cancer victim, school phobic, or whatever. After a cursory physical examination he would quickly hypnotize the patient and suggest that his pain or fear would vanish. He was delighted to find that such a simple suggestion in the trance state would often work a cure.

In 1866 he published his own book on the subject, which allegedly sold but one copy. Who bought the copy? Surely not Liébeault's wife, for at the time she, like many of the neighbors, saw the country doctor as a crackpot. No one knows for certain who bought it, but maybe it was Liébeault, who did it to see his name in print.

Slowly Liébeault's fame spread to the University of Nancy. There Hippolyte Bernheim (1840–1919), Professor of Internal Medicine, already renowned for his work on lung illness, heard reports. A few of his colleagues had drifted to Liébeault's office out of curiosity to see the old doctor at work, and they had told Bernheim about Liébeault. Growing more and more curious, Bernheim went to hear and watch Liébeault in the little shed where he performed his hypnotic practices, and as Braid did with Lafontaine, Bernheim became fascinated with what he saw.

Soon Bernheim decided to experiment with his own patients. By the following year, after hypnotizing hundreds of patients in a very short time, the internist had formulated a new theory based on the idea of suggestibility. In 1884 he presented a paper in Nancy that cast doubt on Charcot's tripartite idea of hypnosis. Bernheim posited that suggestibility had led to the startling phenomena of the Salpêtrière, that the three stages of catalepsy, lethargy, and somnambulism occurred because the Salpêtrist doctors had certain expectations of their patients, which the patients had to fulfill. Furthermore, he posited that suggestibility led not just to hysteria but to many other diseases, such evil suggestibility being called autosuggestibility. The hypnotist could, however, harness the force of suggestibility in a positive way and so effect a cure.

Unlike Liébeault's book, Bernheim's works on hypnosis were widely read and translated into many languages (into German by

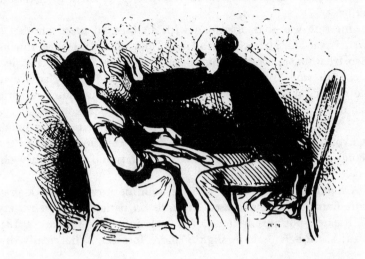

Animal Magnetism by Honoré Daumier, or "Sleep, sleep," by Liébeault. (Bibliotèque Nationale, Paris)

the young Sigmund Freud in Vienna). Soon strangers, both doctors and other learned men, were flowing into Nancy to meet Bernheim and Liébeault (who had moved into the city proper in about 1863) and to study them at their work.

Liébeault's consultation room was a little shack, two by nine meters. The floor of the room was made of red stone and the walls were whitewashed. A number of windows looked out onto a garden, from which the doctor's house could be seen. From nine to noon daily Liébeault consulted with twoscore peasants and other residents of Nancy. Their ailments ranged from cirrhosis with jaundice to anemia, chest pains, headaches, bronchitis, and tics. He would invite each patient to seat himself in an armchair while the other patients sat watching, a group caricature in the manner of Daumier. He would place himself at the patient's left, peer into his eyes, and then suggest to him that he was growing sleepy, that his eyelids were growing heavy. "Sleep, sleep," he would say softly and warmly with conviction, and the patient would fall into a state resembling sleep. Liébeault would tell his patients in this state that they would get better, that their pain would diminish, their appetite and sleep would improve, that their force would return.

One case was that of a man with an infected knee, another a twenty-year-old girl with headaches and abundant flow during menstruation, another an old woman with an ulcer on her leg. Liébeault would mingle hypnotic suggestion with easy advice to the spouses and parents of his patients, in the charming and firm manner of a general practitioner.

Liébeault would let his visitors, medical or lay, try their hands at hypnotizing a few of his patients before they took leave of the benign old doctor and proceeded to the hospital, where they observed Hippolyte Bernheim.

A handsome small man with an aquiline nose and thick gray hair, Bernheim likewise used hypnosis on patients with a variety of diseases, not just hysteria. His technique was similar to Liébeault's, though perhaps slightly more forceful. What really dis-

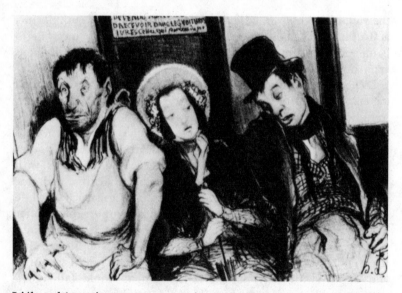

Liébeault's patients: a group caricature. Honoré Daumier, *Interior of an Omnibus*. (Bibliotèque Nationale, Paris)

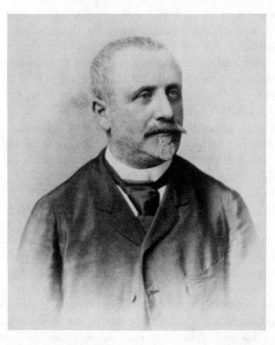

Hippolyte Bernheim, world expert on hypnotism. (Medizinhistorisches Institut, Zurich)

tinguished Bernheim from Liébeault was his more vigorously scientific turn of mind. Liébeault hypnotized any and all, never carefully documenting their diseases. Though Bernheim saw suggestibility at work in many illnesses, he distinguished between illnesses and published his results according to specific illness categories. Thus he could show good results by way of hypnosis in the treatment of hysteria as well as organic affections of the nervous system, other vague nervous problems, gastrointestinal diseases, certain chronic pain problems, and rheumatism.

One story shows the laxness of Liébeault's scientific method versus that of Bernheim. To humor the mother of a boy with diarrhea, constipation, and vomiting, Liébeault had begun to use "magnetized" water—that is, water into which he had touched the tips of his fingers—in the treatment of the boy. Since he saw that drinking this water seemed to produce good results, the old doctor was on the verge of believing, not in suggestibility, as Bernheim defined it, but in animal magnetism, in the manner of Mesmer. When Bernheim got wind of Liébeault's doubts about suggestibility, he recommended that the old doctor use regular water and just tell the mother of his patient that it would help the boy. Liébeault found good results with this method as well, so he readopted Bernheim's notion of suggestibility.

In his book *Suggestive Therapeutics* (first edition, 1884) Bernheim wrote that hypnosis is not an unusual state brought on only in a few hysterics or neuropaths. Rather it is a form of sleep. As a rule, children are very quickly and easily hypnotized, but so are many adults. Those who cannot be hypnotized are "preoccupied, unable to give themselves up: they analyze their own feelings, are anxious, and say they cannot sleep." He believed it was wrong to see all hypnotizable subjects as "weak-nerved, weak-brained, hysterical or women." He perceived that he could hypnotize "common people, those of gentle disposition, old soldiers, artisans, people accustomed to passive obedience" more readily, but that he could also hypnotize "very intelligent people belonging to the highest grades of society, who are not in the least nervous." After describing his own system of grading of hypnosis—which essentially involved the depth of the hypnotic or artificial sleep, the amount of connection with the outer world, and the amount of forgetfulness that occurs—Bernheim emphasized that there is only one fundamental difference between spontaneous and artificial sleep—namely, a continuing rapport with the inducer of the artificial sleep, which does not exist in natural sleep.

Bernheim defined hypnosis as the inducing of a peculiar physical condition that increases the susceptibility to suggestion. Although he readily agreed with the existence of a vast category of patients called hysterics and even mentioned that it was necessary to proceed cautiously and avoid touching the hysterogenic zones, he produced statistics showing that Liébeault was able to place about two-thirds of one thousand patients in some level of hypnotic sleep.

Bernheim further debunked the Salpêtrists, who said that by touching muscles they could induce paralyses during the so-called lethargic phase. He insisted that these paralyses were the products of suggestion and that if he were to tell a patient that he would have a paralysis when touched at a certain place, then and only then would the patient be paralyzed. Similarly, he could induce pain and anesthesia by suggestion during the artificial sleep. So too could he employ posthypnotic suggestion. As Bernheim saw it, "a suggestion given during sleep may lie dormant in the brain, and not come to consciousness until the time previously fixed for its appearance."

"There is one thing certain," Bernheim wrote, "that a *peculiar attitude for transforming the idea received into an act* exists in hypnotized subjects who are susceptible to suggestion." Whereas in the awake subject the cortical centers take in any impression like a suggestion, then analyze and often reject the idea, in the hypnotized subject the idea is immediately transformed into an act. A suggestion made under hypnosis *"effects the unconscious transformation of the thought into movement unknown to the will,"* wrote Bernheim. He believed that the entity called the will was probably concentrated somewhere in the frontal lobes, like Jackson's "organ of mind." Hence in induced or natural sleep the frontal lobes grow less active, and the lower parts of the brain take control of the sleeper. While in natural sleep there is no presence of will whatsoever, in hypnosis the will really resides in the hypnotist, and the patient loses his ability to think and act for himself, relying instead on the hypnotist's suggestions. Hence, Bernheim argues, the lower classes of society "where less cerebral resistance is offered" are less evolved cerebrally and so are more suggestible. These are the patients of Liébeault, the peasants.

The celebrated Battle of the Schools, the Nancy school against the Salpêtrière, ensued over the next eleven years, 1882–93. Charcot and his followers could not take all the attacks on their hypnotic practices lying down. The idea that they had been inadvertently suggesting to their patients how they should act implied that they were fools. Furthermore, much of Charcot's reputation seemed to hang on his theory of the three stages of hypnosis and on the theory that hypnotizability implied hysteria. Hence the disciples of Charcot took up the challenge for the sake of their master and entered into an acrid polemic with Bernheim and his small but growing group of followers.

As a result of this battle the subjects of hysteria and hypnosis gained great popularity. The debate between the Nancy school and the Salpêtrière was waged in medical journals, international conventions on hypnosis, in newspapers and magazines. Journals even came into existence precisely to sing the battle cries of the two schools. One author on hypnosis, Max Dessoir, compiling a bibliography of medical literature on the subject in 1887, noted 801 titles, most of which were written between 1884 and 1887.

Gradually the Nancy school won adherents while Charcot's position grew untenable. Bernheim had produced thousands of cases of hypnotized patients, while Charcot had only a handful of the "old reliables" at the Salpêtrière. Moreover, Charcot had raised an edifice of explanations on the shaky foundation of clinical work based on such subjects as Blanche and Louise. Because of his clear equation of hypnosis, hysteria, and traumatic neurosis, his theses were potentially refutable. Bernheim, however, never really constructed a thoroughgoing system and so was not as vulnerable as Charcot. Much of his thinking rested on the amorphous idea of suggestibility. Bernheim and his supporters were also an amorphous group that disagreed with different parts of Charcot's systems and frequently with one another. They disputed his equation of hysteria with the artificial trance hypnosis; they disputed his three stages of hypnosis, as well as his equation of traumatic hypnosis with hysteria; and they even disputed his four stages of hysteria.

Finally, Charcot's ideas lost prestige because he committed multiple methodological errors, while Bernheim's practice was more solid. Charcot did not always hypnotize his own patients; he barely talked with them; he did not understand the phenomenon of mass contagion at the Salpêtrière; he never used a control group (that is, persons with no illness). Bernheim hypnotized his own patients; he discussed their problems with them; he often worked with outpatients; he worked with a control group.

Regardless of the weakness in Charcot's arguments, he did a heroic task by centering so much medical attention on hysteria, hypnosis, and the various layers and phenomena of the mind: catalepsy, lethargy, somnambulism, psychic trauma, ideas as pathological agents. Furthermore, in the late eighties and early nineties, as his critics grew more virulent and devastating in their attacks, his disciples continued to busy themselves with observations and experiments to prove the original Charcotian thesis. Their work eventually took on a life of its own, separate from Charcot's central ideas. Through such toil a new vista in the history of neurosis was opening before the eyes of the Salpêtrists—namely, the vista of the mind. As the experiments on the few model hysterics grew more and more lavish, a concentration on the more psychological aspects of hysteria and hypnosis developed. Precisely by making Blanche and a few other hysterics so important in the theory of hypnosis, Charcot and his followers began in-depth studies that proceeded by isolating splinters of the mind and exploring further and further into the inner mind, the levels below normal consciousness.

For example, in one experiment, performed in 1891, two of Charcot's younger disciples, Georges Guinon and Sophie Woltke, placed the Queen of Hysterics in a hypnotized state. Then they held some fragments of colored glass before Blanche's eyes and recorded her responses. The first splinter was red glass, to which Blanche responded with joy; then a bit of blue glass, which made her sad; then yellow, which caused fear to spread across her features; then dull green, which evoked surprise and admiration. In rapid succession she was made to smell sulfur, eau de cologne, and chloroform. To each she responded with a strong emotion.

When awakened she was asked about what she had experienced. At first she was demure, refusing to answer. Then, pressed by the questioners, she recounted all the bizarre things that she had seen.

First she was in the arms of her lover (the red glass), "full of contentment and pleasure." Then suddenly she saw the sea (the blue glass) and was pulled into a cave and felt weighted down with sadness. In the cave she saw a torch (yellow glass) whose flames mounted upward. Then in an instant she was transported to a ballroom filled with flowers and green plants (the dull green glass), and she could only admire. Suddenly the scene changed again and she found herself in a tomb surrounded by the dead (sulfur), and she grew frightened. Next, miraculously, she was in a garden, in the middle of clumps of flowers (eau de cologne), and she grew contented. Finally she noted a peculiar odor like that from moist earth, and the air became unbreathable (chloroform). She thought she had nearly died. She swooned and awoke.

Guinon and Wolke repeated these experiments on other hysterics; they collected similar data but with different hallucinations, depending on the personality of the patient. So the individual personality came into greater and greater focus.

In many respects Charcot and his followers really followed the Nanceans, if not in their postulates, at least in their practices. Their differences were not really as great as their rhetoric would lead us to believe. Charcot had his three stages of hypnosis; Bernheim had his own six stages, ranging from catalepsy through somnolence into somnambulism. To a large extent Bernheim admitted the existence of hysteria along Charcot's lines, although he did not accept the four stages of hysterical fits. And on occasion Charcot admitted the therapeutic property of hypnosis, but he was pessimistic—rightly so—about its general therapeutic possibilities.

As the eighties passed, however, Charcot's hypotheses appeared more and more mistaken to the medical world. His glittering reputation grew tarnished, and many adherents began to desert him. The three phases of hypnosis were not reproducible outside of the Salpêtrière. His statements equating hypnosis with hysteria seemed ridiculous, as human beings other than hysterics were not only hypnotized but also made more healthy while under hypnosis. His various disciples tell in their memoirs of his growing list of enemies, of his supposed plan to revamp his theory, of his worsening angina, and finally of anonymous letters telling him that he would die of a stroke or a heart attack.

In the summer of 1893, Charcot—supposedly having just confided in the young Guinon his plans to rework his theory—set off with two of his young men for a restful sojourn in the sunny south of France. On this vacation Charcot grew quite philosophical, often considered a sign of senility in doctors. He discussed at great length with his disciples his long-standing love of art and architecture. A number of rather touching accounts of Charcot's last few days tell of his finding solace in visiting famous Gothic cathedrals and enjoying French country cooking and quiet. Finally one morning he was found dead, having suffered heart failure in his sleep.

Charcot died under a heavy cloud. Even the edition of his *Oeuvres Complètes* ceased to be published in 1893. His monograph on spiritualism, along with a few other post-1882 papers, never appeared in this collection. Nor did his personal papers, his sketches and caricatures. His thesis, which seemed unbelievable to many, had fallen to pieces. Some of his supporters, such as Pierre Marie, swiftly abandoned the study of hypnosis and returned to a more meticulous study of obvious organic illnesses whose individual signs and symptoms were not so slippery. They tried to follow the dictum of Jackson that neurologists should work with what was firm and solid and give up hope of helping diseased minds. Within a few years after Charcot's death hypnosis and hysteria had become less popular as medical and newspaper topics. The journals on hypnosis had folded by 1900. Perhaps these subjects required controversy to remain popular; perhaps the dynamic personality of Charcot was needed to keep the subjects at the forefront of official medicine. Most likely the times had simply turned, the whole controversy being symptomatic of an epoch obsessed with rococo elaborations of the human mind. By 1900, articles on the subjects of hypnosis and hysteria had fallen off to a trickle.

The lasting dichotomy between Nancy and Salpêtrière was not only theoretical—it could be seen as a conflict between urban modernization and traditional rural life. The Salpêtrists believed the city produced more hysteria than the country, which was a logical idea if one subscribed to the old Degenerate myth. For Charcot the hysterics were rendered neurologically degenerate by Paris and its machinery, its alcohol, and its vices; so the hysterics were always described as grand hysterics, whose disease was much more profound than the petit hysterics on whom Bernheim worked. The extraordinary feats of the grand hysterics when hypnotized were called grand hypnosis, since—to Charcot's way of thinking—the phenomena of lethargy, catalepsy, and somnambulism implied grave neurological imbalance. Bernheim meanwhile saw the country people, the peasants, as more gullible and suggestible. This belief too relied on another old myth, that of the Noble Savage, the simple rustic who, if placed in the hands of a more sophisticated person—ideally, a benign doctor—could be made to do and think practically anything. The gullible soul, once hypnotized, might be led anywhere, even if his nervous system was still intact.

For a time Bernheim's star was ascendant. His theory of suggestibility was all the rage. The grand hysterics of the Salpêtrière

faded into the shadows like ghosts and gremlins at the first glimmer of the dawn of true science. Nearly everyone believed that
Charcot had created in his own mind the grand hysteria and the
grand hypnosis and that hysterics themselves had simply gone
along for the glory and the suggestibility.

Yet this interpretation seemed incomplete. Years later, in the
1920s, Dr. A. Baudouin, who had been one of Charcot's young
disciples in the nineties, sought out Blanche Wittman to learn
more of the truth. Baudouin was still befuddled over the grand
hysteria and the grand hypnosis, which had been so prominent in
the 1870s through the 1890s but had disappeared by 1910.

Blanche had never left the Salpêtrière. No longer a patient, she
had become a radiology technician. X-rays had just been discovered by the Curies, and Blanche found herself a niche in which she
could be somewhat productive. Baudouin wrote that Blanche had
ceased to have her crises "when the time had passed in which these
experiences were à la mode." However, as her ill fortune would
have it, she had become a victim of her new profession. She had
contracted the "abominable cancer of the radiologist." As the cancer had spread, her limbs, one by one, had been amputated.

Baudouin sought Blanche out as she lay dying and asked her to
explain her past crises, hysterical and hypnotic. He specifically
asked about the accusation that the hysterics under hypnosis simu-
lated symptoms and so duped Charcot. Her reply was: "There is
no truth [in the accusation]. It is a lie. If we were put to sleep or
had a crisis, it was impossible for us to do otherwise. Besides, fits
and so forth were not pleasant . . . Simulation! Do you think that
it was possible to trick Charcot? Sure, there were many who tried,
but he could throw a simple glance at them and say, 'Keep
quiet!' "

Blanche and the other hysterical women truly suffered from a
psychocultural disturbance. The emotional pain of the Victorian
hysteric revealed itself in the amazing symptom picture described
by Charcot. This grand hysteria is with us no more, precisely
because the psychosocial context—that is, the lot of Victorian
women—has vanished. Told by domineering men to be quiet and
bear their pain, women had no option but to faint and throw
their fits. If Charcot inadvertently recapitulated much of the male-
female Victorian tension in his observations and experiments, it is

not surprising. If his close studies of Blanche, Geneviève, and Louise only exacerbated their conditions, we cannot find fault with him. The Caesar of the Salpêtrière, the Napoleon of the Neuroses, the Master was himself a man blind to the prejudice of his times.

SEVEN

A Proliferation of Perversion, an Epidemic of Murder

IN 1861 the actress Sarah Bernhardt was in Moscow playing the part of the tubercular Marguerite Gautier in Alexandre Dumas's *La Dame aux Camélias*. A Russian doctor who attended the play one night reported that in the fifth act, at the most dramatic moment, Bernhardt began to cough. The audience sat with their eyes glued to the stage, their breathing halted. Then, in a flash, an epidemic of coughing swept across the Moscow opera. For several minutes all of Moscow polite society was reduced to coughing like tuberculars, unable to attend to the words of the actress.

The Russian doctor later told this anecdote to a French doctor, who recounted the story in a French literary magazine, the *Revue des Deux Mondes*, in 1873. That moment when the great actress had induced an epidemic of coughing intrigued many doctors in the late nineteenth century, and the story was repeated in other periodicals and in some medical works. It seemed a compelling and convincing example of how one human could induce involuntary behavior in another.

Hippolyte Bernheim had stressed that a suggestible person, under hypnosis, possessed a *"peculiar attribute for transforming the idea received into an act."* Since he perceived hypnosis not only as a tool that could be used on hysterics but also as having more general application, and since he saw suggestibility as an attribute shared by "common people . . . old soldiers . . . people accustomed to passive obedience" as well as those "very intelligent people belonging to the highest grades of society," Bernheim and the Nancy school opened the way for some of the most bizarre and frightening twists and turns in the history of neurosis.

If suggestion could induce a subject to get better, that is, if the hypnotist could implant in the subject the idea that a particular pain or worry would disappear, there seemed good reason to believe that evil ideas could likewise be implanted in the mind. Bernheim even demonstrated this hypothesis. After hypnotizing certain of his subjects and suggesting that they perform evil deeds, he saw sane but suggestible men and women transformed into murderers while in a trance. One hypnotized subject

> carries out everything according to my command. I make him steal a watch out of someone's vest pocket. I make him follow me in order to sell it, and I take him to the Hospital Pharmacy, an imaginary pawn-shop. He sells it at the price offered, and follows me with the appearance of a thief. . . . I showed him an imaginary person at the door and told him that he had been insulted by him. I gave him an imaginary dagger and ordered him to kill the man. He hastened forward and ran the dagger resolutely into the door.

Bernheim hypnotized other subjects and suggested to them that an idea he would implant in their minds would have power over them even after they awoke from the trance. Then he would tell them that many weeks hence they would hallucinate in his presence that a feather was a cudgel or a piece of paper was a gun or a knife. Bernheim would tell them that on a specific day in the future they would suddenly be overcome by an urge to avenge themselves for some imaginary insult on someone Bernheim had brought along with him. This urge to murder, Bernheim suggested, would immediately become an act. Then, with a snap of his fingers, he would awaken the unsuspecting subjects. They would come out of their trances and go about their business, seemingly themselves. The idea implanted by Bernheim lay gestating, however, slowly growing. Days or even weeks later, at the appointed time, with Bernheim, the "enemy," and the "weapon" at hand, the subjects would hallucinate the weapon, remember the insult, and instantly beat, shoot, or stab to death their enemy.

Bernheim, and especially his follower Jules Liégeois, a law professor at the University of Nancy, used the data from these experiments in actual legal cases then being tried in European courts. They believed that a villain's ability to induce a suggestible person to perform an evil deed was not only an intriguing hypothesis but an actuality in late Victorian society. The two described in their medicolegal works how in one case—that of Dr. X—an evil physician had mesmerized a woman into cuckolding her husband with him. Awaking from her trance of infidelity, the poor creature had resumed her life as a sweet and obedient wife. Then later she had found herself pregnant, even though her marriage was a celibate one. As a result the poor thing went crazy and was locked up in an asylum. There she languished for months, coming to her senses only after the birth of her child, when she identified the evil Dr. X as the father. In another case—that of Eyraud and Gabrielle Bompard—a desperate wretch of a man had so fascinated his lover that he had come to rule her weak will. Acting in a kind of hypnotic trance, the poor Gabrielle had gone on a spree of crime under Eyraud's tutelage. This spree culminated in a senseless murder and a crazy coach ride through Lyons, with the corpse leaping and bounding in a box hidden in the careening vehicle.

During those years when the debate between Charcot and Bernheim over hypnosis was all the rage, many Victorian doctors saw the neurotic as capable of doing or believing practically anything, given the wrong suggestion. Also, many late Victorians saw this suggestibility, or nervous weakness, as spreading throughout society. Modern civilization, with its nerve poisons, its coffee, tea, alcohol, and tobacco, its enervating affluence and devastating poverty, was blamed for the spread of nervousness, as were those instillers of wicked ideas—novels, plays, operas, short stories, newspapers. Fictional and real-life stories could suggest to the gullible reader various strong emotions and passionate acts, which, once implanted in the mind, would be hard to resist.

This fear of civilization and its accouterments was really little more than a reworking of the Noble Savage myth, with the new notion of suggestibility added. Intelligent Victorian men and women could thereby perceive how the good if simple man could be led astray.

An excellent example of this widespread notion that suggestibility catalyzed many criminal acts appears in the medical work of a French doctor named Paul Aubry (1858–99). In his *La Contagion du Meurtre* (1894) he wrote that the human condition was on the decline, that suicide, murder, and anarchism were on the rise, precisely because a generalized weakness in many human nervous systems was leading more and more people to consider and then commit crimes. The world was witnessing a contagion of murder, declared Aubry. If one-third of women and one-fifth of men were hypnotizable and therefore prone to hysteria, as Albert Pitres, a follower of Charcot's, stated in his book on hypnosis, the population of the world was in a desperate situation. Moreover, Bernheim's idea that suggestibility was not limited to hysterics further increased the number of potential criminals roaming the streets of Europe and America.

Aubry evoked the name of "our immortal Pasteur" to argue that only two conditions were necessary for a contagion to occur. First, there must exist the "penetration of a morbid element," an evil idea. Second, there must be a prepared terrain—the suggestible, hereditarily weakened human who is prone to imitating his fellows.

Aubry plundered all of history to find examples of epidemics of murder and other mad activity—the flagellants of the Middle Ages, the witch hunts of early modern times, the Great Terror of the French Revolution when many people were senselessly beheaded. He perceived another epidemic of murder in the bloodshed of the Paris Commune of 1871. Slowly Aubry inched forward into the late Victorian period.

He mounted to a crescendo of societal frenzy in his journalistic account of the deeds of the crazy anarchists between 1874 and 1894. He recounted the gruesome assassinations following explosions, arsons, and riots in every corner of Europe. Documenting how one violent act succeeded another within days, he argued that one anarchistic deed implanted an idea in the mind of another

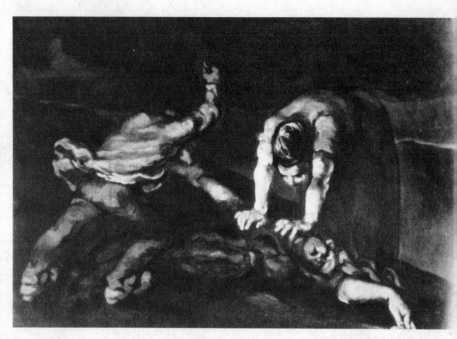

The Murder by Paul Cézanne. (The Walker Art Gallery, Liverpool)

anarchist, who was too weak-brained to stop the eruption of violence in himself. Just as the epidemic of coughing had engulfed the Moscow opera, Aubry envisioned an epidemic of violence threatening to destroy the world, with the popular press playing the role of the evil hypnotist.

Aubry's description of these anarchistic acts delineated a growing fear, reflected in the headlines of the tabloids, that afflicted the bourgeoisie and upper classes. The political plots of madmen throwing bombs into cafés, the assassination both of an American president and a Russian czar in 1881, the explosions that shook Westminster and Victoria Station in London within days of each other in 1883, represented an outbreak of criminal ideas becoming deeds in every corner of the Western world.

Aubry contended that those who are already neuropathic, or nervously weakened, could be "infected" by the already insane to commit such acts. He cited examples of gullible individuals whose nerves were shocked by the introduction of evil ideas. Culled from tabloids and cheap novels, in which desperate characters, real or fictional, were performing wretched deeds, these ideas, implanted in weak brains, lay ripening, like posthypnotic suggestions, waiting to spring forth and become deeds.

For example, a Madame Lombardi from Geneva, who killed her four children in 1885 and then attempted suicide, later wrote in her autobiography that all her troubles began the day she read an article in a Swiss tabloid about a man named Dimier who had been condemned to death for killing his wife. Shortly thereafter the troubled Madame Lombardi saw a second article, this one about a woman who had killed her children. She described the article as acting like a hypnotist, infecting her with evil ideas. Though she claimed she tried to fight off the urges, eventually they exploded, driving her to kill her offspring.

Another example was a fifteen-year-old F. Lemaître, who first stole from his boss and then, when the stolen money was gone, kidnapped a child and cut the child's throat with a knife. In a personal statement this adolescent murderer wrote, "I have read many novels and in one of them I found a description of a scene similar to the one which I committed." Lemaître also spoke of his having followed with great interest the murder trial of one Menesclou. Lemaître wrote, "Menesclou poisoned me."

Aubry cluttered the pages of his book with other examples of adolescents who read of crimes in novels and newspapers and whose imaginations were thereby fired. These adolescents suffered miserably as the foreign ideas grew in them like parasites. The weak ones struggled to be good, to cast off the suggestions introduced by the popular press—but in vain. The nervous system was too weak, the suggestion too strong. The idea became a deed.

Aubry's theory intermingled the Noble Savage myth, the Zeus myth, the Genius and Degenerate myths. The newspaper article served as the Charcotian shock, the bolt of lightning that brought the evil idea to life (the Zeus myth), while civilization was responsible for the institution of the popular press and its baneful influence over children (the Noble Savage myth). Once implanted, an evil idea, or some variant, could become hereditary (the Degenerate myth). The Genius and Degenerate myths coalesced to explain how a Robespierre or a Napoleon could be inspired by evil urges and, simply through their powerful presence, infect every degenerate nervous system in France to go on a rampage of beheading or of war, whipping the world into a frenzy. Aubry's book was a good example of quasi-scientific myth-making in which many frightening intellectual threads grew tangled.

This myth-making reached its culmination at the end of the century in the great works of the Italian doctor Cesare Lombroso and the German doctor Richard von Krafft-Ebing. In Lombroso's *Criminal Man* and *Criminal Woman and the Prostitute* and in Krafft-Ebing's *Psychopathia Sexualis*, the uncontrollable violence and sordid sexuality of nervously deranged men and women interplay with a complex society moving toward decay. While Lombroso was especially concerned with murderers and prostitutes, Krafft-Ebing chose as his subjects sexual perversion and homosexuality.

Both men were especially avid believers in the Degenerate myth and unwittingly accepted parts of other myths, notably the Noble Savage and Zeus myths. Both men displayed glaring prejudices about criminals and prostitutes, women and homosexuals, which betray them as men of the period, antiquated thinkers. Hence both men are pretty much forgotten. From the writings of these two men, especially those of Krafft-Ebing, there emerge the outlines of yet another dated myth about how a neurosis was born, which can be called the Onan myth. This quintessentially Victorian concept, which underscores the danger of masturbation, at times beclouds these doctors' theorizing. Yet Lombroso and Krafft-Ebing were able to step outside the frenzied fear of nervosity, the spread of murder, and the proliferation of sexual perversion, to undertake meticulous studies of their subject matter. Or perhaps it was more a matter of putting the energy of this frenzy to constructive use.

Before the advent of these men, official medicine and much of polite society had perceived the criminal, the sexual pervert, and the homosexual as essentially evil, not really sick—as sinners without salvation. Though Lombroso and Krafft-Ebing made major mistakes—some as a result of naïveté, others based on prejudice—in their conjectures about the causes and treatments of these behavioral "disorders," they nonetheless did highly important work in making the murderer, the prostitute, the fetishist, the flagellant, and the homosexual proper subjects for the student of neurosis. Furthermore, though their writings were cloaked in the

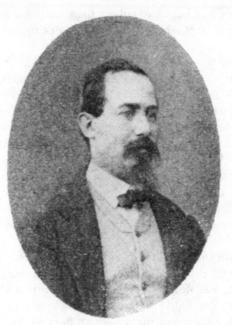

Cesare Lombroso, world expert on criminals and prostitutes. (From Gina Lombroso Ferrero, *Cesare Lombroso, Storia della Vita e della Opere*)

language of cold and impersonal neurology, their search for truth pushed them relentlessly toward an understanding of these sufferers as human beings.

Cesare Lombroso (1821–1910) was a richly eccentric personality whose foibles are buried in obscurity and untranslated Italian biographies. An Italian born in Verona, Lombroso dreamed as a youth of seeing Italy free of Austrian rule and medical science free of superstition and belief in a spirit world. Fired with a love of learning by his proud and beautiful mother, Lombroso studied medicine, especially neurology, with a passion. Still, the flame of patriotism burned bright in Lombroso in the 1860s, as Italian unification and freedom seemed to be creeping nearer, and he enlisted as an army doctor. Even as the Austrians were beating a retreat and church bells acclaimed the great day of independence, Lombroso was already putting his experience in the army to good medical use. He had begun to collect the skulls of soldiers slain in battle, and thus began his study of the workings of the human mind.

Following the rout of the Austrians, Lombroso left the army and set to work as a prison doctor. Almost in the manner of Mary Shelley's Dr. Frankenstein, who collected body parts from charnel houses to perform his experiments, Lombroso examined hundreds of bodies and brains of criminals who had been executed. Hence it happened that one cold November day in the late 1860s he was deputized to do the postmortem on Vilella, a famous Italian brigand. "This man," wrote Lombroso, "possessed such extraordinary agility that he had been known to scale steep mountain heights bearing a sheep on his shoulders." When the young criminologist opened the skull of Vilella he found something extraordinary.

Vilella's brain contained an extra piece of neurological tissue in the median cerebellum, a chunk usually found only in inferior animals. "This was not merely an idea, but a revelation," wrote Lombroso. "At the sight of that skull, I seemed to see all of a sudden lighted up as a vast plain under a flaming sky, the problem of the nature of the criminal—an atavistic being who reproduces in his sperm the ferocious instincts of primitive humanity and the inferior animals." That moment of scientific revelation, when he saw that the brain of a criminal resembled the brain of lower animals, sparked his imagination, realigned his thinking, and motivated his research from that day forward. For the next forty years Lombroso's untiring mind strove to demonstrate a link between criminals and inferior animals. Between 1870 and 1910, working alongside his two daughters and sons-in-law, who developed a profound reverence for him and interest in the subject of criminology, Lombroso applied himself vigorously to his central, riveting theory of the etiology of much criminal behavior.

Lombroso's criminal was a kind of Neanderthal man, a missing link between civilized man and the lower order of animals. In *Criminal Man* (first edition, 1874) Lombroso wrote of how, in the course of natural selection, certain monsters have always come into existence. Usually these monsters are stamped out by spontaneous abortion or infancy death. However, if the monster is physically strong, he survives, grows, and even reproduces. These monsters

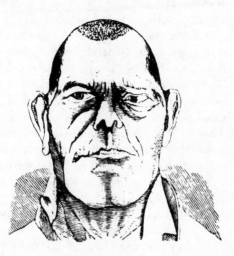

The head of a Born Criminal. (From Cesare
Lombroso, *L'Homme Criminel*)

are like cavemen in the world of high civilization. They are Born
Criminals.

Lombroso, his sons-in-law, daughters, and his growing host of
followers argued that one-third of all criminals were born to be
criminals. Their physical makeup made criminality inevitable.
Put simply, Lombroso took the Lamarckian ideas central to
Morelian degeneracy and, weaving in a little Darwinian natural
selection, conjured up his own version of the Degenerate myth.

Lombroso carried out precise physical examinations to find signs
of degeneration—or, as he called them, signs of atavism—in these
Born Criminals. His precise technique, beginning with examinations of the head and face of Born Criminals, revealed that many
had enormous jaws. Lombroso felt that these jaws were a throw-
back to a period when savage cannibalism was practiced. Criminals, he found, have better than average eyesight, supposedly a
result of the predatory nature of the savage life of their ancestors.
The ears of 28 percent of his criminals stood out from their heads,
he found, "as in chimpanzees." The nose "is frequently twisted,
upturned, or of a flattened Negroid character in thieves; in

murderers it is often aquiline like the beak of a bird of prey. Not infrequently we meet with the trilobate nose, its tip rising like an isolated peak from the swollen nostrils, a form found among the Akkas, a tribe of pygmies of Central Africa." The lips of rapists and murderers he found to be "fleshy, swollen and protruding as in Negroes." The teeth were usually huge, irregular, and far apart, as in gorillas and orangutans. The examination of the thorax of criminals revealed an increase or decrease in the number of ribs, "an atavistic character common to animals and lower or prehistoric human races." He found the upper limbs of criminals generally longer, "an ape-like character." The palms were prone to have simian creases, the toes farther apart, as in apes that use the toes for climbing trees, and "the foot is often flat, as in Negroes." In short, Lombroso posited that the entire body of the Born Criminal showed multiple signs of degeneration.

However steeped in Victorian racism his theory obviously is, Lombroso was unaware of his prejudices and carried his studies even further. A close examination of the brains of criminals, the starting point in the autopsy of Vilella, proved crucial. Autopsies of many executed criminals showed multiple anatomical anomalies similar to those Lombroso had found in Vilella: peculiar cerebral convolutions and multiple pathological findings, such as adhesions, scarring, atrophy, and softening. Beyond this gross examination Lombroso also studied the brains of criminals microscopically. To his great delight he found that in Born Criminals "there is a prevalence of large, pyramidal and polymorphous cells, whereas in normal individuals, small, triangular, and star-shaped cells predominate." Furthermore, in criminals, "the number of nervous cells is noticeably below the average."

Lombroso thought he had found the cause of the outbursts of madness that lead to vicious acts: the brain of the Born Criminal is at fault. His neurons are to blame. These microscopic anomalies explained for Lombroso the lack of moral sense, the lack of remorse, the cynicism, the impulsiveness, treachery, cruelty, and vanity that he saw as characteristic of the criminal. He quoted one criminal as proof of this impulsivity: "To give up stealing would be ceasing to exist. Stealing is a passion that burns like love and when I feel the blood seething in my brain and fingers, I think I should be capable of robbing myself, if that were possible." Inherent cruelty he illustrated with a quote from a murderer turned executioner who said, "My chief pleasure is beheading. When I was young stabbing was my sole pastime."

Lombroso's hypothesis is simply that all of these immoral tendencies are inherent in the Born Criminal because his nervous system and his body are constructed more like those of a savage than a civilized man. This explains the criminal's love of tattoos, a custom that has "fallen into disuse among the higher classes and only exists among sailors, soldiers, peasants and workmen." Likewise, Lombroso posited that criminal slang and graffiti were simply the products of an apelike nervous system.

A typical Born Criminal cited by Lombroso was Rizz, who as an infant bit his mother's breast viciously. As a child he imbedded needles into his siblings' pillows so that when they lay down, they were stabbed. His later crime of murdering his fiancée seemed like a predetermined outcome. Another criminal, Rav, attempted to strangle his brothers and sisters in their cribs, and his later self-inflicted scars were equally inevitable.

Though some of his ideas about the criminal as caveman seem absurd today, Lombroso went even further, offering a similar argument about women and prostitutes. In his and Ferrero's *Criminal Woman and the Prostitute* he pictured woman as inferior to man in all of her organs, including her brain, and inferior sexually, having a weaker sexual appetite. Arguing against the Angelic Invalid myth, which saw woman as more sensitive than man, Lombroso believed that man is more heroic, and therefore more sensitive, than woman. "Heroic resignation requires a great force of the will," he believed, "and certainly this quality is not found commonly among women. Habitual resignation leads one to suspect an obtuseness in sensitivity, or . . . relative insensitivity which permits women to tolerate pain more readily." He also believed that "women feel less because they think less." He argued that female prostitution came into existence to fulfill man's greater sexual desires. To Lombroso, women's love for men is based not on a sexual drive but on devotion, which "develops between an inferior being [like the dog] and a superior being [like the master]."

It was precisely this kind of inferiority that Lombroso saw as making women more suggestible. He extended this idea of suggestibility in the direction of religion. "Religious faith," he wrote, "is nothing other than suggestion. No one has seen God, the Saints, or their miracles . . . rather the weakness [of women] predisposes much to the suggestion of the strength [of a male God]." Male priests, he argued, come to dominate religiously inclined women. Furthermore, priests themselves are usually effeminate men, whose dress is quite similar to women's clothing. Likewise, women are greater liars, he argued. Truth is a more manly act, as the words "testimony" and "testicle" came from the same Latin root, *testis*.

As preposterous as Lombroso's ideas may seem, they were always

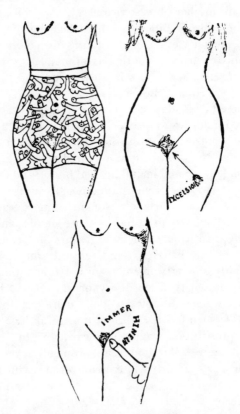

Tattoos on the bodies of Born Prostitutes.
(From Lombroso, *L'Uomo Delinquente*)

founded on exhaustive studies of real criminals and prostitutes. For instance, after scores of examinations he noted a diminished response to smelling salts among many female criminals and prostitutes, compared to noncriminals. He then noted an even greater decrease in response to pain. This decreased response was even more marked, he noted, in the clitoris of prostitutes. From these data Lombroso reached the conclusion that these Born Prostitutes were "true sisters of marble," an age-old saying that Lombroso thought he had now scientifically proved. Lombroso's Born Criminal and Born Prostitute were human beings who, from the time of their birth, could not stop their urges to commit immoral acts because their brains were firing in a faulty pattern. They were savages whose souls were not civilized and who could never be expected to change. They were epileptics of a sort, whose seizures led, without free choice, to crime.

Lombroso admitted, however, that these "born savages" committed only about one-third of the criminal acts in civilized society and composed only about one-third to one-half the prostitutes. Hence he perceived a larger, more amorphous group—more interesting to the student of neurosis—composed of those he called the Criminal by Occasion and the Prostitute by Occasion. They "suffer from a milder form of the disease, so that, without some adequate cause, criminality is not manifested . . . a healthy environment, careful training, habits of industry, the inculcation of moral and humane sentiments may prevent these individuals from yielding to dishonest impulses, provided always that no special temptation to sin comes in their path."

These nervous sufferers are not born to criminality or sexual evil. Rather they are prone to the ways of Sodom and Gomorrah if they come under the influence of a Born Criminal or Born Prostitute. Once again the concepts of contagion and suggestibility as outlined by Bernheim and Aubry loom as important. Lombroso elaborated several cases of such suggestible people.

One was Charlotta, "hysterical and disequilibriated, but with an extraordinary culture." At the time of the death of her father, a colonel, Charlotta was entrusted to the care of X, a princess, aged fifty, who was "already lascivious with men." In a brief period Charlotta had become the inseparable friend and factotum of the evil princess. The two even slept together. Whenever the young

Charlotta tried to rebel, the evil princess would whip and slap her into servility. On one occasion Charlotta actually strangled a dog that tried to bite the princess' daughter. On another occasion she placed her mouth over that of the daughter and sucked out a diphtheric membrane from the choking girl's throat.

Somehow Charlotta wrenched herself away from the princess. The evil X then attempted to murder the girl. In the ensuing trial for attempted murder and sexual corruption, the lurid letters of the princess were entered as evidence. They revealed a twisted mixture of sexual attachment and disdain, which characterized the evil princess' hold on the hysterically susceptible young Charlotta.

In those letters the princess compared her relationship with Charlotta to that of another notorious late nineteenth century couple whose amorous adventures ended in murder: Eyraud and Gabrielle Bompard, in whom, as we have seen, Bernheim was interested. Whereas Bernheim believed that Eyraud was a kind of evil hypnotist who had led the weak-brained Gabrielle into sin, the more misogynistic Lombroso perceived Gabrielle as one of those *belles dames sans merci* of the nineteenth century who twisted the sensibility of the violently enamored male. Eyraud showed some minor signs of degeneracy, such as long arms and a small head. But Lombroso saw him as a Criminal by Occasion, a man susceptible to crime who needed Gabrielle, a lascivious Born Prostitute, to tempt him to sin. As the princess did with Charlotta, Gabrielle implanted an evil thought in Eyraud. The two lovers then concocted a scheme to murder a rich man named Gouffre. Packing the corpse of the dead man in a trunk and placing the trunk in a carriage, "after driving about the streets of Lyon with Gabrielle like a madman, Eyraud left the body of his victim in a spot near which people were constantly passing," and so was arrested and convicted.

Both cases, those of Charlotta and the princess, Eyraud and Gabrielle, represent a typical late Victorian mix of sex and murder, lust and hatred. If it were not for the evil suggester, responsible for the slow but steady corruption of innocence, the suggestible one might grow healthy. But once the degradation begins, there is little opportunity for moral, or neurologic, salvation.

Though one psychiatrist in England wrote, "Of one hundred

young girls, born honest, at least ninety-nine in the struggle against evil, would prefer to die of starvation than live as prostitutes," Lombroso disagreed. He believed that the widespread nature of so many neurotic illnesses such as hysteria and epilepsy, and of bad habits such as smoking and drinking, implied that many nervous systems needed only an evil idea to come along and be implanted. Since one-third of women and one-fifth of men were hypnotizable, according to Pitres, since so many were suggestible, according to Bernheim, since alcoholism was on the rise throughout Europe and America, and newspapers and novels only increased the susceptibility of hereditarily weakened men and women by suggesting ways they could act viciously, a proliferation of sexual corruption and an epidemic of murder seemed inevitable to many medical men.

Lombroso always anchored his wild theories in sober observations made by Darwin and his followers. "The dog," believed Lombroso, "left to run wild in the forest will in a few generations revert to the type of his original wolf-like progenitor, and the cultivated garden rose when neglected shows a tendency to reassume the form of the original dogrose." Beginning with these observations in nature, Lombroso proceeded to describe experiments in which ants, dogs, and pigeons became irritable and savage when subjected to heat, injuries, alcohol, or chloroform.

> This tendency to alter under special conditions is common to human beings, in whom hunger, syphilis, trauma, and still more frequently, morbid conditions inherited from insane, criminal or diseased progenitors, or the abuse of nervous poisons, such as alcohol, tobacco, or morphine, cause certain alterations of which criminality—that is, a return to the characteristics peculiar to primitive savages —is in reality the least serious, because it represents a less advanced stage than other forms of cerebral alterations.

Citing rickets, cretinism, monstrosity, and hairiness as other forms of degeneracy, Lombroso restated in Darwinian terms the arguments of B. A. Morel's *Degeneration*, in which nervous degeneration—going through the stages of hysteria, epilepsy, criminality, sexual perversion, and imbecility—always ends in extinction.

Lombroso's work provided an extremely biased but very typical late-nineteenth-century view of criminals and prostitutes as products of a counterevolutionary process. Once again, cities and modernity were to blame for bombarding the nervous system with too many temptations, too many toxins. Lombroso's argument about transmission of degeneracy, especially regarding the Occasional Criminal, could not really be equated with Darwinian natural selection. Lombroso really was arguing along Lamarckian lines. If the nervous sufferer could resist, he could grow healthy, morally and neurologically. But were he to succumb, his children would become criminals and bordello queens. His grandchildren would be born maniacs and axe murderers. His great-grandchildren would turn to incest, alcohol, opium. Their brains were forever tainted, until the last generation died out in an asylum or a prison cell.

Lombroso may have been one of the most unoriginal writers in psychiatry, borrowing his theoretical concepts from Morel and Moreau, but he was much respected in his time. Though many critics argued that his scientific style was overly anecdotal, too befuddled in ill-defined terminology, and ultimately not grounded in good statistical analysis, and some critics even questioned the notion of the Born Criminal, Lombroso continued to heap up scientific material that appeared to prove clearly and irrevocably the validity of the Degenerate myth of neurosis. His data seemed to make the myth a well documented reality.

From 1870 to 1900 other doctors throughout Europe undertook similar studies, spurred on by Lombroso. Many quoted him and emulated his approach. Others disagreed with various aspects of his theories, especially his emphasis on heredity and nervous inevitability. Some placed greater emphasis on the environment. Frequently, however, they continued to rely heavily on the Degenerate myth or some variation of the Noble Savage or Zeus Myth.

One doctor who followed along lines laid out by Lombroso was Richard von Krafft-Ebing (1840–1902), whose thinking on the subjects of sexual perversion and homosexuality had at least as profound an influence as Lombroso's thought on criminality.

Krafft-Ebing was born in southern Germany in 1840. Educated at Heidelberg University, he chose psychiatry as his lifework, employing it to shed light on jurisprudence, an interest sparked by a relative named Mittermaier, who was an aging law professor there. In 1863 Krafft-Ebing left this medieval university with its steep roofs and crenellated turrets overlooking the Rhine and traveled to Berlin to study psychiatry. At the outbreak of the Franco-Prussian War, he enlisted on the Prussian side as a surgeon. Shortly after Wilhelm of Prussia was proclaimed Emperor of the Germans in the dazzling Hall of Mirrors in Versailles, Krafft-Ebing accepted a less august post at the University of Strasbourg, the alma mater of Liébeault, which was now in German hands. He quickly immersed his fertile intellect in the study of forensic psychiatry even as he continued his academic wanderings around the German-speaking world.

Krafft-Ebing also developed another great interest in life, namely music. While working first at Ilenau and later Graz, two mental sanatoriums in the Alps, he would play the piano for his patients. Partial to Beethoven and Schubert, he noticed that playing their melodies eased his patients' pain. This therapeutic activity, so similar to the kind of medicine practiced in Thomas Mann's *The Magic Mountain*, also calls to mind the romantic and organistic connection of body and soul made by Krafft-Ebing's intellectual forebears Mesmer and Johannes Müller. Yet the doctor avoided the lure of romantic medicine and gave himself so utterly to his more frankly scientific lifework that in later years his piano collected dust while he probed furiously the great questions of his first two loves, psychiatry and the law.

Krafft-Ebing wrote important textbooks on psychiatry and forensic psychiatry, as well as prominent monographs on hypnosis and nervous exhaustion, all of which played a role in his rapid rise to international fame in medicine and his appointment as Professor of Psychiatry and Nervous Diseases at the University of Vienna in 1888. The German neuropsychiatrist also wrote the first great Western work on sexual perversion and homosexuality. His music therapy never ripened as a method of treatment, but his compassion did. Endowed with a "sympathetic nature, penetrating eyes, and a persuasive voice," to quote his colleague Professor Wagner von Jauregg, he learned how to find the proper words of sympathy and comfort for everyone he knew privately or treated professionally. He turned his compassion in the direction of so-called

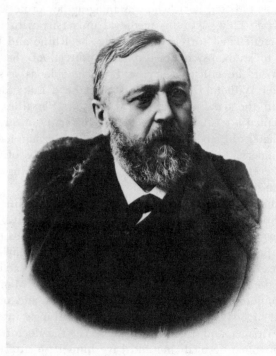

Richard von Krafft-Ebing, author of *Psychopathia Sexualis*, world expert on sexual perversions and homosexuality. (From Anton Mansch, *Medical World Gallery of Contempories in the Field of Medical Science*)

"perverts" and homosexuals, or, as the Victorians called them, "inverts." He collected his data into the book called *Psychopathia Sexualis*.

Psychopathia first appeared as a slender work of fewer than one hundred and fifty pages in 1882 and, going through twelve editions, gradually developed into a stout tome of more than six hundred pages by 1902. Though he meant the work for the medical world and even wrote the more lascivious sections of the case descriptions in Latin, the book fell into the hands of many secret sexual "perverts" and "inverts," many of whom were prominent European doctors, lawyers, and government officials. So the book came to have a much wider audience. Unhappy readers, the "perverts" and "inverts" who wanted to be rid of their problems, wrote to him, telling their stories and asking for advice and help. And so the book expanded, with new biographical material added from one edition to the next.

What precisely were "perverts" and "inverts" to Krafft-Ebing and his Victorian audience? "Inverts" were all homosexuals, the now dated term implying that the individual's sexual feelings were turned inward on himself or toward his own sex. "Perverts" included any persons whose sexual nature was twisted, from Jack the Ripper, a "lust murderer," to a dissatisfied married woman who had affairs, that is, a "nymphomaniac" to Krafft-Ebing and the Victorians.

It seems curious that the Victorians did not generally regard beating servants or children as perverse but did see sexual promiscuity as pathology. This momentary bewilderment on our part can be dispelled if we remember that the Victorians tended to argue along lines that accepted racism, sexism, and class inequality as part of the natural order. Still, Krafft-Ebing, for all his blind spots, forged ahead in his monumental study.

Probably one of the most memorable contributions to the field of psychiatry, as well as to human knowledge generally, that Krafft-Ebing made in *Psychopathia* was to coin and popularize the terms "sadism" and "masochism." Although we moderns may perceive these words as part of our everyday vocabulary, seeing little moments of sick sadism or masochism in many male-female or child-parent interactions, to the Victorian much of what we would today perceive as aberrant behavior seemed part of the natural order and therefore not sick at all. The master-serf relationship still existed in eastern Europe and Russia as late as 1860. The master-servant relationship thrived throughout the Victorian period in Europe and America. Similarly, man-woman and adult-child relationships often indicated mastery and submission, which were considered good and natural. Krafft-Ebing's original formulation of these terms did not encompass the more subtle forms of mental domination and submission that we might refer to as sadistic or masochistic today. He meant a mingling of frankly lustful and openly violent, even murderous, feelings.

Krafft-Ebing coined the term "sadism" as an allusion to the

notorious Marquis de Sade (1740–1814), a French nobleman who had lived a sordid life before being locked away in various mental institutions and prisons, such as the Bastille and the Bicêtre. All the while he was writing novels and essays concerning sadistic topics. His novels, pornographic to the Victorian sensibility, became coveted underground commodities.

In his most famous novel, *Justine, or the Misfortunes of Virtue* (1791), the reader is introduced to two sisters, Juliette and Justine. When these daughters of a noble family are left penniless orphans, Juliette gives herself over to vice, while Justine follows the path of virtue. Juliette sets herself up as a prostitute. She becomes the kept woman of various wealthy men and so grows rich herself. After marrying for money she poisons her husband. She increases her wealth and social position through treachery, destroying many men by her extravagance. Juliette enjoys a fun-loving life as an extraordinarily wealthy woman and comes to possess a great deal of personal freedom.

Meanwhile her sister, Justine, devotes her life to virtue and innocence. Of course her life proves a picaresque wandering from the clutches of one sexual pervert to another. Various men trap her, beat her, commit sodomy with her, involve her in quasi-religious sexual orgies. One man takes pleasure in bleeding young women to death in the midst of his orgies. Another performs beheadings, and still another stranglings, as ultimate titillations. Her last abusers are two judges who perform extensive and debauched acts with her and with each other. They then send her off to die on the scaffold.

On the way to her death Justine meets Juliette. The long-separated sisters recognize each other and fall into each other's arms. By applying her own powers, political and financial, Juliette frees Justine and saves her from death. Sadly enough, poor Justine, on the verge of happiness, is struck dead by a bolt of lightning.

The term "masochism" came from the near contemporary of Krafft-Ebing's, Leopold von Sacher-Masoch (1830–95), a Professor of History at the University of Prague who wrote novels in his spare time. Sacher-Masoch was married to a woman whom he persuaded to take the name of Wanda, the protagonist of his most famous novel, *Venus in Furs* (1870). In real life he and his wife involved themselves in play masochism lifted from the pages of his novels.

Venus in Furs centers on the character of a young masochist, Severin. Poor Severin has wild and enduring fantasies about being a servant to a beautiful mistress. Upon meeting a pretty young widow, Wanda, he sets out to convince her to become his Venus in Furs, his harsh and punishing mistress who will deride him, tantalize him, whip him, and even make passionate love with another man to humiliate him.

At first Wanda finds Severin's fantasies disgusting. She simply wants to marry him and be his loving wife. By degrees, however, Wanda begins to give in. She is induced to deride him with rough language and then to whip him. Soon she finds that such desires to punish are natural to her. She accepts him as her servant. The two, cruel mistress and lowly servant, set off for Italy, where Wanda takes great pleasure in humiliating and whipping poor Severin. The pretend servant is so much in love with Wanda that, though he begins to find her cruelty painful, he sees no alternative to submission.

Ultimately Wanda meets a dashing young Greek nobleman with whom she falls desperately in love. Severin witnesses the courting, and then, tied down by Wanda one last time, he is nearly flayed to death by the gloriously handsome Greek as Wanda watches with glee. The loving pair then departs, leaving Severin wretched, despairing, crushed, but somehow aching for more.

In *Psychopathia Sexualis* Krafft-Ebing simply spun out the threads of sadism and masochism as laid out in Sade and Sacher-Masoch. He cited numerous cases in which grotesque and awful adventures, in the manner of *Justine* and *Venus in Furs*, were played out time and again by real men and women of the Victorian period.

In the first chapter of *Psychopathia*, which is entitled "The Psychology of the Sexual Life," Krafft-Ebing revealed the moral biases that guide his thinking throughout the book. History, he believed, shows that man has been evolving upward, socially and morally, and that nineteenth-century European society was at the height of this evolution. In primitive societies women were mere objects of sexual satisfaction. Mohammedanism elevated women somewhat from the level of slave and sexual object. But only

Christianity elevated the moral instinct by "raising women to social equality with men and elevating the bond of love between men and women to a religio moral institution." Moral evolution, for Krafft-Ebing, had to occur in the direction of emancipation from sensuality. Through marriage, men and women share "in that pure love from which springs the noblest joys of human life." It seems difficult to find any room in *Psychopathia* for healthy sexuality between men and women.

In typical Victorian fashion, Krafft-Ebing shifted from declaiming about moral progress to expostulating on moral decadence. Arguing that nervousness is the vehicle of decay, he spoke of decadence occurring contemporaneously with "effeminacy, sensuality and luxury" in the life of any race. Citing Babylon, Nineveh, Rome, and the France of Louis XIV and XV, he envisioned "large cities as the breeding places of nervousness and degenerate sensuality."

The subject matter of the bulk of *Psychopathia* is sexual aberration, as the Victorians defined the term. The cases cited include lust murders, rapes, fetishism, sadomasochism and necrophilia. Imperceptibly, however, almost insidiously, Krafft-Ebing crept into the description of homosexuality. His depiction of lust murderers, many of whom are degenerates in the Lombrosian sense, appeared alongside cases of homosexuals, many of whom are doctors, judges, and government officials without any external signs of degeneracy. This intermingling of the lust murderer and the homosexual reveals Krafft-Ebing's world view, namely, that one "perversion" is simply a more degenerated variation of the other.

Arguing that the physiology of the nervous system is at work in the pathology of sexual perversion, he developed a schema of the sexual neuroses. He used neurological jargon to differentiate one group of sexual perversions from the next. His schema included "paradoxia," or sexual excitement in childhood or old age; "anaesthesia," or lack of interest in sex; "hyperaesthesia," or abnormally intense libido, lustfulness, and lasciviousness; and, finally, "paraesthesia," or "perversion" of the sexual instincts.

He explained all of these sexual neuroses in terms of abnormal neurological responses in nervously deranged humans. In "hyperaesthesia," for instance, a normal stimulus would set off an abnormally strong reaction. In this connection, he described the case of King Henry III of England, who at a feast of the King of Navarre accidentally dried his face with a garment moist with the perspiration of the wife of the Prince of Condé, Maria of Cleves. Henry developed an illicit passion for her, since the stimulus of smelling her sweat supposedly sped upward through his weak nerves and set off a sexual passion that knew no bounds. Likewise, in a "paraesthesia," or "perversion," such as masochism, the nerves seemed at fault. For instance, in the cases of two celebrated sixteenth-century Carmelite nuns, Maria Magdelena of Pavari and Elizabeth of Genton, who intensely enjoyed being whipped, the Viennese professor believed that the usually painful sensation of being beaten sped inward in the nerves of these nuns and then, mixing in the sexual centers of their brains, produced not pain but pleasure.

Krafft-Ebing gave the first three, less interesting, categories short shrift. The "paradoxias" included children and old men and women who went on sexual rampages. The "anaesthetics" were primarily women not interested in sex with their husbands; theirs was usually thought to be a hereditary problem, not an inter-personal one. The third group, the "hyperaesthetics" included satyrs and nymphomaniacs, men and women whose nerve strengths in the sexual centers of their brains were too intense for them to handle.

It was within the fourth category of sexual cerebral neurosis, "paraesthesia," however, that Krafft-Ebing developed his central ideas. Beginning with sadism, he alluded to the "degenerate Caesars" who "took delight in having youths and maidens slaughtered before their eyes." Then he described the history of "that modern monster, Marshalls Gilles de Rays who murdered and mutilated 800 children. He would lock the children in his castle, then murder and burn their bodies, preserving only a num-ber of heads of particularly beautiful children . . . as memorials." Krafft-Ebing referred to Lombroso for two cases in which blood-thirsty murder mixed with the sexual act. One of the killers con-fessed, "I opened her breast with a knife, cut through the fleshy part of the body . . . I was so greedy that I trembled and could have cut out a piece and eaten it"; and another admitted, "I am fond of women, but it is a sport for me to choke them after I have enjoyed them." These lust murderers were decidedly Lombrosian cavemen whose nervous systems were so awry that they were criminals without any hope of salvation.

Always, however, Krafft-Ebing mixed these horrifying stories with more harmless cases in which the supposed perversion presents a comically macabre picture to the modern sensibility. For instance: "The story of a prelate by Taxil . . . is of great interest as an example of necrophilia. From time to time he would visit houses of prostitution in Paris and order a prostitute, dressed in white like a corpse, to be laid out on a bed. At the appointed hour he would appear in the room which, in the meantime, had been elaborately prepared as a room of mourning; then he would act as if reading a mass for the soul, and finally throw himself on the girl who during the whole time was compelled to play the role of a corpse." Another case involved a respectable man who was never intensely excited sexually except when a spectator at a funeral; still another related to a sadist who would perform coitus only when imagining the bleeding finger of a servant girl from his childhood. There are numerous cases of poor souls who found sexual satisfaction only in fetishes such as "high boots and short jackets (Hungarian fashion)." In one case a man immersed himself in fantasies of "being whipped by handsome young persons aged from twenty to twenty-two, wearing tight trousers. My fantasy was filled especially with young soldiers and hussars." Krafft-Ebing heaped up cases of men who enjoyed being ridden and whipped like horses by "cruel mistresses."

And, finally, there is the story of a Parisian gentleman

[who] was accustomed to call on certain evenings at a house where a woman, the owner, acceded to his peculiar desire. He entered the salon in full dress, and she, likewise in evening toilette, had to receive him with a very haughty manner. He addressed her as "Marquise," and she had to call him "dear Count." Then he spoke of his good fortune in finding her alone, of his love for her, and of a lover's rendezvous. At this the lady had to feel insulted. The pseudo-count grew bolder and bolder, and asked the pseudo-marquise for a kiss on her shoulder. There is an angry scene; the bell is rung; a servant especially prepared for the occasion appears and throws the

count out of the house. He departs well satisfied and pays
the actors in the farce handsomely.

These tales occasionally smell of Chaucer and Boccaccio; certainly they reek of grotesque comedy. It does seem at times that Krafft-Ebing is pulling the reader's leg, though apparently this was not his intention. Indeed, Krafft-Ebing mingled these more ludicrous tales with ones of merciless pederasts and child seducers and men whose lives were ruined by their own desires to be whipped and flogged or by their addiction to *puellae publicae*—prostitutes. Such people, especially the men, were frequently the products of nervous or insane parents, Krafft-Ebing found. They sometimes showed signs of degeneracy as depicted by Lombroso, but they invariably possessed "neuropathic eyes." What Krafft-Ebing meant by this curious term is hard to say. Perhaps he meant bedroom eyes, to use a modern phrase, or simply frightened eyes. These "perverts" and "inverts" were ruining their lives because of their uncontrollable urges. Their happiness sacrificed, their marriages wrecked, they came to Krafft-Ebing seeking relief. The doctor peered at them with his own "sympathetic eyes" and listened to their desperate stories.

One sufferer loved high-buttoned and high-laced boots of all varieties and disdained nude female bodies. He found no relief anywhere except with paid women with whom he could enact his fantasies. Another loved licking the laced boots of hired women and found no satisfaction in coitus. Still another, a Russian prince, got satisfaction only by having his mistress defecate on him.

All these poor sufferers found it necessary to conceal their "paraesthesias," their perversions, from the world. Many even married and tried to play the role of the strong Victorian father. Some even begat children—new neuropaths, new perverts, Krafft-Ebing believed. Always their urges reerupted and drove them to the bordello seeking relief for their *idées fixes*.

Krafft-Ebing believed that there were two ways of becoming a homosexual or, more generally, a pervert: through heredity and through acquisition. He distinguished the congenital form from the acquired form of homosexuality by a list of criteria. First, congenital homosexuals (known not only as "inverts" but also "urnings" after the god Uranus, who loved boys) manifested their tendencies earlier in life, in childhood, while acquired homosexuality manifested itself in young adulthood. Second, the love of the congenital homosexual was an exaggerated love, strong and compelling, while the acquired case had more self-control. Third, many congenital cases showed signs of anatomical degeneration as defined by Lombroso—that is, peculiar shapes of the ears and nose, shortness of stature, overly long arms, and so on. Fourth, they frequently manifested other neuroses, such as hysteria, epilepsy, and nervous exhaustion. Fifth, the congenitals were often brilliant in art and music, or prone to madness. Finally, an examination of the congenital homosexual's family tree revealed many neurotic and psychotic individuals among his forebears.

Krafft-Ebing followed a Lamarckian line of argument in developing his notions of how an acquired case of homosexuality becomes hereditary. "The hereditary factor might be an acquired abnormal inclination for the same sex in the ancestors," he wrote, "found fixed as a congenital abnormal manifestation in the descendants." Arguing that acquired physical and mental attributes can be not simply improvements but also defects, Krafft-Ebing envisioned that "defects" such as homosexuality could be transmitted to a descendant. "Since individuals affected with contrary sexual feelings [homosexuality] not infrequently beget children . . . a transmission to descendants becomes possible."

How does one acquire homosexuality? The answer is simple: onanism. "Nothing is so prone to contaminate under certain circumstances, even to exhaust, the source of all noble and ideal sentiments, which arise of themselves from a normally developing sexual instinct, as the practice of masturbation in early years. It despoils the unfolding bud of perfume and beauty, and leaves behind only the coarse, animal desire for sexual satisfaction." Masturbation renders the youth timid and cowardly in the presence of women, surmised the doctor, and therefore prone to find satisfaction not with women but with men. He saw masturbation as literally weakening the ejaculatory centers in the brain so that normal coitus does not excite the masturbator anymore.

Krafft-Ebing then generalized to all "paraesthesias," both "perversions" and "inversions." He cited many examples of young men, prone to masturbation since adolescence, who became perverse early in life and went to bordellos to satisfy their twisted wishes or exhibited sadomasochistic tendencies with mistresses. This is the heart of the Onan myth of neurosis—that through incessant thinking about sex the neurotic makes a transition from masturbation to promiscuous activity to perverse or homosexual activity. For instance, in one autobiographical statement a male physician-patient wrote that his loss of semen literally sapped his strength, so that he failed to perform adequately with prostitutes. He grew despondent. One night an older man picked him up at an opera and his love of men was born.

Krafft-Ebing contended that the homosexual man could readily cross over into being a transvestite or even into deluding himself into believing in his own femaleness. In one case a young man wrote of his masturbation, his failures with *puellae publicae*, his eventual marriage and failure to perform "his duty" on the night of his nuptials, and his coming down with nervous exhaustion. He tried many different treatments, including baths and eventually cannabis.

> I took three or four times the usual dose of it, and I almost died of hashish poisoning. Convulsive laughter, a feeling of unearthed strength and swiftness, peculiar feelings in brain and eyes, millions of sparks streaming from the brain through the skin—all the feelings occurred . . . all at once, I saw myself a woman from my toes to my breasts . . . I closed my eyes . . . but who could describe my fright, when, on the next morning, I awoke to find myself feeling as if completely changed into a woman or, when on standing or walking, I felt a vulva and mammae!

This poor soul remained a woman in his own eyes, believing that he was cohabiting with his wife in a lesbian manner, and it all could have been avoided if he had not masturbated.

Krafft-Ebing arranged his cases in order of the severity of their "degeneration." First come the young university graduates who masturbate and so become nervously exhausted. They are seduced by males into becoming homosexual. Next come men who have propensities for "butchers, fakirs, drivers, circus riders, and boat captains." Worse still are men who loved dolls in youth, preferred playing with girls, become involved in mutual masturbation with males, and disdain sex with women. Still more degenerate are those who love to dress occasionally in clothes of the opposite sex. Finally there are the inveterate transvestites, those who can fool even their lovers. For instance, "a certain Eliza Edwards, age 24 . . . was discovered to be of the male sex. Eliza had worn female clothing from her 14th year, and also had been an actress." In another case Count Sandor V. proved to be Charlotte Countess V., who had been raised as a boy by her Hungarian nobleman father. Drawn to actresses, and eventually falling in love with a girl named Marie, the fake count wrote her torrid love letters. The transvestite deceived the poor girl into returning her love. Charlotte loved riding and swordplay, and carried on a gallant courtship. She was uncovered only when she was jailed for swindling Marie's father out of five hundred francs. Krafft-Ebing's own examination of Charlotte revealed a young creature with a remarkably narrow pelvis and vagina and masculine-shaped thighs, which peculiarities the doctor attributed to the patient's degenerate heredity.

Piling case upon case, Krafft-Ebing constructed a book that became popular among individuals such as those he wrote about, usually men who were living lives of quiet desperation, who could find no doctor, no confessor, no confidant with whom to discuss their desires or their actions. They read his book and found a glimmer of hope.

Krafft-Ebing did offer hope. The approach he used was to treat the neurotic symptoms with water cures and electricity, then to work on the fixed ideas, the compulsions, the fetishism or homosexual urges, through hypnosis and suggestion.

This sexologist recorded a group of cases in which he and a few of his colleagues treated men who were prone to masturbation and to homosexual urgings and actions but wished to be saved and be happily married. The hypnotic technique was that of Bernheim. The posthypnotic suggestions were to abstain from masturbation, to find sex with men distasteful, and to enjoy sex with women. Krafft-Ebing treated with varying success miserable men searching for marital satisfaction. Some simply gave up onanism and love for men but "had to discontinue treatment owing to business" before turning to women. This flimsy excuse Krafft-Ebing seemed to accept, never perceiving it as a flight from treatment. But one patient who had loved muscular men of the lower classes, was cured after forty-five sessions of hypnosis, and returned "after 6 months as a happy bridegroom." Another, who loved finely formed cab drivers, also married and related that he had even performed the "duty" on the night of the nuptials.

As is clear from the fact that his first suggestion was always abstention from masturbation, Krafft-Ebing believed in the Onan myth. He envisioned the following paradigm. The Victorian adolescent was bombarded all day with corrupting mental images, stray illicit ideas, temptations to smoke, to drink, to go to prostitutes. These combined with various worries—about school examinations, an uncertain career, a declining family fortune. Betaking himself to his bedroom, the poor fellow lay down to sleep, only to be accosted by the urges, the cravings, the fantasies that had been introduced to him by his day away from home, by perusing the tabloids, or by being propositioned by prostitutes.

If the adolescent was strong and resisted his desires, he could become a man and could sire manly boys and womanly girls. Krafft-Ebing perceived his hypnotic technique as a means of rein-stilling this will power in his patients. But if the adolescent gave in and masturbated, he gave life to his urges, his cravings, his fantasies. In this way the onanist placed himself on a downhill course. Krafft-Ebing believed that the act of masturbation literally weakened certain brain centers. Hence masturbation made the adolescent more susceptible to further masturbation, further fantasies, and even made him more prone to acting on his fantasies, his urges, his illicit ideas, which, the doctor believed, invariably drifted in the direction of "perversion" and "inversion." In this way a neurosis was born.

To be sure, the Onan myth of neurosis was not really new with Krafft-Ebing at all. The masturbator had long been perceived, along with the alcoholic, the opium addict, and many others, as a degenerate. As far back as the early eighteenth century, medical writers had considered the masturbatory act harmful, causing ill-nesses as disparate as imbecility and hemorrhoids. In the nine-teenth century, doctors in Europe had come to believe that onanism caused nervous degeneracy. Krafft-Ebing simply followed in this tradition.

What is so curious is that he relied so heavily on this misguided myth yet transformed it into the paradigm outlined above, in which both psychology and compassion are crucial. Krafft-Ebing connected the idea of suggestibility with sexuality through the concept of personal struggle or conflict. To masturbate or not to masturbate? is the Hamlet-like question of the adolescent. This myth—though couched in the language of neurology—of "paraesthesia" and "ejaculatory centers in the brain" nonetheless crept one step closer—closer than the Charcotian Zeus myth, with its concentration on an idea and a fear—to placing psychology at center stage in the medical understanding of neurosis.

In a similar vein, the larger sociological vision of a proliferation of perversion and murder may have been a mirage, but the murderers, perverts, and homosexuals were real. Such doctors as Aubry, Lombroso, and Krafft-Ebing were probably just uncovering sufferers who had always been there but were being ignored by doctors. A massive underbelly of prostitution, sexual perversion, and pornography had long existed, but the Victorians had an uncanny way of officially not talking about them. Doctors, as representatives of official society and science at that time, were also men on the rise in their careers and in society. Hence they were tempted to turn a blind eye to the suffering of the social outcasts who surrounded them. This split existed throughout Europe in the Victorian period: the upper and middle classes disdainfully faced the lower servant and uncouth classes.

In uncovering this underbelly, and in perceiving that crime and sexual "sin" were abundant in their own class, the doctors might have recoiled, might have simply fallen back on disdainful speechifying or damning such unbridled sensuality. However, doctors such as Lombroso and Krafft-Ebing were too intrepid, too honest, to take this posture. What made Krafft-Ebing and even Lombroso original was their humanization of their patients—the criminals, sexual perverts, and homosexuals—in their personalized case descriptions. However naïve and riddled with sexual, racial, and class prejudices their works decidedly are, however embedded in myths their theories may be, by categorizing their suffering patients as neurotics Lombroso and Krafft-Ebing established them as humans.

Perhaps they still saw some as subhumans—the Born Criminals and Born Prostitutes of Lombroso and the lust murderers and congenital homosexuals of Krafft-Ebing. Still, there were thousands of neurotics—belonging to that larger, more amorphous, gullible, suggestible, middle class—who could, both Lombroso and Krafft-Ebing felt, be healthy if reared by good parents or if hypnotized by good doctors.

These two doctors were essentially launching a social and psychological revolution, a revolution of empathy. Though their tools of diagnosis and treatment now seem dated—Lombroso's skull collection a dusty rogues' gallery, Krafft-Ebing's *Psychopathia* an anthology of Gothic tales—these doctors nonetheless believed that the sufferers whom they studied should not be led to the scaffold and beheaded or strapped to an operating table to be castrated, as men had believed for centuries. Rather they deserved to be perceived as mentally distressed human beings in need of doctorly, and simply human, understanding.

EIGHT

Prometheus the Democrat

*I*N the same years that the two neuroses hysteria and sexual per-version seemed hot items in Europe, a third great neurosis became all the rage in America. It developed alongside yet an-other myth about how a neurosis was born, which can be called the Prometheus myth. The formulator of this new myth was George Miller Beard (1839–83) of New York, and the illness cate-gory around which his thinking crystallized was nervous exhaus-tion, or neurasthenia.

Dr. Beard defined it as an American illness, one that was pretty rare in Europe. This startling definition betrays certain character-istically American values that were shaping Beard's thinking. In order to understand neurasthenia, it is necessary to linger on some differences between America and Europe that were in the back of the doctor's mind.

Many Americans accepted the biases of Europeans regarding race, sex, and class, but in America the ideals of democracy, equal-ity, and liberty took root in a way unparalleled in Europe, success-fully combating the older points of view. Certainly democratic thinking was spreading in all of the Western world—leading, for instance, to a revolution every few decades across the Continent, the freeing of the slaves in the British Empire in the 1830s, the end of serfdom in eastern Europe in the 1860s. But in America more thoroughgoing freedom and equality were open to the multiplying citizenry because there was no old order to overthrow.

Perhaps the most prominent intellectual difference between America and Europe evolved in the thinking about heredity. In Europe, the growing middle classes, fighting to raise themselves to equality with the landed and noble classes, often purchased patents of nobility to hide their past. But in America, a man born of humble roots who rose to prominence could hold his head high precisely because he had begun with so little and achieved so much. Every free man, it seemed, might possess a great talent that only needed room to develop. Abe Lincoln, Jay Gould, U. S. Grant, John D. Rockefeller rose from humble backgrounds to command huge armies, form massive business empires, wield great political power. Every American springing from his mother's womb, however humble, seemed a kind of noble savage whose entrepreneurial or political capacities could lift him to new heights of creativity and power. In Europe the bourgeoisie was one the rise but found itself blocked by the classes above and pressured by the classes below. Invariably men on the rise in Europe felt more cramped by their heredity and the powers that be. Only in America did heredity seem infinitely malleable.

The New World also possessed a frontier. Europeans had their own frontiers of sorts, their empires. But in Africa and Asia they ran up against proud people with rich histories. To subject and rule them, the Europeans often applied their notions of race and class superiority. But in America, aside from a few red Indians, who could be massacred or banished to reservations, the landscape seemed empty and free and infinitely fecund. The civilization that the Americans set out to construct rose from the ground. The concept of degeneracy, so ubiquitous in European theorizing, had less importance. America beamed unbounded hope and spiraling optimism to the rest of the world, heady fantasies of freedom, unending social evolution, opportunity, and abundance for all—if only one was willing to forget the past, dig in, and work.

Finally, and very important to thinking about neurasthenia, America was rapidly coming to see itself as a land of inventors. Of course, England not long before had been called the workshop of the world, and new inventions, such as the railway, light bulb, and telegraph, rapidly grew popular in all of Europe. But in Europe, traditional approaches to manufacturing and long-entrenched folkways held sway more powerfully, leaving less room for a free-wheeling style of thinking and living.

These three characteristically American values—emphasizing equality and deemphasizing heredity; stressing opportunity and downplaying degeneration; trusting in individual ingenuity to invent machines that could transform the world—all helped to mold Beard's notions about neurasthenia. This ebullient doctor minimized the importance of heredity, defined the cause of neurasthenia in a positive light, namely overwork, and optimistically applied the physical force behind many of the new inventions—electricity—to the treatment of this neurosis. Neurasthenia held forth exciting new prospects and fantasies that would reshape thinking about all the neuroses.

The son of a New England fundamentalist minister, the young Beard was raised to disdain most pleasures. Confused over his upbringing and his morals, Beard set off for Yale. While an undergraduate there, he, like so many men of his generation, felt a compulsion to choose between two truths: religion, the way of the past, or science, the gospel of the future. Beard suffered severe emotional turmoil during these years, but he also developed physical symptoms, including ringing in the ears, pains in the side, acute dyspepsia, nervousness, vague fears, and lack of vitality. For a long time he accepted the strictures of his austere upbringing against alcohol and tobacco and castigated himself for his own lack of ardor in religious matters. Then, while still an undergraduate, he came across an electrical generator. Acting intuitively, he applied the leads of this generator to his own body, his sides, his stomach, wherever his symptoms appeared. He pushed the lever and gave himself a good dose of electricity. To his amazement his various symptoms soon vanished. At that time he made the great decision of his life: to become a scientist. He chose the field of medicine.

What today we might call in part Beard's identity crisis was to have far-reaching effects in the understanding of neurosis. After beginning his medical training at Yale in 1859, Beard was ripped from his studies by the American Civil War. Conscripted into Mr. Lincoln's navy as a surgeon, he did his duty for the Union with

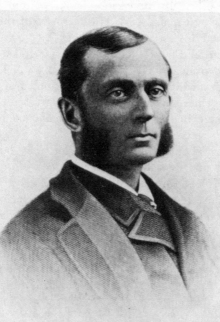

The bare-faced Dr. George Miller Beard, world expert on neurasthenia and electrotherapeutics. (From *Archives of Neurology and
Psychology*)

dispatch but without distinction. He was probably already mulling over greater matters than a mere civil war. At war's end he
moved to New York and completed his medical training at
Columbia University, and hung out his shingle in New York City.
Now in his mid-twenties, with a grave, placid face, Beard, whose
tendency to chuckle and joke never seemed to fit his face, remained a mercurial thinker whose mind was extraordinarily
active. He would polish off an article in a day or a book in months
and publish it without revision. Then he would be off in other
directions, on other intellectual ventures. Some were strictly medical, some quasi-historical, some psychiatric, and some verged on
charlatanism. He was a rare mixture of homegrown anti-intellec-
tualism on the one hand and quick-moving intellectual adven-

turism on the other. In his various books written between 1870 and 1883 he investigated the hysterical aspects of the Salem witch hunts, explained in scientific terms the feats of a well known medium onstage in New Haven, offered some folksy bits of home medicine, then presented a significant theory of electrical therapeutics. A celebrated member of the profession, Beard was friendly with William James and also went to Paris to see Charcot at the Salpêtrière, where Bourneville and Regnard's book describes him hypnotizing a hysterical woman.

Never caring about money, the doctor was, however, clever enough to stay one step ahead of the bill collectors. He used the deafness he developed in later life to foil various collection agents who caught him unawares. Pleading deafness, he would pretend not to understand their threats, until finally they went away, exasperated. In spite of his financial woes Beard remained a sunny, chuckling optimist until the day he died, and he injected this optimism into his study of neurasthenia.

Beard especially warmed to the study of electricity during his medical partnership on Madison Avenue with Alphonso Rockwell in the 1860s and 1870s. He and Rockwell had been looking high and low for new patients in the late sixties when they came across an itinerant electrotherapist named Miller, who applied electrotherapeutics fairly indiscriminately to anyone with a problem. Since Miller was retiring, the two doctors, intrigued, purchased his electrical machinery and took over his clientele. Soon Rockwell and Beard catalogued their experiences with electricity in a book entitled *A Practical Treatise on the Medical and Surgical Uses of Electricity* (1871), which a few years later would appeal greatly to the academic medical community of Germany. But before Beard was discovered by German medicine and proclaimed a genius, he and Rockwell fell out, arguing over whether to represent the author in their book as "we," Rockwell," or "Beard." When the partnership dissolved in 1874 Beard foolishly sold Rockwell the copyright of the electricity book, which eventually netted Rockwell a large sum.

At this point Beard decided to give up medicine and become a popular orator, for he had always loved an audience. Fortunately for the world, when he rented a large public hall and spoke on popular science, only a handful of people attended. Discouraged,

Beard returned to medical practice in 1879. Only then did he fasten on the important subject of neurasthenia.

In the latter days of the nineteenth century, the idea of nervousness had gained momentum in both the medical and the popular imagination. Inspired by the writings of Cheyne and Cullen, Pinel and Trotter, hordes of doctors produced complicated theories about nerves. Charcot and Krafft-Ebing in their works on hysteria and sexual perversions had relied heavily on notions of nerves unbalanced by both environment and heredity. Yet in codifying illnesses they narrowed the scope of their subject matter markedly, leaving a large, amorphous but very real cluster of nervous symptoms for someone else to organize. That man was the inimitable Dr. Beard.

In 1869 Beard categorized many neurotic symptoms as manifestations of nervous exhaustion, or neurasthenia. These symptoms included tenderness of the scalp, headaches, loss of hearing, short-sightedness, mild depression, morbid fears, phobias and obsessions of all kinds, sleeplessness, increased blushing, bad dreams, dyspepsia, excessive sweating, tremulousness, generalized weakness, cramps, heart palpitations, increased ticklishness, "flying" neuralgias, chills, cold feet, cold hands, tooth decay, excessive yawning, impotence, and vaginismus. Beard constructed long, long lists of symptoms that essentially unified a wide array of nonpsychotic symptoms in psychiatry under the classification of neurasthenia.

Of course this illness category was far too wide to hold together its contents for very long. Mixed in with this potpourri of so-called neurasthenic symptoms were those of specific illnesses with discrete causes, which now are known to have little to do with disordered nerves: many infectious illnesses, allergic disturbances, and endocrine disorders. Given Beard's era, without X-rays, without biochemical tests, without electroencephalography and cardiograms, it is not surprising that he overextended his field. Nonetheless the neurasthenia idea made a mighty step in an important direction—toward tying these symptoms as genuine illnesses with a physical substrate, a literal loss of nerve strength.

Before Beard's neurasthenia idea, many of these vague and mild symptoms warranted the name of "nerves." But doctors often had seen these nervous patients as imaginary sufferers, as lazy, as

malingerers or ne'er-do-wells. After Beard, these symptoms seemed
to be, once and for all, the stuff of real disease.

Beard was quick to admit that he himself suffered from neurasthenia. The idea that a doctor could suffer from a neurotic illness
he delineated made it less morally and socially unacceptable than
Charcot's hysteria or Krafft-Ebing's sexual perversion. Beard wrote
that about one-third of his patients were doctors and four-fifths
were of the "higher orders" of American society. So it quickly
became not only acceptable but also fashionable to suffer from
neurasthenia.

Beard's first book on this subject, *Neurasthenia*, appeared in
1880. As a result of it and its two sequels, *American Nervousness*
(1881) and *Sexual Neurasthenia* (1844), thinking about nervous
exhaustion, electricity, and evolution caught the mood of late
nineteenth century America and won wide acclaim, both among
doctors and the lay public.

In these books Beard stands forth as possibly the most entertaining, readable and down-to-earth writer and thinker on neurosis. In
American Nervousness he disparages the value of statistical analysis and argues his points through personal vignettes, decidedly a
style that would appeal to the lay reader.

Beard also possessed many typical nineteenth-century prejudices
and biases. Constantly speaking of the "higher orders" of the
"brain-workers" versus the muscle workers, he also believed in
both the greater nervous weakness and the superior beauty of
American women versus their European sisters. In *American
Nervousness* Beard tells a ridiculous anecdote about a white man
who came to the aid of a black man somewhere in the South. The
black man had been trying unsuccessfully to lift a trunk. The
white man leaped to his aid and with a quick effort lifted the
trunk and carried it up a flight of stairs. The black man is said to
have turned to the white man and exclaimed, "You can lift a
heavier trunk than I can, but I can work longer than you. I can
tire you out." Beard used the story to show that white men are
more able to channel their energy quickly in a particular direction
than black men and so are more in danger of nervous breakdown.
Beard's trilogy, in its folksy style and also in its white-male American biases, captured both the popular and the medical imagination of the period.

But, more important, it was his ideas about electricity, nervous exhaustion, and evolution that made his reputation as a medical thinker. His ability to tie these various threads together in a coherent theory convinced many doctors to diagnose neurasthenia and patients to believe they were its victims from the 1880s onward.

Beard borrowed some of his thinking about electricity directly from Thomas Alva Edison. Beard at first doubted Edison's genius. However, after the inventor delivered a paper to a New York scientific society in 1872 about a new force that he had discovered, Beard stoutly defended him as a man who had observed "new principles until now buried in the depths of human ignorance." Edison had observed some peculiar sparks escaping from an electrical generator. During his partnership with Rockwell, Beard had, in fact, conducted some experiments with Edison at Menlo Park concerning these sparks. Then in 1876, in an article entitled "The Alleged New Force," Beard stated that through his own work with electricity he had noticed those peculiar sparks escaping from an electrical generator, which suggested to him a new force. The doctor claimed boldly that these sparks, neither electricity nor magnetism, may have been the life force itself!

Beard never experimented any further with this preposterous notion. Indeed, a close friend and fellow student of neurosis, Charles Dana, made it clear that Beard hated experimentation as much as he hated statistics. Yet he never gave up the idea of identifying the new force as the life force. Though the phenomenon described by Edison and Beard later proved to be electromagnetism, Beard had already gone a long way with those ineluctable sparks. He applied them in his idea of neurasthenia to characterize victims of a diminished nervous force. Since Charcot, Vigouroux, and others were contemporaneously applying both magnets and electricity to hysterics and other neurotics, it is not hard to see the imaginative link in Beard's mind. A person with a nervous tendency is driven to think, to work, to strive for success. He presses himself and his life force to the limit, straining his circuits. Like an overloaded battery, or like Prometheus exhausted from reaching too high for the fire of the gods, the sufferer's electrical system crashes down, spewing sparks and symptoms and giving rise to neurasthenia.

Another elusive link in Beard's theory of electricity, nerves, and evolution resulted from the influence of the British evolutionist Herbert Spencer. In 1881 Spencer had traveled to America to make a speaking tour. Wined and dined all along the Eastern seaboard by the great robber barons, who seemed to see in his concept of survival of the fittest an apology for their own way of life, Spencer was in his glory. Shortly after his return to England his farewell address to his American friends, entitled "The Gospel of Recreation," appeared in *Popular Science Monthly*. Beard read the article and was struck by the similarities between his ideas and Spencer's. Wondering momentarily whether Spencer had pirated his ideas, Beard polished off his own article, entitled "A Scientific Coincidence," which showed an incredible number of similarities.

Spencer had stated that evolution produced both nervous exhaustion and its cures. The heady evolutionary spiral of modern civilization was straining many human nervous systems, especially those at the apex of progress, but the very inventions and the increasing wealth of America could offer humanity possibilities for rejuvenation. Spencer argued in favor of leisure and recreation, the momentary escape of the "brain-worker" from his thoughts, his civilization. Beard, however, stressed the use of electrical equipment to refresh the life force, to give the nerve sufferer a good shot of just what he was lacking—electricity—so he could throw himself back into the thick of things and think brilliant new thoughts, make extraordinary new inventions, and thus lift man one step higher on the evolutionary ladder.

Beard claimed that Americans, as the most progressive race on the face of the earth, were most prone to nervous irritability and therefore more susceptible to nervous exhaustion. If the English were phlegmatic, the Germans plethoric, then the Americans were nervous, because of their fast pace of life, their teeming urban environment, the inherent insecurity of their frontier lives, the harshness and changeability of the climate, in both the East and the West. Modern civilization, with its "steam power, the periodical press, the telegraph, the sciences, the mental activity of women," was the noxious agent that was very active in American society, catalyzing many, many cases of neurasthenia.

Beard described only one case of neurasthenia in any detail in his first two books on the subject. The patient was a strapping fellow, thirty-six years old, who stood five feet ten in his stocking feet and weighed a hundred and seventy pounds. His complexion was fair, his eyes blue, his hair blond. By dint of personal effort he had learned three foreign languages and rarely took vacations from his work in the mercantile trade. He came to Beard complaining of general fatigue, melancholia, constipation, and morbid fears over the catastrophes that might befall him in his professional enterprises. To cure his illness the doctor sent the man west to Yellowstone, San Francisco, and China for a long rest, which lengthened into eighteen months. The man returned to New York jolly and asymptomatic. This blond-haired, blue-eyed fellow, run down by worry and overwork and cured by leisure, is clearly the prototypical neurasthenic, Prometheus the Democrat in the flesh and nerves.

Like many earlier European thinkers, Beard believed that neurasthenia was on the rise. Exact statistics are not available, he admitted, but they are not necessary. He also claimed that the general tendency to nervousness was on the increase. But unlike many European thinkers, Beard took his argument in a positive direction. He defined this nervous tendency as belonging to persons born with a fine organization—as opposed to those with a coarse organization—frequently associated with superior intelligence, and more often appearing in men than in women. People with a nervous tendency have fine, soft hair, delicate skin, and nicely chiseled features. Their muscular systems may be large or small, but their brains are exceptionally active.

Other signs of fine organization include an increased sensitivity to alcohol and narcotics. Whereas a man of 1830 "who could not hold more than one bottle of whiskey was thought to be effeminate," according to Beard, an American circa 1880 who could not drink nearly as much alcohol was the norm. Beard cited as a proof of this hypothesis an incident about an English clergyman he had once met on an ocean liner.

> To see how an Englishman can drink is alone worthy of the ocean voyage. On the steamer with me, a prominent [English] clergyman of the established Church sat down beside me, poured out half a tumbler full of whiskey, added some water, and drank it almost at one swallow. He was an old gentleman, sturdy, vigorous, energetic, whose

health was an object of comment and envy. I said to him: "How can you stand that? In America, we of your class cannot drink that way." He replied, "I've done it all my life, and I am not aware that I ever was injured by it."

In relating the notion of evolution to nervous exhaustion Beard was turning the old Degenerate myth on its head. One can imagine a European degenerate as pictured by Morel—weighted down with his tainted nervous system, his ancestors all alcoholics, hysterics, opium addicts—on the verge of entering a mental hospital, to die as an idiot. Then, instead, at the last moment, he boards a tramp steamer and sets sail for America. Here he steps into the hubbub of the American scene. He finds the climate more variable than that of tired old Europe, hence more stimulating. He finds the rough-and-tumble scene much to his liking, more invigorating. He can think his own thoughts. He can perform any deed imaginable as long as it is within the law. He can throw himself into any enterprise. He can found a newspaper or go into politics. He can invent the light bulb and make a million dollars, become a best-selling novelist, even head west to mine gold. For Prometheus the Democrat, anything is possible in the whirligig of America. The Degenerate's feeble physique, overly defined features, and delicacy of manner, which had been vices in Morel's and Lombroso's works, became transformed in Beard's books into virtues, signs that the neurotic was a son of the noble Prometheus himself.

Beard argued that Americans are a superior race because of their delicacy. American teeth decay more easily, and therefore Americans have better dentists than those in Europe. Americans are more prone to taking drugs, and so have larger drugstores, veritable "palaces" because of necessity's dictates. Americans may speak more rapidly, but they communicate more effectively. Ultimately Americans have more—and more disastrous—nervous breakdowns than Europeans, and certainly more than blacks and savages, because they are more highly evolved. But obviously American know-how has kept apace with neurasthenia by reaching new heights in its treatment, via electricity. Beard prophesied that American alcohol and drug problems would sometime in the future become nearly unmanageable. But even in prophesying so gloomily, he betrayed a pride in the high-strung nature of the

American race, which would push forward the evolution of the human race.

Beard also borrowed bits of the Genius myth and the Angelic Invalid myth. Like George Cheyne, Beard limited neurasthenia to those of the "higher orders," the "brain-workers" who use their minds to create new ideas. But Beard's notion of the "higher orders" was more fluid. Inherent in his scheme was the American notion of the poor boy endowed with a nimble mind who set out to make his fortune and rise above his class. Furthermore, his Angelic Invalid was no angel at all but either a man of great ingenuity who worked too hard or a woman of great beauty and vivacity who socialized too much. Beard likewise depicted the Genius in an optimistic light; his brain was simply working too hard and too furiously.

Beard seemed to follow the central ideas of the three other myths about neurosis—the Noble Savage, the Zeus, and the Onan myths—but he also recast them in a more optimistic light. In *Sexual Neurasthenia* he described hundreds of cases of men suffering from nocturnal emissions and onanism whom he successfully treated. Counseling them to marry, and administering electricity and various tonics, he was able to help many of them return to an active life. In his two earlier books, *Neurasthenia* and *American Nervousness,* his basic supposition had been quite similar to that of the Noble Savage and Zeus myths, namely, that civilization and its plethora of strains and shocks were the major cause of nervous exhaustion. But Beard consistently believed that these factors could be overcome and the human race could move forward in its evolutionary spiral.

Arm in arm with this evolutionary process came the peril of nervous exhaustion, the two striding forward as the smiling and frowning twins of modern history. If American punctuality was wrecking thousands of nervous systems, it was clocks that were making America a great nation of busy and efficient entrepreneurs. While the telegraph speeded up business and so caused many nervous systems to collapse after a failed venture, it was precisely the nervous energy of the entrepreneur that was revolutionizing the American and the world economy. Even though Thomas Edison's scientific discoveries were constantly exhausting the nervous force of America and Europe, it was also true that

Edison's work would change everyone's way of life around the globe. Finally, if the newspapers headlining the great Chicago fire strained the world's nerves, these same newspapers sent glad tidings of Pasteur's conquest of rabies to every corner of the earth. The greatness of science and civilization were not to be turned back. Out of this hubbub, Beard believed, a great nation, a great civilization of noble and free human beings was forming.

Beard based his optimism about America specifically and Western civilization generally on his ability to cure the many he diagnosed as neurasthenic. He prescribed various cures, such as electricity, rest, massage, work, diet, exercise, and mild cautery, and a range of medication, such as strychnine, marijuana, and arsenic. Beard thought that cautery as well as strychnine and arsenic acted reflexively by speeding a local irritation through the nerves to stimulate the central nervous system. He also employed opium, alcohol, and caffeine for similar purposes—a surprising treatment, since most doctors perceived these substances as poisons that played a significant role in the downfall of the nervous system. However, Beard claimed that nervous irritability and weakness could be caused by too little as well as too much nerve force. Therefore certain potentially nerve-irritating drugs, such as caffeine and opium, could cure select cases of neurasthenia. He treated each case individually. In one case he might recommend rest and in another work. He might administer arsenic to calm the nerves or caffeine to agitate them. Beard sincerely believed that the underlying difficulty, regardless of the symptom picture, was a physical irritation or weakening of the nerves. Whatever the actual treatment, its purpose was to restore the nerves to a healthy balance.

Reflecting his fascination with Edison and the most advanced technology of the times, Beard imagined the nervous system as a series of cables and light bulbs. The current moved backward and forward through the cables and the bulbs blinked on and off as a human being thought, walked, slept, ate. Since human brain tissue was being strained by the stresses of civilization and evolution, this thinking and walking, sleeping and eating were becoming more stressful activities. Hence the "lights" burned too long and too brightly, and nerve force was drained off too quickly. The lights began to dim, and the electrical energy diminished. The symptoms of neurasthenia—tenderness of the scalp, headaches, loss of hearing, shortsightedness, mild depression, and so on—were the outcome.

Beard's impact on the medical world was very immediate. His cures seemed to work, though a disciple of Hippolyte Bernheim, reviewing the history of neurasthenia, might arch his eyebrows and mutter under his breath the catchall word "suggestibility" to explain much of Beard's success. Other doctors in America and even in Europe took up the electrical theories and the electrotherapeutic techniques and likewise seemed to get good results. Similarly, the general public—which may have been suggestible—grew fascinated with nerve strength, nerve weakness, and neurasthenia. Many articles, some scientific, some popular, appeared in magazines on these wonderful subjects.

Though Beard's life was cut short in 1883, throughout the eighties and nineties the interest in neurasthenia mounted in the Western world, not reaching a peak until the first two decades of our century.

During the period when Beard was electrifying his patients, 1870 to the early 1880s, another American, beginning with some similar ideas about nervousness, was developing the second great cure for neurosis. The doctor was named Silas Weir Mitchell (1829–1914) and his rest cure became as popular in the treatment of neurasthenia as Beard's electricity. A prominent physician in Philadelphia since the Civil War, Mitchell had been in charge of neurological injuries there during the war. At that time he had learned of a common nervous condition following forced marches and pitched battles. Mitchell attributed this condition to the straining of the body and mind by overactivity. He found that rest and a good diet worked wonders for the soldiers, and he filed away this discovery in his mind, to be used again years later.

After the war Mitchell began to gain acclaim through his popular novels while establishing a medical practice in affluent Philadelphia. His practice became as popular and fashionable as his literary works. His clientele consisted primarily of women who complained of feeling tired and worn down, lacking will power and purpose.

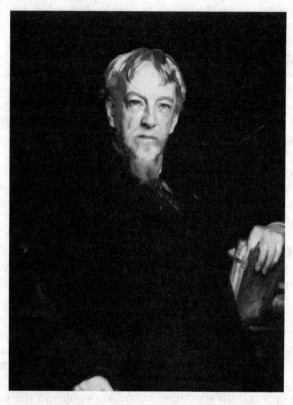

Dr. Silas Weir Mitchell, gentleman and poet, originator of the Rest Cure. John Singer Sargent portrait of S. Weir Mitchell, M.D. (Collection of the Mutual Assurance Company, Philadelphia)

Mitchell developed into the star of the prestigious Hospital for Orthopedic and Nervous Diseases in Philadelphia. He collected around him a group of young doctors and soon stood forth as a medical figure similar to Charcot. Though he never made comparable neurological discoveries, he nonetheless brought many of the new ideas about neurology to America and developed an excitement at his hospital that brought him many admirers, both doctors and patients.

Possessing a "powerful, strange head, splendid inward-looking eyes and a beard so fine that it did not hide the outline of his jaw," the Philadelphian cut a picturesque, almost majestic figure. Hobnobbing with such medical and literary notables as Oliver Wendell Holmes, Sr., Sir William Osler, and Henry James, Mitchell combined medical, social, literary, and personal distinction.

Though he had a charming, subtle bedside manner, behind which lay a shrewd intuition, he exhibited an almost ruthless male chauvinism and Victorian roguishness. One woman who pleaded paralysis was essentially inert, perhaps depressed. Mitchell took her for a ride in his carriage. Some distance from her home he drew his team to a halt and sternly bade the woman alight and walk home. This she did. Though cured, she never particularly cared for Mitchell again. With another woman who refused to get out of bed, pleading an indisposition, Mitchell used a similar method. First he tried to persuade her to walk by telling her that he intended to crawl into bed with her. She did not believe him. Even after he had undone his coat and vest she remained motionless. It was only when he started to unbutton his trousers that she leaped up angrily. In such conduct the charming Philadelphia ladies' doctor portrayed elements of both a no-nonsense Victorianism and a more modern, acute psychological insight.

Both these stories, however, make it seem that Mitchell was trying to expose his patients as malingerers. In fact, his major contribution to the subject of neurosis resulted from his accepting many of his invalid patients at their word. He believed they were truly indisposed or paralyzed, neurasthenic, or mildly hysterical. What they needed was a good rest to get over their problems, and what he did was to systematize rest as a way of getting the batteries charged, the life force flowing again. This was the famous Rest Cure, the cornerstone of Mitchell's real successes.

In a 1904 article Mitchell recounts how the cure evolved. He tells of treating an invalid woman, a Mrs. G. of B. in 1874, "a lady of ample means" who had become "exhausted by having had children in rapid succession and from having undertaken to do charitable and other work to an extent far beyond her strength." When this Angelic Invalid came to see Mitchell, she weighed under a hundred pounds and complained of headaches and nausea. She appeared pale, even anemic. She had been to numerous spas, "passed through the hands of gynecologists, worn spinal

supporters and taken every tonic known to the books." Although
many doctors had called her a hysteric, Mitchell preferred the
popular diagnosis of neurasthenia, with its exhaustion principle.
One evening, after having listened to her pitiful story during three
or four visits, he almost gave up hope. That night his experiences
with Civil War soldiers came to mind. The next day when she
visited him again he decided to suggest a regimen of rest. But the
woman dreaded simple idleness, since she had found that some
exercise was necessary for her to hold down her food. Remembering some old successes with massage, Mitchell then trained a
masseuse to rub and stimulate her muscles. This way he felt she
got both rest and passive exercise, but not too much movement
that might overtax her nerves and so undo the good of the cure.
By degrees he added treatment with electricity in the manner of
Beard and placed special emphasis on a bland but fattening diet.
"In two months," he wrote triumphantly about thirty years later,
"she gained forty pounds and was a cheerful, blooming woman fit
to do as she pleased. She remained, save for time's ravage, what I
made her."

In 1878 Mitchell published a manual called *Fat and Blood:
And How to Make Them* in which he outlined the specifics of the
Rest Cure. Under this regimen the wealthy, sensitive sufferer was
ordered to bed in a secluded spot in the country. For at least six
weeks she was sequestered from family worries and the overstimulation of city life. Only three persons could influence her: the
masseuse, the nurse, and the physician. The masseuse massaged the
patient daily, soothing overworked muscles and tired nervous
tissue and also stimulating appetite and helping the patient to
sleep better. The nurse literally spoon-fed, clothed, and tucked in
the patient, not coddling her but not castigating her either, speaking in a low soft voice, helping her with her various bodily functions. And the physician, the mastermind of this process, sat by the
patient's bedside and let the patient talk and talk. Mitchell ca-
joled his patients out of their hypochondriacal fascinations and
lightly reminded them of home and hearth. This technique he
supplemented with large quantities of cow's milk and small doses
of electricity. Other medication was prohibited by Mitchell.

The treatment manual insisted first on total bed rest, with no exercise for the first two weeks except some passive movement initiated by the masseuse. Then, as the third week turned to the fourth, the patient began to sit up; a week later she was allowed to walk a few steps around the room, and gradually to walk increasing distances. As active exercise increased, passive movement tapered, and as the milk diet diminished, solid foods became the daily fare. Much to Mitchell's pleasure, his patients were quick to get out of their beds, quick to eat, and were happy to return to their families.

Mitchell's treatment manual· went through many editions in many languages. His fame spread, not only in America but in Europe. As the title *Fat and Blood* implied, Mitchell's first version of how the cure worked emphasized insufficient fat and weak blood. Once Beard's neurasthenia idea caught on in the 1880s, Mitchell quickly salvaged the treatment but changed the theory by no longer talking of tired blood and lack of fat but rather of exhausted nerves. Mitchell, some doctors said, was a charlatan, because he popularized ideas about nerves and rest. But the public, especially women, came to him in droves, looking for and finding solace in the Rest Cure.

Mitchell's longer, more delicately written work on nervousness, *Lectures on Diseases of the Nervous System, Especially in Women* (short title, *Nervous Women*), draws extensively on his experience of many years with scores of invalided Victorian ladies. *Nervous Women* intersperses cases of neurologically crippled women with those suffering from the illness "our ancestors called . . . the vapors." His sample of patients is restricted to the "women of the upper classes," but his theory is that they all suffer from exhausted nerves caused by unhappy love affairs, loss of social position and money, and "the daily fret and worrisomeness of lives which, passing out of maidenhood, lack those distinct purposes and aims which, in the lives of men, are like the steadying influences of a flying wheel in the machine." Mitchell was taking up the Beardian idea that exhausted nerves caused these neuroses, but he specifically applied it to women. In a sense he was updating the old Angelic Invalid myth. Postulating that his nervous patients, usually genteel ladies, had overworked themselves either as mothers or as socially active women, he preached rest, relaxation, and retreat from the world of cares. In some respects, Mitchell was very sympathetic to woman's lot in life. In fact he attracted just those women in whom "change in social cirumstances, love affairs, disappointments, of what the French call *vies manqués*, combined with physical accidents to create invalidism. These invalided women unite in themselves neurasthenic states and a bewildering list of hysterical phenomena. These are 'the bed cases,' the broken down and exhausted women." Hence he attributed their symptoms entirely to exhausted nerves brought on by a woman's suffering.

In the next breath, however, he displayed an entirely different perception of these women. In fact he was disparaging. He wrote that these women were "the pests of many households, who constitute the despair of physicians, and furnish those annoying examples of despotic selfishness, which wreck the constitutions of nurses and devoted relatives, and in a conscious or half-conscious self-indulgence, destroy the comfort of everyone about them . . . there must be in every country thousands of these unhappy people. They worry doctor after doctor, go hopelessly through the various cures, and at last end in therapeutic inactivity."

A sophisticated man, Mitchell seemed capable of embracing a contradiction. On the one hand he accepted the nerve-exhaustion idea, which validated the illness as being due to a woman's lot in life. On the other hand, in his description of the patients themselves as pests, selfish, self-indulgent, he revealed a glimpse of Victorian misogyny. But Mitchell himself was unusually intrigued by and respectful of intelligent women, as his literary correspondences with a few prominent Philadelphia ladies attest, and this attitude undoubtedly extended to his patients.

In his *Nervous Women* Mitchell divided his cases into two major groups: the genuinely ill, true Angelic Invalids, who have, like tragic Victorian heroines, strained their overly refined nerves in the manner of Prometheus himself; and his version of the Victorian Degenerates or villainesses, the malingerers, who mimic disease because they are lazy, spoiled, selfish.

Mitchell's book is filled with cases of women who suffer from true exhaustion and so appear quite noble. The final blow came to one of them in the form of a telegram ("by ill luck the writing looked like that of her dead husband"). For another the shock of falling from affluence to a need to "support herself by giving lessons in music" led to the nervous illness. These women fall hopelessly ill, take to their beds, and languish. They are young, thin-blooded, pale, prone to feverishness. They wait for their hero, their doctor, their Prometheus, to appear on the scene and whisk them off to the Rest Cure. He and his wise nurses take them in tow and firmly rule them during the Cure. By "a slow, steady, hopeful training of the will power through everyday effort" he sees his patients thrive. They are clever young things who simply need a bit of stern counseling from a good solid man, a doctor, and a fine woman, a nurse, to be saved.

Along with these Angelic Invalids, however, are Mitchell's villainesses, the pests, the self-indulgent women, whom he seemed to see as morally corrupt. In *Nervous Women* he balanced the concept of immoral, "half-conscious" shamming and uncontrollable weakness of the nerves in certain women with the idea of hereditarily weakened nerves, "a morbid birth gift . . . in its worst shape it is made or acquired by misuse of alcohol or tobacco or tea or coffee." Hence Mitchell departed somewhat from the sunny optimism of Beard's neurasthenia idea. He moved from the Victorian Angelic Invalid myth, a female version of the Prometheus idea, back to the more pessimistic idea of degeneracy, of alcohol and coffee and opium, of vice and indulgence being at the heart of some cases of nervous exhaustion.

As an example of his female Degenerate type he described a woman with tremors who had been stumping all the doctors and who in fact was secretly drinking alcoholic cologne. He wrote:

> I confess that I too would have been deceived as to this case had it not been for a practice now become with me a deeply confirmed and increasingly active habit of noticing in a room not only the patient but everything else. Missing a bottle of cologne from its usual place, I was apt to make use of its contents, hence I said, "Where is your cologne?" "My maid upset it," she answered. "She had set it on the table yesterday; she is very awkward, and did the same thing last week." My eyes naturally turned to the table, which was of antique mahogany varnish. Now, I have observed that when cologne falls on varnish it per-

manently whitens it, but this table was clean of spots . . .
I was suddenly sure that she was drinking cologne, and
this proved to be the case.

Once confronted with this evidence, the woman apparently gave
up her invalidism.

In another case, that of a woman who supposedly was unable to
walk and to eat and complained of a tender spine, he examined
her soles and discovered that they were

> dotted with black marks; coupling this with the fact that
> she had complained of a wood fire as having smoked, I
> concluded that she had been afoot in the night and that
> the dark marks came from 'blacks' on the floor, the result
> of a defective fire draft. A moment later, observing some
> crumbs on a bolster, I asked her to sit up that I might
> examine her spine. As she·arose, I threw aside her pillow
> and saw under it two oranges, several slices of bread and a
> banana. To my amazement, she said coolly, "Well, I am
> caught; I thought you would do it soon or late."

She too was cured.

Even these women, these self-indulgent and malingering types,
Mitchell perceived as nervously weak, hereditarily or otherwise,
and therefore morally susceptible to the urge to deceive family
members and so rule the household tyrannically. He was nonetheless quite optimistic about his ability to cure them. Like Sherlock
Holmes, Mitchell had an uncanny way of finding out precisely
what was wrong with his patients and curing them. His patients
would then write long letters to Mitchell, confessing the factors
leading to their nervous and moral downfall. One young woman
concluded: "I carried on a sort of starvation process, physical and
mental. Why that process should have brought me into such a
condition, I must leave with someone wiser to unriddle"—namely,
Dr. Mitchell. Mitchell saw even these cases of self-indulgent,
hereditarily tainted women as unconsciously motivated. Most were
only hurting themselves; others were honest Victorian women
broken by circumstances, deserted by their men, their loved ones
dead, their households collapsed.

They were all extremely interesting to a medical man. They

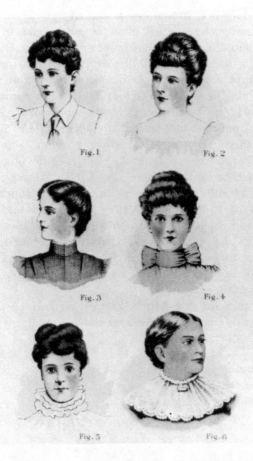

Six blushing Victorian women, the nerves to their facial blood vessels exhausted. (From T. J. McGillicuddy, *Functional Disorders of the Nervous System in Women*)

were often prone to blushing and swelling, to paleness and episodes of palpitations, to slowing down of their heart rates, to quaking and aching, lying in bed for days and years; they were victims of back pain, of anorexia, of fainting fits, and the shakes and chorea. The medical explanation for the blushing and swelling was a pat one: "every hysterical woman is liable to a certain want of tone in the surface vessels" because the nerves to the blood vessels are too weak. In one case a woman immediately entered a trance whenever she smelled musk or even spoke of this odor, her heart pounding away at an immeasurable rate. She seemed a veritable Yoga expert in her ability to send her heart rate soaring. Then it would slow down to below forty, and she would lie in a state resembling death for up to four days. Another woman, thirty-five years old, was "embittered by losses of property, by the ill treatment of her husband, who finally deserted her." She had had four pregnancies and was supposedly the victim of an incredible disorder of her nerves supplying the muscles of the blood vessels to her abdomen, being thereby weakened. Hence she was prone to developing a swollen enlargement in her belly, which reddened and grew warm to the touch. Doctors gathered around her in the genteel boardinghouse she ran in New York, amazed by the hysterical pregnancy she underwent every month. This case so intrigued medical men that a medical illustrator painted her as she lay in bed. The doctors who could cure such cases seemed heroes of great proportions to the public.

It is no surprise that Mitchell's two versions of the woman neurotic, the Victorian heroine and the self-indulgent hereditary

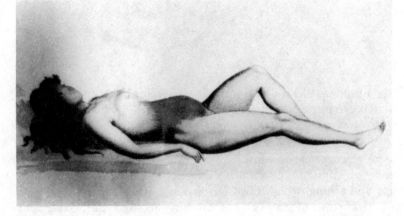

A martyred Victorian woman, a patient of Weir Mitchell's, her abdominal nerves exhausted. (From McGillicuddy, *Functional Disorders of the Nervous System in Women*)

Degenerate, should appear in the pages of his novels. Probably his best representation of the two types can be found in his *Roland Blake* (1886). In this book Mitchell sketched many factors in the causes of nervous illness and the elements of the Rest Cure.

Roland Blake is a New Hampshire Yankee who through his remarkable bravery and transcendental idealism spends his life rescuing individuals from the clutches of death. Much of his bravery occurs during the Civil War. His final act of heroism is rescuing the beautiful but sheltered heroine, Olivia Whynn, from the clutches of the evil Octopia Darnell.

Octopia is a chronic bed patient, a southern belle who has little hysterical fits of shaking and finds music and light jarring to her constitution. She is evil. She has ruined her brother Richard, the villain of the novel, by spoiling him as a child, which has made him vain and dishonest. She has already begun undermining her own health through, as Mitchell so nicely puts it, in a combination of medicine and morality, "a slow moral, molecular disintegration."

Octopia turns her evil attention to the young and orphaned Miss Olivia, "whom she could drag within the morbid circle of her own demands for sympathy." She tries to control Olivia's actions, insisting that the young heroine sit patiently with her in her sickroom for hours. Octopia knows that Olivia's father has committed suicide because of business failure, and she sets out to blackmail Olivia's grandmother into supporting her. Also, she tries moral chastisement to put the independent-minded Olivia under her power. She scolds Olivia, accusing her of being disrespectful and unfeeling. She insists that the heroine hold her hands and read endlessly from the newspapers, always editing out the bad news of Northern victories over the Southern armies. Ultimately Octopia tries to insinuate herself permanently into Olivia's life by insisting that she marry the infamous Richard, who has meanwhile become a traitor to both North and South. To Mitchell, this is the model of a household that breeds nervous illness, an evil web that spawns vanity, moral decay, and nervous decline.

By marrying Richard Darnell, the kind-hearted Olivia would be dragged into this morass, never to escape. She cannot help tormenting herself because she has been "on the verge of a denial of the god of self-sacrifice instinctively adored by good [Victorian]

women." She falls more and more into the clutches of the evil
Octopia and Richard and escapes only through an act of the will,
a flight into health. Insisting that she must go with her grandmother to the country, she slips off to Cape May and so begins a
kind of Rest Cure.

Learning of Octopia and Richard's plans, Roland Blake flies to
Cape May to save Olivia. There he and Olivia, now isolated from
the evils of the Darnells, meet, walk along the sands, exercise in
rowboats; she paints and he keeps an eye on her painting equipment. They eat well and lose themselves in nature, far away from
the New York City of the wicked Darnells. Their love ripens. In
the meantime, interestingly, Octopia, frustrated in her own evil
designs, grows self-reflective, and eventually she marries a well-
meaning man. Ultimately Olivia and Roland walk off into the
sunset arm in arm.

In *Roland Blake* Mitchell imaginatively sketched the Victorian
heroine, the good woman whose innocence is nearly wrecked, and
the evil one, Octopia, the tainted villainess whose self-indulgence
and vice are nearly responsible for her ruin. This is in many ways
an American version of the European tale about a Degenerate who
takes into his hands a young innocent, and by working on her
tendency to imitation, drags her down into the pits of immorality,
perversion, and criminality. What distinguished Mitchell's degenerate and susceptible victims from the European versions of
Lombroso and Krafft-Ebing is the degree of hope the American
doctor felt he could offer. Although Krafft-Ebing did cure a few
homosexuals and fetishists, he believed that most of his cases were
hereditary and therefore incurable. His posthypnotic suggestions
worked on only a few. Mitchell's Rest Cure, on the other hand,
seemed remarkably salutary for wide numbers of sufferers. His
Philadelphia clinic became a true Mecca for nerve patients, and
many remained healthy for years afterward.

Mitchell shared Beard's class prejudices about neurasthenia and
his optimism. Both men spoke of a hereditary component in nervousness, but Beard considered it a sign of mental superiority, the
hallmark of the evolutionary process, which occurred in "the
higher orders" and "the brain workers." In his choice of patients
Mitchell likewise implied that the problem of nerves remained to
a large extent an upper-class problem. The two Americans also

agreed that their favorite techniques, electricity and leisure, could and would work wonders on the human nervous system and so restore the nervous sufferer to strength and vigor. Once restored, Beard's blond-haired Prometheus and Mitchell's rest-cured Angelic Invalid could throw themselves wholeheartedly into the thick of life and so aid in the making of a great American nation. Prometheus the Democrat could become a great inventor, a doctor, a statesman. The American Victorian heroine, leaning on her hero Roland, could walk off into the sunset and beget healthy sons and daughters who themselves might be in danger of neurasthenia, but who also held in their bodies and minds great promise beyond belief.

NINE

Prometheus Goes to Europe

I N *American Nervousness* George Beard proclaimed that the
North American way of life was spreading abroad. Perceiving
the European style of living as slower, more traditional, he believed he saw signs that the tempo of Europe was quickening. In
one respect Beard was correct, even prophetic. Long before the proliferation of such proud American inventions as Coca-Cola and
designer jeans, the doctor envisioned a modern world uprooted
from its past, free of traditional values, galloping forward on the
backs of commercialism and materialism. In another respect, however, Beard was a bad historian—like many Americans—in not
recognizing the roots of American hurry and commercialism.
Behind his ideas about "brain-workers" as the movers of modernity
and those most likely to suffer neurasthenia there lay an uncriti-
cal, even enthusiastic acceptance of a code of action that was not
so very modern, that in part found its roots not in America at all
but in Europe, three hundred years before the birth of Beard. His
ethical standard for the "brain-workers" was basically the so-called
Protestant ethic, which encouraged the middle-class virtues of hard
work, individual responsibility, sobriety, single-minded striving
after material rewards—everything that made for a good capitalist.
In casting aside his own fundamental Protestantism and embracing science as a young man, Beard had never actually expunged

from himself the moral standards of his father. He had merely transformed his religious ethic into a secular one.

These middle-class virtues blossomed in America. Finding an empty landscape and freedom for boundless expansion, the capitalist strove to make his schemes a reality. Beard's original conception of neurasthenia and his fascination with electricity as a cure were both products of this humming atmosphere, which stretched from sea to sea.

Meanwhile, in Europe, where the Protestant virtues had been born and nurtured, the capitalistic ethic competed in a more cluttered landscape with other standards, some ancient, some quite new and intriguing. One of them, which assumed an antimaterialistic, perhaps even passive point of view, might best be called the Catholic ethic. Identified with the figure of Christ and many saints, this ethic preached love of one's fellowman, turning the other cheek, and bearing one's cross of pain while believing in a reward beyond the grave. This ethic will be examined more thoroughly later. Another code, which will be examined in this and the succeeding chapters, can be called the modern perspective. Often identified with the artist, this code stressed personal turmoil and pain, underscored the centrality of the individual imagination, and ultimately insisted on the need for personal solutions.

Needless to say, individuals accepting either the Catholic ethic or the modern perspective might cringe and grow troubled, even pessimistic, when confronted with the world of the expanding market and muscular empire building. When the doctors who had inculcated so much of the Protestant ethic studied these cringing, troubled, and pessimistic individuals, they were frequently tempted to classify them as neurasthenic and even degenerate. In labeling these anguished persons as intractable neurotics, European doctors reintroduced the notion of heredity as preeminently important in the breeding of these diseases. They also assumed a therapeutic pessimism as they gradually lost faith in the power of scientific inventions to work miraculous cures. Hence European doctors who first took note of the neurasthenia concept necessarily transformed this simple American notion into one that was more complex, troubled.

When the neurasthenia concept was exported to Europe, the sunny optimism of Beard and the genteel airiness of Mitchell took on a more somber tone. European doctors had complex reasons for adopting the neurasthenia notion. To be sure, two English physicians, Hugh Campbell and William Playfair, simply tried the techniques of Beard and Mitchell on their patients now diagnosed as neurasthenic, found them improving, publicized their results, and so turned the heads of other doctors. But, more important, other European doctors found the idea of neurasthenia useful theoretically in explaining their scientific observations. For instance, in his debate with Charcot over the railway neuroses, Oppenheim argued that hysteria and traumatic neurosis should not be equated, since many traumatized patients did not develop the hysterical symptoms outlined by Charcot. Rather, they looked more like Beard's neurasthenics. Charcot countered this criticism by widening his purview. He came to believe that all traumatized neurotics were hysterics, neurasthenics, or some combination. Krafft-Ebing, in his studies on "perverts" and "inverts," likewise relied on thinking about nervous exhaustion to explain how masturbation sapped the adolescent's nervous system, leaving him prone to homosexuality, fetishism, and other disturbances. Similarly, many doctors argued that what Bernheim diagnosed as suggestible could be equated with nerve weakness. Therefore neurasthenia quickly became the final common pathway down which a neurotic tumbled toward criminality, hysteria, homosexuality, perversion— essentially any dire neurosis. This paradigm, popular in Europe, held that anyone hereditarily weak in nerves was further weakened by the "steam-power, the periodical press, the telegraph, the sciences, mental activity of women," of which Beard had spoken, and could be transformed into any kind of neurotic, if he failed to watch his step.

To be sure, neurasthenia itself remained largely a disease of the upper classes. The Europeans also frequently accepted the evolutionary and electrical notions of neurasthenia and believed that some nervously strained men and women were salvageable through rest and electrotherapeutics. In fact the Europeans embellished these techniques and added still others, such as hypnotism and vacations to spas and the seaside. Though they developed a rich and diversified armamentarium with which to fight the enemy, what characterized the European literature on neurasthenia was a pessimism, a sense that rest and electrotherapeutics were not as helpful as Beard and Mitchell had led the world to believe. Behind the wan gentility there crouched twisted nerves.

Nearly every great neurologist in the 1890s wrote a textbook on neurasthenia. Nearly everyone applied the diagnosis to masses of patients. Charcot and his followers apparently diagnosed one-third of their patients as neurasthenics. Krafft-Ebing and his German colleagues pounced on Beard's idea and diagnosed the disease even more frequently. Although the idea of linking evolution, electricity, and nerves was somewhat simplistic, Europeans seemed to like it. French and German, British and American patients and physicians grew enthusiastic about seeing themselves as highly evolved and forever evolving. But they also believed that certain neurasthenics were cases of devolution of the nervous system. Hence doctors everywhere turned to neurasthenia to explain many symptoms that hitherto had been considered melancholic or hysteric or hypochondriacal. Now all were nervous and neurasthenic.

Neurasthenia was the illness of many Americans in the novels of Henry James; they fled to Europe for solace and a slower civilization. Neurasthenia became the malady of the great, the sensitive, the overworked, the "brain-workers"—all those at the ethereal tip of the social evolutionary ladder aching to rise one step higher. It is a wonder that all Westerners did not take to their beds and refuse to get up, blaming everything on neurasthenia.

In fact, many did, and neurasthenia spread across Europe. Physicians called it a modern illness rather than just an American one, an illness related to industrialization, urbanization, overstimulation in the evolutionary spiral, too many curious and lurid ideas, too many periodicals and novels and inventions. Some Germans liked to blame it on the French, believing that one of the underlying causative factors of German neurasthenia was the French Revolution, with its strange and illicit notions of liberty and equality.

The Europeans, however, always balanced the evolutionary theory of neurasthenia, the Prometheus myth, with the degeneracy theory, the Degenerate myth of Morel, updated by Lombroso and Krafft-Ebing. Their version of neurasthenia was much less self-congratulatory, much more anxiety-laden than the American version. They were not so sure that evolution was going in the right direction.

The literature of neurasthenia is vast, and it is impossible to do a thorough review of it all without giving the contemporary "brain-worker" a case of eye strain, headache, and perhaps generalized prostration. Beard himself would have been elated had he lived to see the publication of Franz Carl Müller's *Das Handbuch der Neurasthenie*, the ultimate German textbook on the subject, in 1893. This textbook, written jointly by a host of medical worthies, contained a review of the literature on neurasthenia, discussions of such other diseases as hysteria and syphilis with which neurasthenia could be confused, and a description of the plentiful modes of treatment. A glance at the twenty-seven-page bibliography of this work reveals an astonishing array of tracts. However, Beard would have been too busy to take time to read much of this literature.

The Europeans clothed the illness in more scientific garb than Beard had ever done. Through experiments on animals and men, many doctors seemed to believe they had proved the physiological reality of neurasthenia. They also saw it as flourishing not just among the better classes and intellectuals but also among the working classes. They blurred the identity of the illness with that of syphilis, tuberculosis, drug and alcohol addiction, and so implied that it was an insidious, terminal disorder. They multiplied their therapeutic regimens to fill hundreds of pages and still felt that neurasthenia was barely controllable. Hence the initial idea —that it was a nervous illness among the better classes, caused by overwork and usually cured by rest and electricity—became a confusing knot of malevolent symptoms that ultimately left poor Prometheus bound to his bed and nagging his relatives, who themselves must have been tempted to become neurasthenics.

Though Beard's work on electricity was imprecise and his thinking about the alleged new force was never fully developed, a Frenchman named Charles Féré, a follower of Charcot's, proved much more meticulous in measuring and describing the life force. Using four instruments to measure body changes (a dynamometer for muscle strength, a plethysmograph for lung capacity, a sphygmograph for blood pressure, and a galvanometer for changes in skin conductivity), Féré introduced certain sensory impressions (light, sound, heat, or pressure) into the sense organs of normal human subjects. He showed changes in all of his measuring machinery, and hence in the physiology of the human being. Also, he found that "intellectual work is accompanied equally by an exaggeration of the circulatory tendency [blood pressure], in the frequency and amplitude of respiration, a greater abundance of secretion, and an increase in the dynametric force." Similarly, he found that the pulse and blood pressure and the various secretions (such as saliva and sweat) were all affected by emotion.

Féré's solid-seeming work was taken up by another follower of Charcot's, a doctor named Fernand Levillain (1858–1910). This Frenchman argued in his *La Neurasthénie: Maladie de Beard* (1891) that hyperexcitation by various stimuli—sensory, emotional, or intellectual—heightens the workings of the body and is necessarily followed by a period of weakness. This physiological cycle was seen by Féré in his normal subjects, and Levillain believed it was the source of the nervous excitability, succeeded by weakness, seen in the neurasthenic. By showing how nerve weakness brought on by various stimuli could be measured through changes in breathing, sweat, pulse, and so on, Levillain felt he had demonstrated the physiological explanation of how nerve weakness occurs.

Two other medical researchers, Mosso of Italy and Anjel of Germany, devised perhaps more clever means of measuring the physiological changes that supposedly took place in the body of the neurasthenic who was using his nervous system. By means of an amusing apparatus called Mosso's ergograph, the movement of the index finger could be registered as it lifted a weight attached to it by a thread. In the case of the healthy person, if the finger was given ten seconds between each exertion, then it readily regained its force and could continue this exercise indefinitely. In the neurasthenic, the ten-second interval between exertions was not enough for the finger to regain its strength. Even the neurasthenic's index finger seemed weaker than that of the healthy person, Mosso believed. Likewise, Anjel believed he could show that the vasomotor apparatus of the neurasthenic was more excitable and more easily exhausted than that of the healthy person. Measuring the arm before and after intellectual work, either reading or calculations, he demonstrated that the volume of the neurasthenic's arm (and therefore the amount of blood circulation through it) diminished more drastically and more rapidly than that of the healthy person challenged with the same intellectual work. These experiments were described, paraphrased, and quoted in many textbooks and monographs throughout the Western medical world, thereby legitimizing the notion that the physiology of the neurasthenic was profoundly aberrant.

What doctors could not cull from their experiments, which were still relatively primitive, they simply made up. For instance, three German doctors, Krafft-Ebing, Rudolf Arndt (1835–1900) of Berlin, and Paul Julius Moebius (1835–1907) of Greifswald, posited a biological framework to the Pandora's box of nervous woes. Arndt explained neurasthenia in terms of an actual embryological defect in the brain tissue of the neurasthenic. Krafft-Ebing believed that poorly developed nerve centers and connecting links, or radiations and reflex processes, are at the etiological core of the various head, back, cardiac, and other symptoms. Moebius believed that a kind of metabolic poisoning must be taking place in the neurasthenic and that eventually a true chemical lesion would be found. All three concurred that this neurosis had underlying, yet-to-be-discovered biochemical causes, about which they were willing to hypothesize, or fantasize.

The theory of overexercise and overstimulation in the neurasthenic seemed solid to the Europeans, and they also supported the basic Beardian notion that civilization was a major factor in making neurasthenia widespread. Yet most Europeans also reiterated the importance of heredity. Many French works on neurasthenia, in fact, divided it into two major groups: true neurasthenia, or "shock" neurasthenia; and degenerate neurasthenia, or hereditary neurasthenia. Whereas the first was curable, the second, sadly, was not.

The French neuropsychiatrist Gilles de la Tourette (1857–1904) presented excellent clinical vignettes to illustrate this distinction. The true, or shock, neurasthenic type was exemplified by a forty-five-year-old businessman with no family history of nervosity. After a long period of overstraining his nerves in the competitive business world, he withdrew to the country to recharge his batteries. There, however, he devised a scheme that involved investing all of his money to make his fortune. Upon returning to his business in Paris, he increased his work load, traveled extensively to extend his power and money, and strained his nerves beyond belief. After six months he could see the success of his plans, but he suddenly developed the symptoms of neurasthenia: headaches, insomnia, nagging dyspepsia, and mood changes. His family grew concerned. The man consulted Tourette, who diagnosed true neurasthenia. The businessman left his ventures in the hands of a trusted colleague and retired to a country hydrotherapy spa far from his business. His symptoms soon disappeared. He convalesced on a pleasant sea voyage, returned to his business within six months, and took up the struggle again, though less avidly, since his fortune was made. He never overtaxed his nervous system again.

Tourette described a degenerate, or hereditarily neurasthenic, young man of twenty-six, employed in a ministry of the government. His mother was a nervous type, with symptoms similar to her son's. Possessed of a family fortune, with a long history of nervous exhaustion going back to college, this young man had interrupted his education on a number of occasions and had been diagnosed as a "cerebral anemic." He never finished his baccalaureate, and he began to suffer from severe headaches, became taciturn, and showed a lack of interest in friendships. These symptoms freed him from the obligation to serve in the armed forces. While living with his widowed mother his headaches grew worse, and he became a victim of obsessions and hypochondriacal fears.

Tourette's treatment was similar to that in the first case but was not effective. The young man would go from spa to spa across Europe, frequently trying to return to his work, but he would immediately suffer a relapse and go off to another spa. Fortunately he had money to support his neurasthenia. Tourette counseled him to live on the money from the family fortune and not work. Needless to say, he did as his doctor prescribed, and he lived unhappily ever after.

The Germans were even more pessimistic than the French. Krafft-Ebing, for instance, regarded 80 percent of all cases of neurasthenia as hereditary. Moebius was forever searching for the ancestor who implanted the neurosis in his patients. Neurasthenia became simply another of the nervous diseases a doctor could attribute to a degenerate family that, according to Morel's theory, declines and eventually becomes extinct. Arndt even called into question the central Beardian idea that work was the major cause of neurasthenia. He spoke of a true neurasthenic disposition, not like Beard's Prometheus but rather like that of Lombroso's Born Criminal. Arndt wrote, "This weakness is inborn, and insofar as it is not noticed for a while because it is so slight or it is easily overlooked, it is nurtured, and only comes forth more clearly after the working of some mischief," that is, the shock of overwork. "The essence of this illness is the impoverishment and starvation of the nervous system . . . the nervous substance is over-ripe and remains fetal or embryonic. The nerve cells are poor looking and have only short, poorly branched projections." He wrote that the embryonic brain substance of the neurasthenic accompanied a poorly developed vascular system. Hence he coined the term "neurasthenic-anemic tendency." He saw anemia as being a component of the nerve weakness, as going hand in hand with neurasthenia to cause the downfall of the entire body. He considered tuberculosis, general paralysis, tertiary syphilis, rheumatism, cancer, and gout as being the natural progression of the neurasthenic-anemic tendency. He believed that it led, through a number of generations, to madness and imbecility, as Morel had believed.

"To wish to distinguish the neurasthenic from the syphilitic and the anemic as Beard had done is meaningless," Arndt wrote. All the various causes, both general and specific, that Beard had described—overwork, emotional shock, chagrin, sadness, as well as tobacco, alcohol, and opium—Arndt saw as only accelerating an "atomic and molecular process which has already been under way." All flowed from one source, the neuropathic and neurasthenic forebears. Arndt's wretchedly pessimistic rendering of the neurasthenic idea, once so cheery and exhilarating to the sanguine Beard, now smelled of the Old World's complexity, its slow but steady demise.

When the Europeans spoke of civilization as breeding neurasthenia, they added pages and pages to Beard's list of "steam power, the periodical press, the telegraph, the sciences, the mental activity of women." For instance, Levillain spoke of intellectual strain causing neurasthenia, and indeed his tales of young scholars who broke down while cramming for their finals at the Sorbonne imply that he saw studying as dangerous. He lectured parents against telling terrifying stories to their children or instilling too much religious fear in them. He shook his head at modern music, at the dramas of Strindberg, Ibsen, et al., and despised the naturalists and realists for their shocking scenarios. Of course there were the nerve poisons—coffee, tea, tobacco, and alcohol—to be avoided. He pointed out that modern man used all these stimulants to work above his natural level of productivity. "Modern man," he wrote, "tries to hold up and to replace natural energy with artificial mead." Also, Levillain spoke of sensuality and the products of a cosmopolitan world—too much fine and exotic food, too much sex and perfume and luxury—as inciting neurasthenia. "Always and everywhere," he wrote, in "the sounds of noisy carriages rolling across the pavement, the hiss of locomotion, the cry of street vendors . . . electrical lights . . . the most refined perfumes and spices . . . liquor and tobacco . . . not to mention the lack of air . . . one obtains . . . the description of the diverse influences at work during a sojourn in the great cities on those humans predisposed to the development of neurasthenia."

Likewise, Krafft-Ebing preached against the vices of practically everything exciting. He warned strongly against stimulating children with fairy tales and ghost stories, which he thought bred excessive imagination and a risky intellectual curiosity in the young neurasthenic. The incipient neurasthenic was already all too suggestible, impressionable, and imaginative without these extra stimulants. They must be concealed from the child to steer him away from nervous destruction. He cited innumerable cases catalyzed by masturbation, coitus interruptus, too hot baths, too much mineral water, too much rest cure, and he saw women as being all too prone to neurasthenia because of childbirth, their need to mind the sick, and their menstrual periods. He claimed he had seen neurasthenia incited in men by fear of syphilis, anguish over the dangers of masturbation, unhappy marriages, and promotion in the military. Nearly everything could cause neurasthenia, and it is easy to imagine scores of Westerners frightened by their doctors, taking to their beds, even hiding under them, to avoid some noxious agent that might render them nervously exhausted.

Most European writers began to see neurasthenia as occurring as readily among the working classes as among the upper classes. The various machines near which the workingman spent his day chronically shocked his nerves and so undermined his nervous system. The roughness of the workingman's life, his cold and cramped quarters, all set off the symptoms of neurasthenia.

Most authors, however, saw women as more prone to neurasthenia than men because of the inherent fragility of a woman's nervous system. Effeminate men were also exceptionally neurasthenia-prone, as they obviously possessed the fragility of women. All the doctors preached that women should remain in the home, where they would not be incessantly pounded by the hubbub of the marketplace. All of them counseled against equal education for women, since such education could only ruin women's nerves.

Mitchell's ideas and his rest cure were popularized in England by William S. Playfair (1835–1903), a renowned physician in London. In his slender work *Nervous Prostration and Hysteria* (1883) Playfair described a series of prototypical upper-class women whose chronic invalidism was cured by Mitchell's type of treatment. In these stories we catch an amusing glimpse of Mitchell's success, even secondhand, working its wonders in Europe.

In one case, a married woman of thirty-two had had a number of children and had suffered various uterine troubles. After her husband's death, in 1876, and the development of an infection in her pelvis, she took to her bed. Despite the disappearance of her uterine symptoms, she lay paralyzed for four years. Adopting Beard's and Mitchell's ideas, Playfair believed that the etiology was simple: giving birth to too many children, pelvic infection, and the shock of her husband's death had ruined her nerves.

In October 1880 she was conveyed to London "on a couch slung from the roof of a salon carriage on a train so as to avoid any jolt or jar, since the slightest movement caused much suffering," for a consultation with Playfair. The relatives were banished, and once under his care, the patient struggled against the doctor's prescriptions. But without a hitch, the Rest Cure, with its massage, milk diet, and other ingredients, worked. In four weeks the invalid who had been paralyzed for four years walked downstairs and was soon off to Brighton for a brief convalescence.

Another great case was that of a remarkable woman Playfair

first glimpsed as he walked the esplanade at Brighton with a doctor friend. The two men came upon her "reclining at length on a long couch, and being dragged along, looking the picture of misery, emaciated to the last degree, her head thrown back almost in a state of opisthotonos [a spastic position in which the patient balanced on her head and heels], her hands and arms clenched and contracted, her eyes fixed and staring at the sky." Turning to his colleague, Playfair said archly, "I am sure that I could cure that case if I could get her into my hands." The doctors walked on.

A few years later, as luck would have it, a colleague referred this invalid of twenty years to Playfair. He applied the Rest Cure, but an intense struggle ensued, since the patient found the regimen painful. Massage sent her into convulsions. She shrieked and groaned when separated from her friends. She had multiple convulsions on the first night of her treatment. Yet the next day she was quieter. Soon she was eating, and in six weeks she was off on a trip to Capetown. On this convalescent voyage her former nurse, now her close friend, fell ill, and the lady nursed her back to health. The Rest Cure was at times incredibly successful, even in Europe.

Playfair's invalids had much in common with Mitchell's, just as Tourette's neurasthenic businessman seemed similar to Beard's blue-eyed entrepreneur. But the cases that yielded so dramatically to rest and electricity became rarer and rarer, especially when the neurasthenia idea began to include tuberculosis, alcoholism, rickets, and syphilis. One of Beard's major notions had been that somehow the nervous tendency counteracted the tendency to tuberculosis or rickets, that the diseases were mutually exclusive. The Europeans tended to disagree with him on this point. They frequently saw neurasthenic symptoms as the first sign of a long, degenerative illness, and the wan, hereditarily weakened neurasthenic as evolving into a tubercular or syphilitic whose fate was dissolution and death.

However hopeless and predetermined neurasthenia seemed, by the late 1890s the medical world had devised various techniques for battling the forces in society that irritated and dissolved the human nervous system. Many techniques were popular among the middle classes: warm milk and languorous bed rest; hydrotherapy

Three types of electrotherapeutics, tonic to the nerves: I. Faradization, or treatment with alternating current. (From George M. Beard and A. D. Rockwell, *A Practical Treatise on the Medical and Surgical Uses of Electricity*)

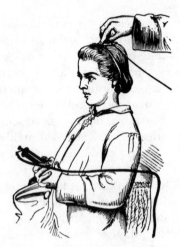

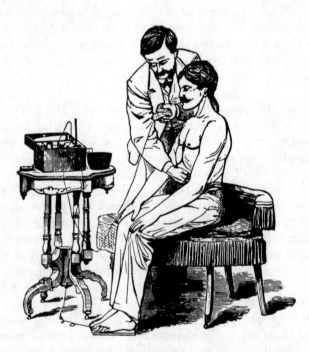

II. Galvanization, or treatment with direct current. (From Beard and Rockwell, *A Practical Treatise on the Medical and Surgical Uses of Electricity*)

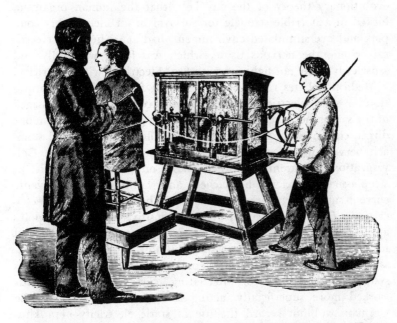

III. Franklinization, or treatment with static electricity. (From Beard and Rockwell, *A Practical Treatise on the Medical and Surgical Uses of Electricity*)

and sojourns at peaceful, pastoral spas; for German burghers, long soporific vacations in dreamy Switzerland, which the German *Handbuch* described in luscious detail; for American millionaires, sojourns in slow-paced Europe, where Henry and Alice James had gone in 1872.

But the technique most in keeping with late Victorian fascination with mechanical magic was electricity, with all its wires and sparks. Books on the role of electricity in treating neurasthenia and allied neuroses sold quickly, and the general public readily accepted this idea. Low-voltage, painless electricity caught on as a cure. Urged by their doctors, patients came to their offices, to sit transfixed in hard wooden chairs while cups were placed on their heads and chests, a lever was thrown, and electricity, that life-giving force, flowed into the nervous system. The popularized evolutionary theory of the day held that the human organism, locked in a horrible struggle for survival in an increasingly complex and overstimulated environment, had at its helm an electrical system, the nervous tissue, which was firing wastefully and senselessly. Why not fight fire with fire? Electricity with electricity?

Medical debates raged over the use of faradization, galvanization, or static electricity to treat various conditions. A "massage" of the sympathetic nervous system through galvanic, or continuous direct, current would, doctors believed, affect the heart and stomach nerves and so eradicate heart and stomach symptoms. Galvanization apparently worked best on symptoms such as sleeplessness, anxiety, headaches, and fainting. The galvanic current supposedly worked wonders for these through the electrical force fields generated between the positive and negative poles applied at various points upon the body, especially the head and neck. The force fields seemed to act almost like an internal massage, relaxing and soothing the tense nerves in the central nervous system. With faradic, or alternating, current, the force fields worked more superficially, acting like a muscle massage. The Germans did not regard the use of static electricity—Franklinization—as being as worthwhile as the two other types, but they still built and liberally used machines that produced this type of electricity. Through a series of spinning wheels, artificially generated static electricity was channeled through a tube into the air as a hail of sparks, which the doctor directed to the patient's body to diminish symptoms. The sparking tube would be applied to the head to decrease migraines, to the abdomen to break up constipation, in the vagina or into the penis to treat vaginismus or impotence. One Frenchman named Boisseau de Rocher invented an internal Franklinizer that he fished into the stomach to treat the gastrointestinal symptoms of neurasthenia. The French generally preferred the static charge, the Germans the dynamic currents. Beard employed galvanic current, Mitchell opted for galvanization as well as faradization. Electricity was applied everywhere and seemed to have good effects on many patients.

Massage was another technique for healing the neurasthenic. Writers on neurasthenia thought it worked by stimulating the nervous and muscular systems, the circulation, and the metab-

olism. Kneading the muscles was thought to soothe the neurasthenic incapable of work but also to stimulate his nerves in a
positive, more tolerable way than hard labor. Certain doctors
frowned on excessive exercise, such as long-distance running or
bicycling, because it might strain the nerves. But gentle exercise
was frequently encouraged. Through massage and techniques such
as isometrics and well planned exercise programs, the doctor could
gradually alleviate nervous exhaustion.

Doctors recommended head massage for headaches, back massage for backaches, abdominal massage for gastrointestinal complaints, chest massage for heart aches. This technique posed obvious problems, however, when doctors confronted patients with
sexual problems such as impotence. Since it was a well established
belief that many neurasthenics, especially sexual ones, were practicing onanists, the doctors got around the problem of genital
massage by utilizing the anatomical fact that the nerves of the
genitalia arose from the back. A good massage of the lower back
could be helpful to many onanists and sexual neurasthenics by
relieving impotence, priapism, anesthesia, and hyperesthesia of the
genitalia.

Dieting was another major treatment. It could be of two varieties, fattening and thinning. The Mitchell approach was seen as
fattening but soothing, as the prescription of milk and only milk
in the early stages of the rest cure cut off the sufferer from his
supply of tea, coffee, alcohol, and tobacco, all seen as stimulants.
The slimming regimens included vegetarian, low-fat, low-
carbohydrate, and low-protein diets. The common factor was ab-
stinence from stimulants, which were clearly central in the
etiology of neurasthenia.

Sea baths were luxuriantly described in the *Handbuch* and
other medical works. The doctors believed that the to-and-fro
movement of the waters against the sand and rocks was hypnotic
and healing. Appealing to the invigorating quality of the salt air
in the lungs and the sedating effect of the warm water on the skin,
they felt that a seaside sojourn both stimulated and soothed the
central nervous system. This dual influence on the nerves ener-
gized all the body organs, promoting health.

The European doctors devoted chapter upon chapter in their
books to hydrotherapy. One approach involved institutions spe-

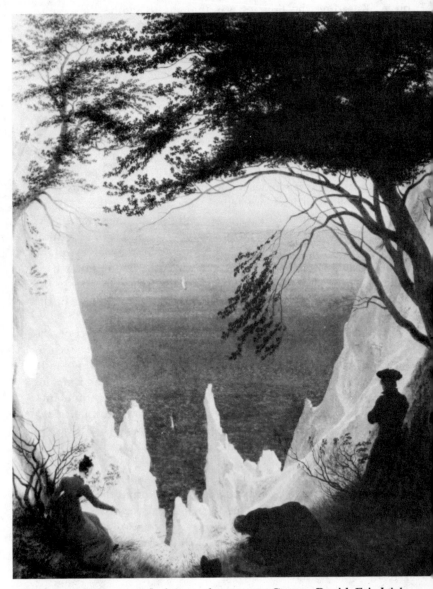

A sea sojourn: a sedative to the nerves. Caspar David Friedrich, *The Chalk Cliffs of Rügen*. (Stiftung Oskar Reinhart, Winterthur, Switzerland)

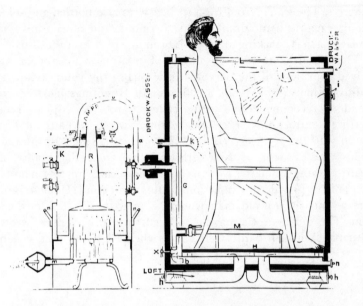

Tea and hydrotherapy. (From Harry Keen, *Triumphs of Medicine*)

cializing in warm and cold bathing, where the patient was wrapped alternately in hot and cold sheets, then sponged and showered, with different parts of the body bathed at various temperatures. A second approach was hydrotherapy in spas such as Carlsbad and Marienbad. At these various spas thermal waters bubbled forth from springs or spewed from belching geysers into the open air. The doctors surmised that the salutary effects of the spas were due partially to the patient's fascination with the sound and sight of the water issuing from some unknown yet richly mysterious part of the earth. They did not doubt, however, that the chemical components of the water—bicarbonate, sulfur, and so on—played at least as significant a role. Medical debates raged over whether the various bubbling waters at Carlsbad, Marienbad, Franzensbad, or Baden-Baden were helpful for one kind of neurasthenia or for another. Other debates concentrated on whether baths in brine water, brackish water, bog water, and other kinds of water would soothe the nerves of various neurasthenic sufferers. The waters from fresh springs were also bottled and sold. Many a neurasthenic drank Vichy, Pyrmont, and other waters as he sat in a nerve-racking metropolis brooding over his ill health.

The penultimate physical means of treating neurasthenia involved injections of the nervous tissue of healthy young animals. Julius Althaus (1833–1900), a colleague of Hughlings Jackson's in London, recommended a drug called Cerebrine Alpha. This sterilized extract was "prepared for me," wrote Althaus in *The Failure of Brain Power (Encephalasthenia)* (1898), "by Messrs. Brady and Martin of Newcastle-on-Tyne, from the brains of healthy young animals." Althaus had good results treating neurasthenia with hypodermic injections of this compound. He described one seventy-six-year-old man whom he treated with this medication. The old neurotic, having suffered since his twenties, wrote Althaus, "You will hardly believe me when I tell you that within

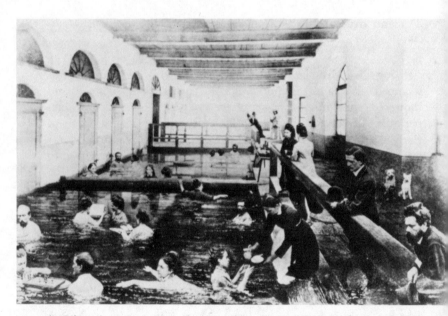

A Victorian Jacuzzi: a neuromuscular massage. (From Georg Osthoff, *Die Bäder und Bade-Anstalten der Neuzeit*)

48 hours after your operation I was quite another man and have remained so ever since." As dangerous as this treatment really was, if a doctor accepted the premise that neurasthenics were lacking in nerve strength because of civilization, it wouldn't be difficult for him to arrive at the idea that a good shot of strong nerve tissue from an uncivilized animal might turn the nervous human being around. The patient, carried away by the doctor's enthusiasm, may have gotten better by way of suggestion.

The doctors were at least dimly aware of such psychological factors. For instance, moral exhortation, a precursor to modern relaxation techniques, involved encouraging the patient to think of pleasing and restful images. In this way he could quell ruminations and recurring worries. Doctors saw the isolation technique that Mitchell introduced into Europe in 1883 as a means of isolating the nervous sufferer from psychically destructive relatives (such as Octopia Darnell). Marriage could achieve the same end by snatching the nervous individual out of a bad environment. Of course the doctors, like the bold Roland Blake, could cure patients through suggestion. They could administer a placebo tablet, or tell the patient that he would notice his headaches or dyspepsia going away, or give him a supposedly magical slip of paper that would ward off impotence or any other symptom.

The greatest weapon in psychological therapy was hypnosis. Though many thought that a neurasthenic was inherently not as hypnotizable as a hysteric or even a healthy person, and though some feared that hypnosis itself could prove to be a great shock to the nerves, Bernheim showed that of 30 cases of neurasthenia, 17 were cured, 12 improved, and only one was not significantly affected by hypnosis. According to the *Handbuch*, an Austrian psychiatrist named Baron Albert von Schrenk-Notzing hypnotized 40 people, of whom 11 were cured, 13 improved significantly, 9 were much improved, and only 9 were essentially unchanged. Bernheim, Notzing, a Dutch psychiatrist named Frederik van Eeden, and others employed a series of hypnotic sittings. In the first, patients passed into a state of light hypnosis. In the second, a deeper state of hypnosis occurred. In each ensuing session the hypnotic trance grew deeper and deeper, and the doctors made curative suggestions to the patients with progressively more conviction and force. One French doctor, Auguste Voisin, was even more

dogged in his use of hypnosis. He would make a hypnotic suggestion, then have the patient sleep for hours. Voisin thought he was
thereby letting the suggestion sink in. Doctors felt that it was
ultimately a matter of helping the patient develop new reflexes—
new, healthy, automatic ways of thinking—to overcome the older,
unhealthy reflexes.

All this theorizing and treatment was helpful for some Europeans—the true, or shock, neurasthenics. Yet much of the per-
plexity about European neurasthenics concentrated on one central
fact, namely, that the bulk of the patients got slightly better but
were never cured. These patients were usually called degenerate
neurasthenics. In fact, it is likely that the treatment regimens became so outlandishly complicated precisely because the symptoms
were so entrenched; they shifted and were alleviated but then surfaced all over again.

The doctors had done their best; they had applied the principles of the American, English, French, and German specialists.
They had wrapped their patients in hot and cold towels, prescribed a trip to the Alps or the seaside, admonished their patients
not to read novels, not to go to the theater, not to move an inch.
Yet the patients still remained ill, often refusing to follow doctor's
orders. Neurasthenia was popular among patients because of the
idea that it was hereditary, and therefore they were not to blame,
since their parents were the culprits.

The doctors frequently found themselves dealing with unhappy
people who translated their psychic woes into physical symptoms
and had little reason to get better, since as long as they were
neurasthenics, little could be expected of them. On one hand, the
doctors perceived the neurasthenic as someone who could get better if he had the will power. On the other hand, they defined
weakness of will as a symptom of the disease—so it was hard to
know where the patient would get the will power. Furthermore,
the patient seemed to use whatever strength of will he had to
defeat the doctor's efforts. The neurasthenic could see himself as
highly sensitive and temperamental, with a finely evolved mind.
Doctors could reply that this showed only a highly degenerate
state of mind. The tension between doctors and patients could
grow quite marked in recalcitrant cases of neurasthenia.

This perplexing lack of will and battle of wills are exemplified in the writing of one important doctor and his celebrated patient, who have left behind extensive documents. The doctor is Adrien Achille Proust, and the patient is his son, Marcel Proust, the famous French novelist.

Adrien Proust (1842–1912) was a professor of medicine in Paris who rose from a humble background and whose fame rested upon his development of public-health techniques to keep the Continent free from typhoid fever. Truly an important figure in the Heroic Age of Medicine, he received the French Légion d'Honneur in recognition of his medical accomplishments. Since so many infectious diseases could be controlled through cleanliness and other practices that kept germs at bay, his major medical interest was in hygiene. Hence when he turned to the subject of neurasthenia, it is not surprising to find that the title of his book, written with Charcot's disciple Gilbert Ballet, was *The Hygiene of the Neurasthenic* (1897) and that he concentrated on ways of keeping cases of the illness from breaking out.

Marcel Proust, his son, was a great nervous sufferer. In early life he was so sickly that he missed years of schooling. His medical problems included asthma, hay fever, insomnia, dyspepsia, and anxiety attacks, as well as addiction to many drugs, such as caffeine to wake him up and barbiturates to put him to sleep. He had received a score of different diagnoses, but all his doctors agreed that the underlying problem was what the French called a neuroarthritic heredity.

In early life, though his parents had tried to direct him into a career as a lawyer or a statesman, Proust had been intrigued with the French aristocracy and with art. Also, his life style became irregular. His asthma and hay fever were less marked at night. So he developed the habit of arising late in the day and staying up until sunrise. As a young man he was part of the chic life of Paris, with its salons, its theaters, its dazzling and opulent style of living.

In early life Proust was a habitual masturbator. By his twenties he was deeply involved in bisexuality. His homosexual affairs in early life centered on young men of his own bourgeois class. But he was also irresistibly attracted to handsome aristocratic men.

After the death of his parents in 1910 and 1912, Proust tried briefly to reform his life style and get over his symptoms by going to a sanatorium. But this was only a halfhearted attempt. Soon he became a recluse, his sexual tastes centering on men of the lower classes—servants and chauffeurs. He also became an inveterate habitué of brothels, where he was involved in various sadomasochistic practices.

During this time he was laboring away on his monumental novel *Remembrance of Things Past*. He withdrew more and more into his cork-lined bedroom and finally took to his bed. Living in his imagination, the novelist composed most of his great work while lying down. Fighting against time—his health was worsening year by year—Proust wrote unendingly. His life ended in the 1920s as the first volumes of the work on which he had been concentrating so much energy for thirty years began to bring him recognition. He died of a pulmonary hemorrhage in the arms of his brother Robert, a surgeon.

Ironically, in *The Hygiene of the Neurasthenic* special emphasis is placed not on the evils of overwork but on heredity. The authors specifically speak of the neuroarthritic tendency, which they saw as a *sine qua non* of neurasthenia. They gave credence to the very old idea that the tendency to suffer from nervous ailments and arthritis or diseases of the joints is hereditary and that the two are frequently seen together. Weakness of mind and of limbs seemed to go hand in hand in certain weak and wan children. Proust and Ballet then spoke of the need to "safeguard the future of the children of neuropathic and arthritic parents." Hence they paid special attention to what they called "the physical and moral education" of the neuropathically susceptible child. They advised parents to raise these children in rural places where life was calm —away from theaters, concerts, and all worldly activities—where pure air and simple food would nurture them.

Turning to moral education, the doctors stressed that children are more suggestible than adults and therefore that moral education must be founded on suggestion. The parent and the doctor must suggest certain positive principles and help the patient avoid potentially harmful influences. The most important task of the parents, in conjunction with the doctor, is to find an occupation, a profession, a task for the neuropathic child. "It is necessary to habituate the child to want to do things and to accomplish what he wants . . . in a word to be able to do what he must. It is for this reason that it is good to impose on him a task" that is not above his limited neurological means. Also, the potential neurasthenic should be shielded from all emotionality and sexuality. All imaginative children's literature should be hidden, children should be prohibited from masturbating, and "at the approach of puberty, his parents should take care to detour these children from all which could attract their attention to the sexual function, from all which could be the cause of sexual excitation."

The link between Adrien Proust's book on neurasthenia and the life of his son can be discerned from *Remembrance of Things Past*. The narrator of this work is a sickly young man who seems to have inherited his weakness from his mother and maternal grandmother. In this fictional account the protagonist, Marcel, initially falls ill out of longing for the pampering of his mother. Growing tenuously healthier, the boy is enthusiastic over the prospect of seeing the famous actress La Berma (based on Sarah Bernhardt) as the tragic lead in *Phaedre*. But his circumspect father forbids him to go, in order that he may avoid overexcitement. The son inevitably suffers a relapse during his great love for a young girl named Gilberte, at about the time his father grudgingly allows him finally to see *Phaedre*.

Marcel begins to recover only when he and his grandmother set forth for the fictional resort of Balbec on the north coast of France. Here he is initially beset by violent if obscure nervous attacks. Slowly he begins to heal as his grandmother and he begin walking along the sea and driving to nearby picturesque sites. Forgetting Gilberte and growing healthy are even easier once Marcel makes new friends. First he meets Madame de Villeparisis, a noblewoman and compatriot of his grandmother. Through her he meets her great-nephew, the handsome young nobleman Robert de Saint-Loup-en-Bray and then the enigmatic but intriguing Baron de Charlus. Finally he meets a bevy of pubescent young girls. Out of this "little band" steps the beautiful orphan Albertine, with whom he falls desperately in love.

There is an elaborate interlude in which Marcel falls in love with a noblewoman, the Duchess of Guermantes, and so ascends into the world of French nobility, and yet another long episode in which he descends as a voyeur into the pits of sexual perversion practiced by the Baron de Charlus. Finally Marcel returns to his love for Albertine. But he shows his neurasthenic tendency by his indecision over marrying the girl. Albertine eventually runs off, and before a reconciliation can occur, she is accidentally killed. Marcel is crushed by a flood of remembrance and remorse and takes himself to a sanatorium. Here he spends many years trying to recover.

From the lives of the two men, the novel by the son, and the book by the father, a unified clinical paradigm can be constructed of how a neurasthenic and his doctor and family interacted. First the father notices that his son is in weak health. The son has difficulty doing schoolwork, staying with a task; he is sickly and misses school days. He is not manly, not athletic. Rather, he has a propensity for art; he is a dreamer. The father tries to protect him from the theater, which he fears will be overstimulating. He tries to ward off the evil influences of society, the vain hopes and foolish waste of time and energy. He wants his son to choose a career. But the son cannot help his own propensities, which he sees as hereditary. He fails to follow the dicta of his parent and so suffers severe consequences, namely, a breakdown of his nervous system. This leads him to go to the sea for rest and recuperation. Rather than finding quiet, he is introduced to new stimulation, odd personages and ideas, and eventually a new love.

By now the son is old enough for the parent-doctor to be less directly influential. The son dreams of being a great artist or of loving a noblewoman. Neither dream seems inherently foolish, but the son never seems to go about either with any firm resolve. He never openly woos the noblewoman, he only fantasizes about her, and his literary scribblings never seem more than squibs and pastiches. He is slowly dragged into the pits of degeneracy. Fleeting love and promiscuous sexuality become central to his prodigal life. His health and his morals are utterly ruined. He lives a life at odds with what his parents meant for him. The commercial virtues of sobriety, hard work, and self-discipline seem to die out in him.

At the death of his father he takes himself to a sanatorium to recover. The mourning son loathes his own dissipated life and tries desperately but vainly to reform. At the sanatorium he meets doctors who speak to him about his life. Unfortunately they are not as clever as he, as well read or sophisticated. He leaves before his cure is complete. He never marries, squanders what is left of the family finances, and spends what energy he has in literary scribblings. He is a degenerate neurasthenic who has lived on the vainest of hopes—the fleeting fantasy of literary fame.

In Proust's case, of course, the results were much more than vain scribblings. The paradigm of degenerate neurasthenia as moral health undermined through faulty heredity and undisciplined education does not seem to apply to this great man. In this exceptional case of a "failed" son who did great things, we see a weakness in the middle-class position of Victorian medicine.

The Victorian doctor who treated the degenerate neurasthenic frequently placed himself, unsuspectingly, in the role of parent. Doctors have always been parental figures in many respects, giving their patients solace, advice, and, especially with the psychologically disturbed, admonishment. Since degenerate neurasthenics were supposedly suggestible human beings who Lombroso and Krafft-Ebing feared were capable of homosexuality, perversion, and murder, the doctor wished to influence them to use their limited energies in safe ways. This was the heart of their struggle. The doctor advised the child to hear no fairy tales; the patient rebelled and became fascinated with the *Arabian Nights*. The doctor advised no stimulation by art; the patient wanted to be an artist. The doctor warned against sexuality; the patient became a dreamy lover of unattainable women, a masturbator.

By admonishing their patients to eschew so much of modernity, doctors may have locked themselves and their patients into a struggle for control over the patients' moral code. Just as Marcel's father would not allow him to see La Berma in *Phaedre*, only reluctantly letting him go to see the play in his adolescence, so too did parents of potential neurasthenics and their doctors only grudgingly allow their effete fledglings to go into the world. They hovered over their patients like moral policemen. Obviously, sexuality was one of the evils most to be avoided and therefore one of those areas around which a battle of control was most bitterly fought. Similar struggles took place over alcohol, tobacco, food, patterns of sleep, friendship, and work.

As in the case of Charcot and hysteria, it would be utterly wrong to say that the doctors themselves created neurasthenia. Within the flowing garment of symptoms called neurasthenia there resided an anxious and depressed human being. But cultural pressures and family expectations surrounding this human being only deepened and prolonged the symptoms. Victorian standards of manhood and womanhood, the importance of choosing a safe career, marrying wisely, preserving the family fortune and name paralyzed the anxious and depressed patients and brought the doctor onto the scene.

In observing the symptoms rather objectively and diagnosing neurasthenia, the doctor was pushing forward the revolution of empathy. According to the neurasthenia notion, based on ideas of evolution and electricity, the patients lying in front of the doctor were low in nerve strength and so were ill, in every sense of the word.

In developing the numerous treatments, the doctor intuitively offered his patients both physical and psychological means to a cure, though he did not always comprehend how the cures worked. He counseled his patients to flee psychocultural stress—family expectations and social demands. He sent them to the country, the sea, the mountains. There they could contemplate the scenery and their own psyches, place their distressing life situations in some perspective, make some internal adjustments, and return in an improved state of mind. The forty-five-year-old businessman from Tourette can now be seen as a man in a mid-life crisis who was helped immensely when his doctor named his distress neurasthenia, sent him off to the country for a rest, and counseled him to lighten the burdens of his business. The invalid lady whom Playfair first viewed in Brighton can now be seen as a woman trapped in an empty high-society existence. By subjecting her to the Rest Cure the doctor ripped her out of this mire and also introduced her to a woman nurse, with whom she became fast friends. The convalescence cruise to Capetown during which the now-humane aristocrat nursed the sick companion only confirmed the former invalid's newfound distance from her old way of life.

Though one cannot be certain how enduring these cures were, one can surmise that they offered the patients a means to escape their defective styles of life, reshape them in solitude, and return to the fray ready to live a more balanced existence.

For many, however, such techniques were only superficial. Their society and family structures were less flexible, their own states of mind more fixed. These were the hereditary, or potential, neurasthenics. Both the twenty-six-year-old patient described by

Tourette and Proust himself are good examples. The battle between parents and young neurasthenics was too fierce. The doctor who appeared on the scene only became another authority figure in this struggle for control. Just as Charcot's scrupulous observation of the hysterics in Salpêtrière only worsened and hardened their preexisting symptoms because of his male-female biases, the expert in neurasthenia unwittingly fell into the role of the Victorian parent, bringing his own anxieties and apprehensions to the child-patient and so deepening his symptom picture.

In neurasthenia one sees mirrored the more general apprehension of the middle class vis-à-vis modernity. The doctor's anxiety was specifically translated into attitudes about how to rear a child in a society undergoing confusing transition. The modern city, the railway, the newspapers, the naturalistic novels of the day, the dramas of Strindberg and Ibsen stood as symbols of encroaching modernity from which the parent-doctor hoped to shield the child-neurasthenic. The values of modernity might, the doctor-parent feared, twist or distort the unformed ethics of the child-neurasthenic. The city sounds and lights, the lurid tales of Zola and Maupassant might weaken the nerves and moral sentiments of the susceptible child and ultimately transform him into a degenerate.

Doctors in the Victorian age seemed unaware that they frequently failed to separate morality from medicine. Since the neurasthenic seemed to need someone to serve as an overseer, the doctor placed himself in the role of theorizing about and trying to enforce what the Victorians called moral health. But in his theorizing he blindly brought to the bedside of the child-neurasthenic his own commercial virtues of sobriety, hard work, will power, domination of the external world—all the characteristics that had helped him to plod forward and become a middle-class doctor.

His patient, nurtured on many of the intriguing ideas of modernity that questioned, satirized, even villainized the money-grubbing and Philistine tendencies of the older generation, was necessarily suspicious of the doctor's answers and prescriptions. Though rarely able to break free from the doctor's position of strength, the patient sabotaged his treatments, redoubled his symptoms, and so nettled the doctor. So the battle waxed more violent. Though the doctor might be annoyed with his weak-willed patient, he at least made money on the deal. Meanwhile the patient lay brooding and self-loathing, another casualty in the heightening struggle between two competing value systems. The human being whom the Victorian doctor saw as entertaining a modern perspective all too readily was diagnosed as a hereditary neurasthenic or, worse still, an incurable degenerate. In the two chapters that follow we shall discuss two forms of this incurable degeneracy.

TEN

Mephisto

WITHIN the crevices of the Victorian psyche there crouched a gnarled figure who came to haunt the pages of many medical tracts. This sinister form was the Sinful Genius, the diabolical artist tempted by Mephisto to sacrifice his morality for the sake of artistic and intellectual insight. In this nerve-twisted figure we see Beard's American Prometheus, the "brain-worker," and the more turgid European Genius and Degenerate remodeled, entwining brilliance and sin so tightly that medical cure via rest, electricity, or moral exhortation seemed impossible. This combination of good and evil enticed many Victorians and, in fact, has much appeal to this day.

What is so remarkable about this prototypical brain sufferer— with his drugs, his alcohol, his sexual irregularities and tempestuous affairs, and, most important, his moments of godlike inspiration—is his historical reality. Scandalous true stories abound of Victorian geniuses who were also great moral profligates. Two such men who warrant special attention were Richard Wagner, the brilliant German composer, and Paul Verlaine, the great French poet. The often dry listing of symptoms and personal foibles in the medical writings on these two men comes to life as lurid details in the biographies of the two Sinful Geniuses.

One summer morning in 1865 in the city of Munich a great German tenor succumbed to brain fever. He was Ludwig Schnorr von Carolsfeld, whose death wrapped the city in mourning and set tongues wagging. Schnorr had been singing the part of the hero of Wagner's *Tristan and Isolde* on the Munich stage, and his sudden death not only ruined the opera, since his voice proved irreplaceable, but also plunged Wagner into self-recrimination. According to newspaper articles and rumors, Wagner had killed Schnorr— not literally, of course, but by way of his music. The physical and mental strain that Schnorr had experienced in singing the near-impossible part of Tristan had supposedly overtaxed his nerves and had led to an early death from Wagnerian fever.

Wagner had been leading a lascivious life in a *ménage à trois* with the Munich Kapellmeister Hans von Bülow and his wife, Cosima, a fact bandied about in the press. While Schnorr was supposedly immolating himself on the altar of Wagner's genius, Bülow was willing to sacrifice his marriage and his reputation for the sake of this heartless composer. Revering Wagner as a demigod, Bülow remained the Munich Kapellmeister and the cuckolded husband for years to come, humiliating himself in both public and private. In the same years the infamous Wagner was incessantly lying to his patron, the young and impressionable King Ludwig of Bavaria, insisting that the stories about his life with Cosima and Hans were lies invented by his enemies. The Dream King, as Ludwig was called, believed this great liar, or more probably perceived such immorality as a small flaw in the imposing form of this Sinful Genius. He gave lavishly to keep the evil composer wrapped in silk and satin dressing gowns, a passion for the great one. Though Wagner had promised all his scores to Ludwig in return for such munificence, he had a nasty habit of selling them to other buyers and pretending that Ludwig had no rights in the first place. All the while Ludwig adulated Wagner and silently paid off the bill collectors who were forever appearing to collect from the spend-thrift composer.

Another man whom Wagner used and abused was the philosopher Friedrich Nietzsche. As a young man Nietzsche became enraptured with *Tristan* and so admired Wagner from afar. By a happy coincidence, when Wagner, fleeing the gossip in Munich with his Cosima, settled in Triebschen, in Switzerland, the youthful Nietzsche—then a professor at Basel—snatched the opportunity to run to the Wagnerian doorstep to bow before the Master.

Acting as a lackey to Richard and Cosima, running errands hither and thither, and, more important, composing philosophical tracts that legitimized Wagner's thinking on art, Nietzsche long remained enraptured of the godlike Wagner.

The list of men Wagner abused and women he seduced is too long to recount. What is so impressive is how willing they were to be seduced, lied to, sadistically treated, and cuckolded. Viewing his genius as sublime, his operas as fruit from Valhalla, they considered it a great honor to serve him. Wrapping himself and his operas in an unreal nimbus, Wagner seemed to agree with his admirers that he was an artistic prophet and that his various operas were God-inspired productions. In his various essays he not only spoke of his art as the artistic form of the future but also inveighed vigorously against all moral and esthetic values that would stifle it. These values he connected most definitely with the Jews, since many of the money collectors knocking at his doors were Jews.

Though Wagner would die like any mortal—in 1883—of a heart attack, though Ludwig would drown in a Bavarian lake, with his psychiatrist, in the 1890s, and though Nietzsche would go mad with neurosyphilis, Cosima Wagner would carry on the work of building a musical and quasi-religious cult. Avid Wagnerites would regard the trip to Bayreuth to hear the *Ring* cycle as a kind of religious pilgrimage. The mystique of the Sinful Genius and the quasi-religious experience at the opera would deepen and reach a culmination, it seems today, in anti-Semitism and Nazism.

In a similar if less fanatical vein, the French poet Paul Verlaine lay in a Brussels prison cell in 1873, paying for his sins. A man of twenty-nine at the time of his imprisonment, Verlaine could well remember how he had met the teenage poet, Arthur Rimbaud, whose brilliant verses would transfix the French-speaking world but who had catalyzed Verlaine's moral downfall.

Before meeting Rimbaud in 1871 Verlaine had already won a small name for himself in the world of letters and was financially secure, as he had married an heiress. Though given to the sinful habit of drinking, Verlaine faced an even more sinister temptation one day when the youthful Rimbaud, a runaway from his strict mother in the provinces, showed up at his doorstep pleading for a haven.

The promising young man won over the sentimental Verlaine. Despite Mme. Verlaine's remonstrances, the two poets were quickly off drinking together, discussing esthetics, and soon had eloped to London. Here their liaison—by then a sexual one with a sadomasochistic twist—reached a pinnacle, and then crumbled. Verlaine ran off, leaving Rimbaud to make his own way and to write some of his best poetry in his English exile. Verlaine returned to his wife, who scolded him, deloused him, and fed him. Soon, however, Rimbaud was again at his door. The married man was tempted, and the whole poetical-sexual liaison was on again. The two poets ran off to Brussels, where they again squabbled, even pummeled each other. Verlaine drew a pistol and shot at Rimbaud. Apprehended by the police, the pair were led before a judge, who held Rimbaud, then nineteen years old, to have been corrupted by the older man. Chastised, the youthful and down-at-the-mouth Rimbaud was given train fare back to France, where he was met by his angry mother, who twisted his ears, gave him a lecture, and took him home to scrub him and shear his locks.

Verlaine was not so lucky. He was left behind in Brussels to pay for his sins. Though he threw himself on the mercy of the old judge, he was sentenced to prison for shooting at the young Rimbaud and, it seems, though not officially, for sodomy, for being part of the Paris Commune, and for alcoholism. Hauled weeping from the courtroom, Verlaine was locked in a Belgian prison.

During the two years of his imprisonment Verlaine suffered terribly. Ironically, though the twisted tale of the two artists reached the newspapers and helped earn for them the name of dirty poets, Verlaine underwent a religious conversion in that prison cell. He began a most sensuous and richly lyrical cycle of poems that culminated in his seeing the depth of his own helplessness and turning humbly to Christ crucified and the Blessed Virgin Mary, pleading for forgiveness.

Though Verlaine would frequently fall prey to both alcoholism and deep depression over the next twenty years, wandering from aging prostitute to aging prostitute and from hospital to hospital in Paris in the 1890s, his unattainable obsession would remain that of Christ led to slaughter, and his lyrical magic would soar higher and higher.

The lives of scores of other artistic geniuses, such as Charles

Baudelaire, Guy de Maupassant, Oscar Wilde, and George Sand, were checkered with personal irregularities. Many were alcoholics or drug addicts, financially incompetent or sexually perverse, homosexual or simply promiscuous. Living this kind of life seemed *de rigueur* for the making of great art. These Sinful Geniuses fascinated and repelled the Victorians, both medical and lay, and they came to be called decadent and *fin-de-siècle*. They lived enviable but unhappy lives that carried them far beyond the boundaries of middle-class morality. Many seemed lost souls, men and women without consciences.

Yet they also seemed cultural prophets, blazing a trail that the common citizen might follow. Nevertheless this cultural prophesy was a complex matter. Did it mean that ordinary people could gain insights into human nature by appreciating the works of these geniuses? Or did it mean leading lives like theirs? Many Victorian doctors interested in degeneracy and genius found themselves in a dilemma over just this question. They were struggling to keep their nervous, hysterical, and neurasthenic patients, especially those of the "higher orders," away from moral and neurological degeneration. The amorality that the artist or bohemian espoused seemed to be enticing patients to make a leap that would —doctors believed—only destroy them. At the same time, however, evolutionary theory seemed to suggest that geniuses, especially political and scientific ones, were precisely the beings natural selection had created to bring about human progress. In a period of great transition, both social and moral, the direction that this evolution was taking seemed extremely uncertain. Thus ideas about genius, degeneration, evolution, and moral health grew confusing in the 1890s.

Building on the original thinking of Morel and Moreau, many doctors analyzed the biographical material of geniuses who were also degenerates. They spilled much ink over the likes of J.-J. Rousseau, who could love only women who were cruel to him, who preached the importance of education while he left his own illegitimate children in orphanages, or especially Napoleon Bonaparte, whose political dominance of Europe seemed predicated on his lack of conscience.

A Hungarian Jewish doctor, Max Nordau (1849–1923), stands forth as probably the most influential medical author on the subject of the Sinful Genius. His *Paradoxes* (1886) and *Degeneration* (1895) lay out much of his thinking and describe a neurotic prototype that can be called the Aspiring Esthetic. Another celebrated doctor, Cesare Lombroso, the Italian criminologist, wrote a significant work called *The Man of Genius* (first Italian edition, 1882). Both doctors spoke the language of neurology, describing genius and sinfulness as arising from faulty neurological tissue. One part of the brain, hypothetically connected to ingeniousness, was firing too much; another part, connected to morality, lay inactive.

Before investigating Nordau's medical works it is worth while to review his moral perspective. He was a complicated and talented thinker, a medical intellectual in a perplexing period of social and moral transition. A sober, logical, and methodical man, born in Budapest in 1849, his father a rabbi named Gabriel Sudfeld, Nordau forsook his Jewish heritage. Choosing to live a cosmopolitan life from an early age, he wrote poetry and fiction with great verve. Concurrently he entered medical school in Budapest and worked for the city newspaper. While covering the World's Fair in Vienna in 1873 Nordau first conceived of universal humanity as his ideal, united with the notion of human progress and cultural evolution. His extensive travels throughout Europe for a few years deepened his love for the great Western ideals of liberty, equality, and fraternity. It seemed only logical that the young Jew-turned-humanist would settle in 1880 in Paris, which then seemed the capital of the Western world.

There he worked as a liberal journalist, a humanistic doctor and playwright and novelist for almost twenty-five years. Taking a second medical degree in Paris, he specialized in women's and nervous diseases but also devoted much of his energy to larger sociological questions of human progress. Between 1881 and 1893 he wrote three works that won him a wide reputation in Europe. Also, he authored a number of plays and novels, almost as complements to his sociological works.

In his *Paradoxes* Nordau laid out his essential postulates about genius and human progress. Cultural evolution is based on the birth of geniuses, he wrote. Natural Selection allows a few great men, and occasionally women, to be born. They often lack the morality of the common man, but, in compensation, they can use their reason more innovatively. To Nordau, reason was much

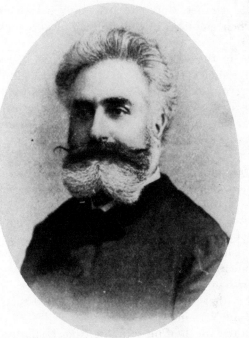

Max Nordau, doctor, novelist, polemicist.
(From Max Nordau, *The Shackles of Fate*)

more important than emotion in the evolution of the human race. He held that reasoning is a faculty of the frontal lobes, the higher parts of the brain, whereas emotion is a by-product of the brain stem and middle parts of the brain. He saw the genius as casting aside old ways of thinking and so presenting a new view of existence to humanity. Though the genius might be misunderstood during his tempestuous life, the human race slowly but inevitably follows him, and hence cultural evolution occurs.

Nordau believed that the political genius is of the highest order, since he not only thinks original ideas but also, through the strength of his will, acts on them, bringing abstractions to life. Nordau believed scientific and philosophical geniuses to be of a second order, having original ideas but lacking the will power to turn them into deeds. The artistic genius he perceived as belonging to a third order, since the artist only helps common people reconcile their emotions to the rational advances taking place in civilization.

A liberal in the Victorian sense, the doctor believed that cultural change should take place gradually and logically, via evolution, not revolution. Science rather than art would be a prime driving force. Also, Nordau believed in the growth of human solidarity rather than in individuality. Hence his attitudes about various changes in society were conservative from our point of view, very much connected to his middle-class morality and out of step with certain more modern attitudes. He did not believe in the emancipation of women, since he saw them as neurologically and physically inferior. Yet he supported the abolition of slavery and the right of all middle-class male citizens to vote. He believed in a middle-class morality based on order, custom, rationality, and especially self-discipline. Despite his Jewish heritage, Nordau accepted much of the Protestant ethic and even married a Scandinavian Christian woman. He was wary of the unbridled excess and individuality that seemed to be preached by artistic geniuses such as Wagner and Verlaine.

Nordau drew much of his thinking from Lombroso. In fact, the Italian doctor's *Man of Genius* was really his inspiration. Lombroso had published his first essay, "Genius and Insanity," in 1864, then expanded his thinking into a 350-page book *The Man of Genius* in 1882.

In his preface Lombroso laid out the cornerstone of his thought. "Just as giants pay a heavy ransom for their stature in sterility and relative mental weakness," he wrote, "so the giants of thought expiate their intellectual force in degeneration and psychosis." Already he was balancing the good and the evil of genius. Mentioning Rousseau and King Ludwig of Bavaria as examples of degenerate geniuses, Lombroso stated emphatically, "Genius is a neurosis . . . and like every neurosis which depends on irritation of the cerebral cortex, it may take on different aspects, according to the spot attacked." Different parts of the nervous system were irritated and so were stimulated more than other parts. Various types of ingenious ideas escaped into the outer world, depending on which brain center was overstimulated. Thus some geniuses appeared in art, others in religion, others in politics, and still others in abstract thought.

Lombroso next set out to distinguish a list of physical and behavioral symptoms of genius, comparable to the symptoms he had catalogued when discussing the Born Criminal. Unlike the criminal type, with his huge jaw, slicing incisors, massive forearms, simian creases, dexterity, and fits of bloodthirsty violence, the genius type was characterized by short stature, congenital malformation, sickliness in childhood, and huge or tiny brains, stammering, left-handedness, and sexual sterility.

Some of these features call to mind Beard's description of the "brain-worker," with his overactive mind and meager physique. But others suggest a more degenerate being, twisted in body and unable to further the evolution of the species. What especially distinguished the Sinful Genius from Prometheus and allied him to the Born Criminal was his lack of ethical principles, which made him a law unto himself. Another equation that allied the Lombrosian genius with the criminal was his epilepticlike fits of inspiration, which Lombroso compared to the fits of bloodthirsty rage in many criminals.

All geniuses, Lombroso believed, struggled against and lamented their languid and lazy natures for long periods of time. They moaned and groaned over their own stupidity and ignorance. Then one day, as if lightning bolts had struck them from the heavens, they were inspired. Veritable epileptics all, like Prince Myshkin in *The Idiot*, they saw in a flash the "promised land" and leaped forward into a brilliant new idea or feeling or act of genius! They wrote and painted feverishly, they saw into the heart of things philosophically or scientifically, or they won great battles in single strokes. This is the heart of genius, believed Lombroso, the moment of inspiration, when a lesion or brain center fired exuberantly.

Since the malady of genius resolved itself into localized irritation of the cerebral cortex, manifesting itself in attacks of inspiration, the Italian doctor was arguing that "motor epilepsy"—that is, the grand mal and the "marches" of Hughlings Jackson—had its "psychic equivalent," that is, the moment of inspiration. Lombroso was correlating inspiration with the "mental automatism" described by Jackson. Via this interesting correlation Lombroso was deepening the myth of the Sinful Genius, transmuting Moreau's genius into a morbid neurological sufferer whose over-activity in the brain was specifically due to the active and violent firing of an epileptic "discharging lesion," to use another of Jackson's phrases. The result was not an automatonlike carrying out of one's work, not as in the case of Jackson's doctor-patient Quaerens, but rather an astonishing act of creation.

To prove the identity of motor epilepsy and the moment of inspiration, Lombroso lingered over the case of Napoleon Bonaparte. Quoting and paraphrasing at length the French historian Hippolyte Taine, he described Napoleon as lured to conquer Egypt by "the mirage of omnipotence; in the East he caught a glimpse of the possibility that he might found a new religion." "Never," wrote Taine, quoted by Lombroso, "even among the Borgias and Malatestas, was there a more sensitive and impulsive brain, capable of such electrical accumulation and discharge . . . and never was there more impatient insensibility . . . his heart and intellect were full to overflowing . . ." His physical compulsions, his frequent fits of weeping, vomiting, and fainting were all explicable within this context.

Seeing himself as a veritable superman, above the usual social laws and mores, "Napoleon wept not on account of true and deep feeling but because, 'a word—an idea by itself is a stimulus which reaches the inmost depths of his nature.' " Lombroso believed that a word, an idea had elicited a fit of psychic epilepsy in Napoleon, a fit that manifested itself in weeping.

Hand in hand with psychic epilepsy came amorality. The feelings so central to any moral stance were foreign to Napoleon. He used his followers and admirers and functionaries for whatever he could get out of them, be it political or financial support. He even induced some of them to overstep the bounds of morality themselves. He then cast them off without gratitude, letting them die en masse in futile battles. He cut off Josephine for the sake of his career and loved to shock noble ladies with "unpleasant witticisms." He "related to the empress herself the favors which more or less spontaneously they granted him." In his description of the amoral monster Napoleon "Taine has here given us the subtlest and precisest pathological diagnosis of a case of psychic epilepsy,"

Lombroso asserted, "with its gigantic megalomaniacal illusions, its impulses and complete absence of moral character."

The Sinful Genius, clearly a minority figure, one in a million, might be evil, amoral, alcoholic, sexually promiscuous, and perverse. But most humans remained neurologically healthy. If not geniuses, they at least had consolation in knowing that they were not necessarily neurotic. Essentially, the Lombrosian genius laid down his life, sacrificed his neurological system for the sake of the common man. Although his own life might be a pack of miseries, although he might die in exile like Napoleon or be beheaded like Saint Paul, or assassinated like Julius Caesar, or crucified like Christ himself, at least later generations of humans would come along, see the originality of the idea or the act of the genius, and evolve. The healthier human beings would inculcate the ideas of the genius into their safer, if less fantastic life-styles. Hence cultural evolution could continue upward, inevitably upward.

Lombroso did discuss such contemporaries as Robert Schumann and Verlaine, but he did not really draw any distinctions between premodern and modern Sinful Geniuses. Nor did he distinguish the scientific or political genius from the artistic genius. He left these subtler points to his young admirer Nordau.

Nordau dedicated his *Degeneration* to Lombroso, even calling the Italian his master. Nonetheless his book is more pessimistic than Lombroso's works—even apocalyptic. In Nordau's book the anxiety-provoking theme of neurological decay mixed with the notion of the decline of Western civilization. Lombroso's optimistic world view clashed with Nordau's belief that history would not necessarily move in a happy direction and that modern art bred immorality in the common man.

Nordau's starting point in *Degeneration* is subtly but significantly different from Lombroso's. While Lombroso saw the genius as the degenerate neurotic, classifying all brilliant men and women as both geniuses and degenerates, Nordau saw the genius and degeneracy as separate neuroses. Diagnosing such time-honored authors as Shakespeare and Goethe as neurotic geniuses, he labeled such Moderns as Wagner, Baudelaire, and Verlaine as neurotic degenerates only, not geniuses at all. Furthermore, while Lombroso perceived the genius-degenerate, whether a religious visionary, a brilliant statesman, or an artistic figure, as an instrument of cultural progress, Nordau applied the word "degenerate" only to those modern artists he saw as counterfeit geniuses. He feared they were leading civilization downhill toward chaos. The Lombrosian optimism had turned into a strident polemic flowing from Nordau's pen, and the Lombrosian neurotic genius seemed a man long dead, replaced by a pack of counterfeits and criminals.

Nordau feared that the unbridled excesses of such artistic geniuses as Wagner and Verlaine and their sensual art could drown the world in chaos. It is this fear that haunts every page of his book. The book includes a long and distressing description of the *fin-de-siècle* world of the nineties, characterized by "a contempt for traditional views of custom." Nordau perceived an optimistic epoch as ending and the old bulwarks of civilization, reason and religion, as tottering. In the interim "false prophets arise . . . men look with longing for whatever new things are at hand . . . they have hope that in the chaos of thought, art may yield revelations on the order that is to follow in this tangled web." In this troubled time, he wrote, men are arising who pass themselves off as geniuses, as visionaries and mystics, and their works are gobbled up by the uncertain and overly susceptible masses, by troubled Aspiring Aesthetes looking for some answer.

He conjured up the image of men and women of the higher classes, as the Victorians were wont to call them, "fold[ing] their hands before pictures at which the common sort burst out laughing." At the opera and the concert hall, "applause and wreaths are reserved for *Tristan and Isolde*, and especially for the mystic *Parsifal*," because the confused and neurotic listener comes looking for excitement and confusion. This nervous excitement, Nordau contended, is the modern counterfeit of an original idea, which was a meaningful answer to the riddle of life. "A dissonant interval," he wrote, "must appear where a consonant interval was expected . . . keys and pitches must change suddenly . . . the listener . . . gets excited as a man who vainly endeavors to understand what is being said in the jumble of a dozen voices." Nordau's Aspiring Aesthete goes home nervously excited but also exhausted. He may see Wagner as a near-religious prophet and may even become a devotee. But the Wagnerian craze only hid the Aspiring Aesthete's empty search for some way of feeling alive.

Likewise, with drama, novels, and poetry. Crying that the

prerequisite for a work to be fashionable in the nineties is obscenity, Nordau lamented the need of the modern reader to feel stimulated. Writers such as Ibsen, Zola, and Verlaine fulfilled this need by inventing perverse and licentious characters who titillate the reader. Feeling is what is important. As long as one feels something, one feels alive.

Nordau was not speaking about just a few shocking poets such as Verlaine and Rimbaud or such outrageous figures as Wagner and Baudelaire but about the whole movement of art circa 1890. Also he was not talking about only the degenerate artist but about the neurotic audience. He was worried that modern art was making modern man more neurotic, more immoral.

He posited that the Victorian physician could not help seeing in the *fin-de-siècle* desperation—both in the artist and in his audience—two diagnostic categories, two diseases. The first is degeneration, counterfeit genius. The second is hysteria, "of which the minor stages are designated as neurasthenia." Thus he restated the ideas of so many of the authors on European neurasthenia and clearly linked his work with that of Krafft-Ebing and Lombroso on criminality and perversion.

In speaking of the degenerate, Nordau spent little time on the physical stigmata associated with nervous degeneration (irregular teeth, protruding ears, and asymmetrical development of the two sides of the face and the cranium). He quickly plunged into describing four mental stigmata of degeneration, namely, the lack of moral sense, emotionalism, lack of will, and "the predilection for inane revery." By concentrating on these symptoms he could use not only the bodies, the neurological systems, and the lives of these artists for diagnoses but also their productions, their pieces of art.

Nordau believed that the diagnoses of hysteria and neurasthenia applied "for the most part to the multitude who will imitate the fashions [the degenerates] design." They are frequently females, impressionable and susceptible types, but also nervous men. "When he sees a picture, he wants to become like it in attitude and does; when he reads a book, he adopts its views blindly."

In explaining the spread of both degeneracy and the neuroses, hysteria and neurasthenia, Nordau simply dusted off the ideas of

Pinel, Trotter, Morel, and Moreau. He discussed the rising abuse of alcohol, opium, and hashish, and the evils of the city. All led, he believed, to one all-consuming problem: nervous exhaustion. Quoting numerous neurologists, psychologists, and psychiatrists, he stated that nervous exhaustion and fatigue could change the healthy man into a hysteric or neurasthenic and that nervous fatigue had become a way of life for most men and women in the last half of the nineteenth century. Railways had multiplied, postal services had expanded by leaps and bounds, novels and newspapers were everywhere. When the poor circumspect Western citizen reads the newspaper, "he takes part . . . in the thousand events which take place in all parts of the globe, and he interests himself simultaneously in the issue of revolution in Chile, in a bush war in East Africa, a massacre in North China, a famine in Russia, a street-row in Spain, and an international exhibition in North America."

Nordau divided degenerate artists into two major categories, the mystics and the egomaniacs. He saw the former as indulging in a writing style that is obscure, overly symbolic, "hinting at mysteries" without delivering. The latter are those whose central theme is the self.

Extensively, in precise language he described how a sensory impression enters the nervous system of a mystic and sets off certain stimuli in certain centers of the brain. By the association of ideas—which he saw as having developed along evolutionary lines—certain neighboring cells pick up the stimulus and fire, and so thoughts rise into consciousness. In the normal healthy man, images enter consciousness in a clear, crisp manner. However, in the mystical degenerate the images are vague and illogical, trailing off into nebulousness "like floating fog in the morning wind." The mystic, Nordau felt, lacked the ability to see firm outlines. The simple stimuli spread in vague and eccentric waves across his brain.

In the brain of the egomaniac, Nordau envisioned an opposite sensory process. Unlike the mystic, who is too sensitive and weak-willed to ward off unneeded impressions, thoughts, and shadows, the egomaniac has a dense sensory system. The healthy infant is originally self-oriented—"a model of egotism," to use Nordau's words—not precisely aware of the outer world. Maturity brings a growing awareness of the outer world: "The 'I' retires behind the

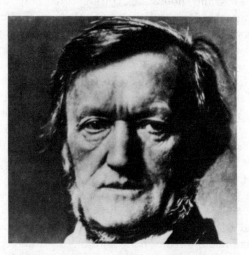

Richard Wagner, the craggy-faced German profligate and composer. (Richard-Wagner-Museum, Bayreuth, West Germany)

'not-I' and the consciousness." Not so in the case of the egomaniac. The gray matter of his frontal lobe is probably not developed well enough or is not vigorous enough for such natural development to take place. They remain like children. The external world, the "not-I," is not well represented in the minds of these degenerates, and "the molecular movement takes place . . . in a less free and rapid, less rhythmic and vigorous manner."

Interspersed with these scientific-sounding analyses are Nordau's discussions of the lives and works of nearly every significant modern artist. He extruded an especially strong venom toward Wagner, whom he saw as his mortal enemy. He lambasted both his ideas, as expressed in his "Art Work of the Future," and his art, especially his mystical *Parsifal* and his artistic brainchildren, the leitmotif and endless melody. The doctor insisted that all of Wagner's creations were simply the product of a wobbly and will-less central nervous system.

Nordau analyzed the writing style of "Art Work of the Future" as a faulty mixture of metaphors and weakly constructed sentences, of verbs and nouns descending into mere drivel. After recapitulating the Wagnerian argument that the mingling of dance, poetry, and music in one art form—Wagner's, the musical drama—was the superior art of the future, Nordau declared that this theory was quintessentially counterevolutionary. Living in a time before the vogue of primitivism in art, he argued by biological analogy that evolution takes place in the direction of differentiation and specialization, not synthesis and confusion. Likewise, he saw as lewd and immoral operas such as *The Valkyrie*, in which brother and sister, Siegmund and Sieglinde, beget a child, the hero Siegfried, or *Parsifal*, in which the Catholic Mass, with its Introit, Confiteor, Offertory, and Communion, is put to music and parodied in the manner of a Black Mass. All this illogic, Nordau asked, is the art of the future? All this retrogression and love of the mystical and the blatantly erotic? Should not the good German burghers "be blushing crimson and sinking into the good earth for shame?" How can the true Catholic priest allow this mockery of the Eucharist to go on! And the public duped! How could this occur in a civilized land?! For all these exclamatory questions Nordau found a simple and obvious explanation, namely, that the Wagner cult, complete with its Bayreuth pilgrimage, is nothing more than another manifestation of the hysteria and neurasthenia so widespread among the German people.

Nordau argued that the wars of 1866 and 1871 against the Austrians and the French helped to ruin the nerves of the poor Germans. "In my belief," he wrote, "it cannot be doubted that every great war is a cause of hysteria among multitudes, and that a larger number of soldiers, completely unknown to themselves, bring home from a campaign a somewhat deranged nervous system. . . . under the action of the two great wars with the development of large industries and the growth of cities, hysteria among the German people has, since 1870, increased in an extraordinary manner." To a people weakened in the nerves and not versed in the subtleties of art, a hypnotic degenerate such as Wagner, backed by the financial support of the handsome if cracked Ludwig II, comes along, wrote Nordau, teaching anti-Semitism, vegetarianism, antivivisectionism, and "Teutonomaniacal chauvinism." Soon the whole of Germany is entering the Wagner cult, in which the music's "powerful orchestral effects produced in them hypnotic states . . . and the formlessness of the unending melody was exactly suited for the vagaries of their own thought."

Nordau also launched an attack on Verlaine. He insisted that "we find, in astonishing completeness, all the physical and mental marks of degeneration" in the skull of this decadent poet. Nordau referred to some portraits of Verlaine that clearly showed, he insisted, the great asymmetry of the head, with its enigmatic bumps, Mongolian physiognomy, pointed cheekbones, obliquely placed eyes, and meager beard. The great poet had passed two years in prison for his illicit conduct, Nordau noted. He was a dipsomaniac and an unabashed vagabond.

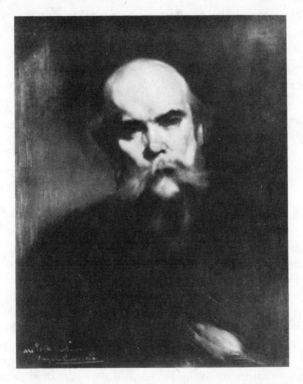

Paul Verlaine, the bump-skulled French *débauché* and poet. (From Gerhart Haug, *Verlaine: Die Geschichte des Armen Lelian*)

Next Nordau discussed the degenerate's poetry, mentioning his religious fervor, which mixed with eroticism, and his tendency to repeat phrases, all signs of Verlaine's mysticism, as evident in these lines:

> O Mon Dieu, Vous m'avez blessé d'amour,
> Et la blessure est encore vibrante,
> O mon Dieu vous m'avez blessé d'amour.

His most virulent attack was against the poet's tendency to combine "completely disconnected nouns and adjectives, which suggest each other, either through a senseless meandering by way of associated ideas, or through a similarity of sound." To illustrate this tendency he quoted one of the poet's most famous poems, "Art Poétique," his poetical manifesto:

> Il faut aussi que tu n'ailles point
> Choisir les mots sans quelques méprise;
> Rien de plus cher que la chanson grise,
> Où l'Indécis au Précis se joint.

> Car nous voulons la nuance encore,
> Pas la Couleur, rien que la nuance!
> Oh! la nuance seul fiance
> Le rêve au rêve et la flûte au cor!

Insisting that this powerful piece of poetry is "completely delirious," Nordau seemingly applied some fairly strict laws of logic, arguing that nuance and color are not mutually exclusive.

Finally Nordau returned to a larger social purview. Just as he saw Wagner as hypnotizing and seducing the nerve-shattered German people, so too he believed that Verlaine's popularity was due to rampant nervosity among the French after generation upon generation of war and revolution. This social tumult, wrote the doctor, stretched back at least to the 1789 revolution and ran forward through the Napoleonic Wars, the revolutions of 1830 and 1848, culminating in the Franco-Prussian War of 1870 and the ensuing Paris Commune and Siege. The outcome of this century of turmoil was a nation of tired and meager nervous systems. Nervous exhaustion, he boldly declared, explains the Frenchman's enthusiasm over so many new fashions in clothing and cosmetics, as well as in poetry. This aspiring aestheticism is nothing more than the result of the breeding of a handful of bump-skulled and syphilitic madmen such as Paul Verlaine enticing the common man into running after crackbrained fashions.

Nordau found unacceptable the experimentation of the Moderns, both in their lives and in their art codes, since they tempted fatigued common people to be like them. Nordau followed squarely along the path of Victorian liberalism, which saw history as progressing toward greater liberty, equality, and fraternity. He also was very much a child of the scientific idea of materialistic determinism.

The reception of *Degeneration* by the intellectual world of the 1890s was a hot one. To be sure, George Bernard Shaw, author of *The Perfect Wagnerite,* took up his pen to label Nordau a degenerate himself. Yet thousands of readers acclaimed the ideas of *Degeneration,* and Nordau was ranked as one of the world's most highly acclaimed intellectuals in the nineties.

However, Nordau's name and his various books are now nearly forgotten. No one reads his *Degeneration* or *Paradoxes* any more, let alone his novels and plays. No one takes his arguments about the Moderns seriously. In taking the Victorian stance against the Moderns, Nordau relegated himself to the halls of obscurity, his books to the dusty back shelves of libraries. His notions of sinfulness and moral health are grounded in middle-class mores. It was significant to him that four degenerates—Nietzsche, Maupassant, Schumann, and Baudelaire—died of neurosyphilis, that a fifth, Verlaine, was an alcoholic and a syphilitic, and that a sixth, Wagner, was an inveterate anti-Semite and in many ways a megalomaniac. Thus he could judge these men's acts, ideas, and works as dangerous. Unlike us, he lacked the ability to separate the artist from his creation. He feared very deeply that the very ideas of suicide, of sexual promiscuity, of unbridled excess described in their works would be imitated by the gullible readers who seemed to be multiplying in the late Victorian age.

Yet it was not only the content of the art that galled Nordau, it was also the form. Nordau insisted on logic in art. He would have argued that the interior monologue of Proust's *Remembrance,* for instance, was a product of a mystic and megalomaniac, that those who were wooed into appreciating it were simply being charmed by a counterfeit genius.

Certainly Nordau's views of literary logic now seem weak. The importance of recording personal experience and searching for an individual solution are taken for granted today. Indeed, from our vantage point, we all must become Sinful Geniuses who sell the happy innocence of our childhoods for the sake of self-insight. Like artists, we all must indulge in personal myth-making.

For Nordau, however, other alternatives still seemed possible. He dreamed of a whole society that was coherent, logical, rooted in the scientific method. In time, however, even he came to doubt these values. His fears of societal illogic, egocentrism, and passionate excess reached a personal crisis during the years following the publication of *Degeneration*, when he became embroiled in the famous Dreyfus Affair. When the Jewish captain was wrongfully found guilty of espionage and imprisoned for life, Emile Zola became one of the first to sound the battle cry against anti-Semitism, militarism, and political corruption.

The swarming minions of Mephisto seeming ascendant, the forces of liberalism were called into action. Nordau joined hands with Zola, one of his former nemeses, and strove to overcome the wicked hordes who worked to keep Dreyfus in chains. In the end Dreyfus was pardoned, but his success seemed so faint, so minuscule. The fearful figure of the Sinful Genius, embodied in Wagner, the strident anti-Semite, and Verlaine, the rootless alcoholic sodomist, still seemed triumphant in a society in which anti-Semitism, militarism, materialism, and nationalism grew ever more virulent.

Over the next few years Nordau slowly relinquished his stance as a fearless internationalist and fiery liberal. First made aware of the young movement called Zionism during the Dreyfus Affair, he became one of its leaders by 1900. He envisioned Western Jewry as breaking free of the declining West and its decadent forms. As the century turned, this man, so hopeful about world history in the days of the 1873 World Fair in Vienna, so self-assured in his polemics against Wagner and Verlaine in 1893, had grown more troubled in his thinking about cultural evolution and human solidarity.

ELEVEN

Christ the Neurotic

IN the same years when new art movements were flourishing in the West, a spiritual renewal was also gaining momentum. To the medical eye these movements, artistic and religious, had much in common, at times even seeming to blend together. The individuals involved in these trends often shared a gnawing sense that logic, reason, and science could not offer peace of mind. They looked to a world beyond the everyday experience of buying and selling, lending and borrowing. In some respects they seemed pessimistic about the direction of this world, fearing that in the widespread materialism of modernity, humanity could lose its soul. Hence they looked in the direction of mysticism and transcendental experience for inner peace. Both movements stressed the importance of age-old symbols, of rituals, mystery, solitude, communion with a spiritual world.

But the religious reawakening did not glorify moral profligacy. It appealed to the troubled sensibilities of many Westerners, especially those of the educated classes. Yet another neurotic type flourished in the late nineteenth century, namely the Religious Self-Tormentor. In his soul he struggled with the forces of good and evil. His language was religious: God versus the devil, the spirit versus Mammon. Sometimes Mammon and the devil even became terms synonymous with logic, reason, science, and modernity.

During the nineteenth century there also developed a fascination with quasi-spiritual psychic experiences, such as clairvoyance,
séances, automatic writing, and hypnotism. Though faith in the
old forms of religion had waned, a desire to believe, to believe in
something, remained. For a scientific man, science itself frequently
fulfilled this purpose. But for many laymen the need to find something in which to believe proved bitter and confusing.

Though many of the religiously troubled sought solace from
their clergymen, others turned to doctors. This is not surprising in
light of the eminence of Victorian science, toward which even the
religiously troubled felt attracted, or at least ambivalent. The
doctors who saw such patients used fashionable analogies to comprehend their emotional pain. Just as the neurasthenic or the
suggestible individual seemed vulnerable to the snares of modern
art, which preached amorality, so too the religiously inclined
person often seemed to admire exotic, even demented personages,
some of them ancient. The models for the Religious Self-
Tormentor were Christ and his saints, who, from a middle-class
purview, looked quite disturbed. Christ had preached turning the
other cheek and loving one's enemies. Christ had died ig-
nominiously on the cross, a triumphant defeat. This approach to
life was at loggerheads with the muscular expansionism of late
Victorian times, the self-assured march toward material benefits
which seemed the course of human history. In short, Christ seemed
a neurotic, the archetype of a great neurotic figure who can be
called the Saintly Fool.

In the person of Saint Francis of Assisi, the Saintly Fool was
stigmatized with the five wounds of Christ. He undertook long
fasts and prided himself on his physical suffering, which he traded
for spiritual comfort. Likewise, in ecstatic trances Saint Theresa of
Avila envisioned the bleeding wounds of Christ, reveling in deep
physical suffering for the sake of spiritual food. Both these saints
and many others seemed degenerates or hysterics to the Victorian
doctors.

Along similar lines, Lombroso believed that Saint Paul's religious inspiration when he fell from his horse and was converted
and Mohammed's visions were based on the firing of an epileptic
lesion. Krafft-Ebing explained the flagellatory practices of some
sixteenth-century Catholic saints as sexual neuroses, as masochism

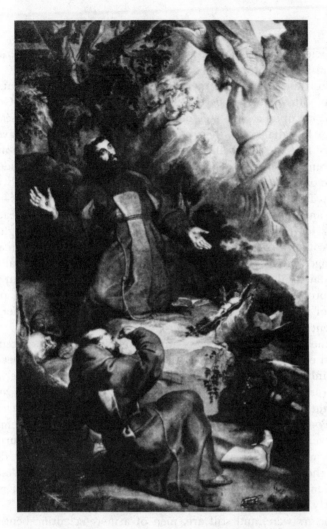

Saint Francis of Assisi in an ecstasy, receiving the stigmata. Peter Paul Rubens, *The Stigmatization of Saint Francis*. (Wallraf-Richartz-Museum, Cologne)

resulting from abnormal reflex arcs playing on faulty brain centers. Charcot and his followers described the ecstatic and crucified poses of their patients in the Salpêtrière as hysterical fits—the so-called period of passionate attitudes—and extended this thinking in the direction of saints. The combination of middle-class values and scientific explanation helped to make religious experience appear highly neurotic.

According to Beard, the seventeenth-century witch-hunts in Salem, Massachusetts, began after a pious doctor named Griggs had come upon a bevy of adolescent girls in the midst of a séance. Griggs had diagnosed their pranks as witchcraft and so played a crucial role in the ensuing trials in which these girls accused many innocent persons of witchcraft. A veritable hysterical epidemic broke out, wrote Beard, culminating in the infamous Salem witch-hunt. Two hundred years later, in the 1880s, three siblings—two boys and a girl—likewise were involved in a séance. Instead of going to trial they were diagnosed as hysterics and brought to Charcot's Salpêtrière. They were isolated, electrically treated, massaged, and cured of hysteria. The realigning of medical and popular thinking over two hundred years had been a slow but very real progression. Much that in 1680 had been the hallowed property of religion seemed by 1880–90 proper subject matter for the student of neuroses.

Some of the doctors were, unfortunately, blind to a central aspect of the religious rebirth: religion, perhaps more than art and certainly more than science, speaks to the human soul. In the wake of triumphant science and technology, as well as urban growth and the disruption of traditional ways of life, the lure of a more emotional, even mystical experience, during which life seems to achieve wholeness and meaning, had widespread appeal. Furthermore, while Darwinian postulates about man's interconnectedness with the rest of nature had discredited the world view of Western religions, an appeal to perhaps a more primitive aspect of man, namely, his need for ritual, gained impetus.

Doctors were, and still are, men of a more scientific bent. Although in their private hours Charcot might be wrapped up in a study of Gothic architecture and Krafft-Ebing enthralled with Beethoven's "Moonlight Sonata," their scientific systems were usually rational, having nothing but disdain for mysticism, ritual, and emotion. The seat of rationality was believed to be in the frontal lobes and the seat of emotion in the lower levels of the brain, so emotions seemed more primitive, less evolved. Hence enthusiasm over ritual and mysticism seemed like mental illness, dissolution of the nervous system.

However, an impressive aspect of the religious revival of the late nineteenth century was its sophistication, its modernity. Its adherents were not only French and Bavarian peasants but also many intelligent, though troubled citizens who needed a renewed sense of meaning, of roots, of unity. Many, especially in France, turned in the direction of Catholicism. England witnessed the growth of the High Church movement. In America, Christian Science developed. This religious revival was affecting many of the "upper orders" from which prominent doctors drew their clientele. Furthermore, certain religious figures, whether saints or disturbed humans, seemed to have godlike powers—to cure the sick, for instance. The doctors, of course, relied on the concept of suggestibility to explain such powers. Yet the extent of the power possessed by great religious figures interested the medical world enough for them to study these humans closely, precisely because the doctors coveted this very power.

Doctors did notice one common denominator in religious experiences, namely, the craving for heightened meaning. This instant of revelation for the religious individual took three basic forms. First, there was the moment of ecstasy, when the religious seer enters into a trance in which he and God commune. Next, there was the moment of healing, when the faith of the ill person is renewed and he is cured of a debilitating disorder. Third, there was the moment of religious conversion. After struggling with his own fears and uncertainties, doubting the goodness of the world, the existence of God and the immortality of his own soul, for inexplicable reasons the religious one enters into a state of barely being connected to this world, a state of painful waiting. Then, as if a miracle were taking place, he rips through the veils of earthly sham, taken over by forces outside of himself. He possesses a heightened sensibility in which he feels his own self and the cares of the world falling aside. For a delirious moment he comes face to face with God. He is cured, he enters into reveries, or he is converted. He is like Moses seeing God as a burning bush on Zion. The moment is short. God recedes. But always he carries the memory with him. The moment shapes the rest of his life.

Various Victorian doctors decided to study each of these three moments of heightened sensibility. A number of Salpêtrists, in particular Desiré Bourneville, became interested in ecstasy. Charcot, in "Faith-Healing," his last paper before his death, concentrated his attention on patients cured by faith. Religious conversion became the subject matter of a very important book, *The Varieties of Religious Experience* (1902), written by the American doctor, psychologist, and philosopher William James. This book, easily the most sensitive and most satisfying work written on the subject, can be seen as the culmination of the other men's works. The doctors moved from the blatantly materialistic to the clearly psychological. Bourneville's work is basically that of a materialist who writes off ecstasy to hysteria. Charcot's paper on faith healing is a more complicated analysis in which neurology, sociology, and psychology mesh. And James's *Varieties* is a delicate examination of the psychological experience of religious conversion.

Charcot placed ecstasy in the middle of the hysterical progression. Two hysterics, Geneviève and Louise, had both experienced ecstatic episodes, along with great misery and passionate sexual excitement, while in the so-called period of passionate attitudes. Their ecstatic and crucifixion poses were preceded by the epileptoid period and the phase of grand movements and were followed by the fourth and final phase of the grand hysteria, delirium. Charcot and his followers had sketched and photographed the hysterics in their various poses.

An atheist, Charcot used this material to discredit religion. The Salpêtrists depicted celebrated religious figures such as Theresa of Avila and Saint Catherine of Siena as victims of hysterical neurosis. Likewise, they viewed the seventeenth-century outbreak of witchcraft in Loudon as an epidemic of hysteria. They studied religious art from the fourth century A.D. on, tracing early representations of ecstasies and of miracles as performed by Christ and his various saints, which they saw simply as cases of hysteria. Christ's casting out a demon from a possessed man in a fifth-century mosaic was really a picture of a man curing a hysteric; a saint in the fifteenth century who cast out a devil from a woman was merely a doctor-priest healing a female hysteric. Saint Philip Neri was doing likewise in the sixteenth century, and on and on, through Brueghel's painting of the dance of Saint Guys' and Rubens' painting of Saint Ignatius curing a possessed woman. Onward Charcot's followers moved into more modern times: the

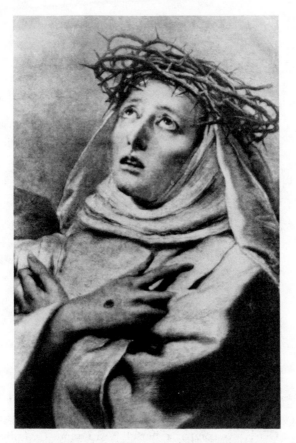

Saint Katherine of Siena, by Giovanni Battista
Tiepolo, or the Saintly Fool savoring her pain.
(Kunsthistorisches Museum, Vienna)

witches of Loudon, the cures of Joseph Gassner in the Vienna
woods, of Anton Mesmer around the *baquet* in prerevolutionary
Paris, the experiences of the Marquis de Puységur in the shade of
the elm tree. The closing pages of many books by the Salpêtrists
include studies of one or two hysterics just then inhabiting the
Salpêtrière.

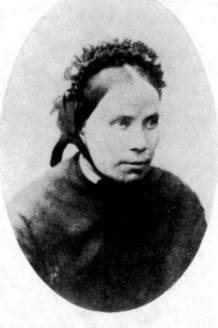

Louise Lateau, the Belgian *stigmatisée*.
(From Johannes Maria Höcht,
Träger der Wundmale Christi)

Geneviève was an excellent example of an ecstatic in the great hospital. Geneviève compared herself to a famous Catholic ecstatic named Louise Lateau, who in the late 1870s was getting quite a bit of newspaper coverage in France. In fact, Geneviève had once set off from the Salpêtrière on a pilgrimage to visit her "sister" Louise Lateau in Belgium (not to be confused with Charcot's own Louise already described). Though the hysterical pilgrim never made it to Belgium, many a doctor—some atheists, some Catholics—did travel there to visit Louise Lateau. There they saw strange and weird sights in the midst of a furor.

The facts of her life possessed the simplicity of sainthood. Born in the tiny village of Bois d'Haine in 1850, she was the youngest of three daughters. Her father, a workman in a nearby ironworks, died of smallpox when Louise was just a child, and her mother was a bed patient for the first two and one half years of Louise's life. Only in 1853 was her mother able to get out of bed and earn a small pittance. Cared for by a wet nurse in infancy, Louise was essentially an orphan. She was sent from home to care for invalid women at the age of seven and thus became accustomed to spending the greater part of her night by sickbeds.

The turning point in her life was a mysterious illness. One day when walking through the fields near Brussels, Louise was attacked by a bull and wounded in the side. Early Freudians would see in this event a reenactment of the Europa and the Bull myth, coinciding with the onset of menstruation. But the Victorian doctors, both Christians and atheists, saw it in a very different light. Christian commentators viewed this episode, especially Louise's lack of regard for the festering wound in her side, as a manifestation of her saintly selflessness. The materialistic doctors saw her wound as a shock to the nervous system and as an explanation for later recurrent outbreaks of bleeding from her side.

The accident brought Louise home to her mother. "Then came a period of sickness, borne with the most exemplary patience; never, even when tortured with racking pains, did she allow a moan to escape her lips," a Christian doctor wrote. Slowly the infected wound in her side healed, and she recovered enough to learn a new trade, sewing. With this skill she and her family, aided by a newfangled sewing machine, began to eke out a living.

In 1866 a cholera epidemic broke out in her village. In this time of woe Louise manifested her sainthood by caring for the sick and burying the dead, risking her life and health and driving herself to the point of nervous exhaustion. By early 1867 she "suffered from intense headaches and pains in the throat and from loss of appetite." By September she was on the verge of death and was administered the last sacraments. After a novena to the Virgin she suddenly awoke and declared that she would live. Soon she was healthy.

Three weeks later, however, she was again ill. She was now prostrated by new headaches, according to a Christian apologist, and by neuralgia in her arms and legs, according to the atheist

Bourneville. In January 1868, she spat up blood and once again verged on death. Her condition worsened into April, the time of Lent and Easter, and she was again administered the last sacraments. Once again she was restored to relative health, and the simple villagers, struck by the long suffering of the girl, were already beginning to think of her as truly a saint, worthy of admiration and emulation.

Then on April 24, 1868, a Friday, she experienced a return of the intense pain in her arms and legs and blood began to flow from her left side. She kept this secret, and the bleeding ceased. But by the first of May, the following Friday, the blood flowed again, and she sought the aid of the village priest. He made nothing of it, and the bleeding stopped by Saturday. On the following Friday she bled from the left side and also from both hands. A doctor was consulted, and he endeavored unsuccessfully to stop the bleeding. Meanwhile the priest had notified his bishop, who brought the Church authorities swooping down on Louise.

On Friday, August 28, an archbishop visited Louise at three o'clock in the afternoon at her cottage. He found her in an ecstasy, bleeding from both her hands. Hearing her name called, "she instantly recovered consciousness," a Catholic doctor wrote. "Finding herself in the presence of the archbishop, she was filled with confusion and, falling on her knees begged his grace's blessing. After a short conversation, [the archbishop] left the cottage and again she passed into an ecstasy."

The Church's authorities quickly established two commissions to investigate Louise. One was theological, its members priests and theologians, its chief endeavor to decide if the case were the work of God or the devil. The other was medical, headed by a doctor named Lefebvre of the Catholic University of Louvain. Its mission was to establish if these phenomena were attributable to nature or to God. Members of the two commissions examined, observed, and questioned Louise in great detail.

For a while Louise was tormented by the thought that she might be possessed by a devil. She even writhed and tumbled like one possessed. Happily, she was soon visited by a vision of Christ, who told her to be still. Afterward, when the priests were questioning her again, she surprised them with her equanimity. Asked about it, she told them of her beatific vision of Christ, and the priests

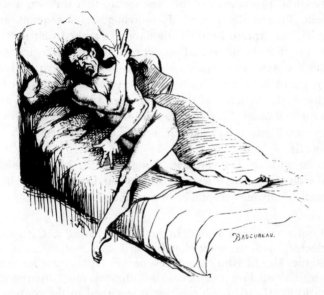

Passionate attitude: demonic attack. (From Désiré
Bourneville, *Louise Lateau, ou la Stigmatisée Belge*)

and theologians soon came to see her as a saint. From then on, all
her Fridays were ecstatic experiences. She had no more contortions
resembling possession.

The Catholic doctors saw no hysteria, no hereditary taint. No
fewer than a hundred physicians, they argued, had examined her
by 1875, and all had failed to make a definitive diagnosis of any
medical disease, thus leaving open an avenue for the religious to
proclaim her a saint. Mystified by the regularity of her Friday
bleeding, the Catholic doctors poked at the bleeding points in her
hands, her side, and her feet. They looked at the wounds under
microscopes and wrote that they had never seen anything like
it—skin that could break open so rapidly, bleed so freely, then
heal so quickly. They all scratched their heads, looked puzzled,
and said it was a miracle.

Meanwhile the Salpêtrists read the literature on the Belgian saint, looked about at their Genevièves, and Blanches, their own Louises, and proclaimed simply and firmly that this was a case of hysteria. Bourneville wrote, "Hemorrhages are frequent among hysterics," to explain Louise's stigmata. He argued that it was not surprising that the pious and poorly educated Belgian girl and the various ignorant villagers should sanctify this "sweat of blood." The pages of Bourneville's little book on Louise are cluttered with sketches of the hysterics of the Salpêtrière in their demonic attacks and crucified poses. Even her ecstasies were little more, in his eyes, than what Blanche had experienced when presented with colors and smells.

In the midst of her ecstasies, along with the bleeding and the crucifixion poses, there were periods when Louise passed beyond the reach of anyone except a bishop or one of his minions.

> Louise remained seated in her chair [wrote a Catholic doctor], inclined somewhat forward, and motionless as a statue. Her bleeding hands rest on her lap, her eyelids are motionless. Her countenance indicates rapt attention: dead to all earthly objects, she is absorbed in the contemplation which seems to hold her above the region of the earth . . . no spectacle can be more impressive than that which is now presented. The bleeding coronet on her forehead; the blood trickling down over her face and falling on her dress; her hands, the blood which is dripping on the floor where it lies in large patches; the circle of bystanders of every rank and condition grouped around, speechless from awe and wonder, and many of them weeping with emotion—all this combines to form a scene which irresistibly presses upon the beholder the conclusion that this is the work of God.

The commissioners had performed primitive experiments to test the authenticity of this ecstatic state. Doctor Lefebvre tickled the mucous membranes of her nostrils and her mouth with a feather: no response. He pricked her face with needles: no response. He applied liquid ammonia to her nostrils: still just ecstasy. It was only when the bishop or someone with ecclesiastical jurisdiction over her spoke to her—in French, German, Latin, or Hebrew, though she knew only French—that she responded. The commissioners had her bishop pass his jurisdiction from one person to another behind Louise's back, and she would only answer whoever had the jurisdiction and fail to notice those who did not. Catholic doctors discussed the idea of catalepsy and hysteria but dismissed these diagnoses. Miracle, they said. Miracle! Miracle! they cried.

Bourneville was intrepid in arguing that this ecstasy was a frequent phenomena in the Salpêtrière, that Louise belonged in the annals of medicine and not sainthood. He believed that every single aspect of the case could be seen in the confines of the Salpêtrière and in the realm of hysteria. Her anorexia was a hysterical symptom; her insomnia, her constipation, all the aberrations in the functioning of her body, he contended, he and his colleagues had seen in various patients in the Salpêtrière.

The Catholic doctors wrote that when she fell into an ecstasy, the scenes of Our Lord's life were enacted before her. "When she sees him kneel or fall, she is irresistibly compelled to do the same . . . when he is roughly handled, she is penetrated with horror." Bourneville responded to this by quoting the case of a patient named Lev, a hysteric, who likewise passed into ecstasies and afterward described apocalyptic visions including brilliant diamonds and stars in various colors. "Our Lord," said Lev, ". . . with long, curly chestnut-colored hair and a large red beard. He is beautiful, large and strong, enwrapped in gold. The Blessed Virgin is in silver."

The atheistic doctors generalized their diagnosis of hysteria into an antireligious polemic. If Louise Lateau was truly a hysteric par excellence, and the Salem and Loudon girls of the seventeenth century were just mentally ill, then religious phenomena in general were based simply on the ignorance and suggestibility of the Christian masses and on the churchmen's thirst for power. For ages the various Christian churches, intimately connected with royalist causes, had enjoyed great political privilege. However, with the secularization of society and the loss of much temporal power, the Christian churches had to turn to other techniques for keeping the gullible multitudes in tow. The focusing of so much attention on the poor hysterical Louise Lateau was an example, the materialist doctors argued, of how the Catholic Church still appealed to the miraculous to keep its flock on the straight and narrow.

While science was holding the Victorian citizenry in awe through its own miracles—the light bulb, the telegraph, the railways—and winning many over to a belief in logic, reason, and science, the religious forces had to retrench. One place in France became the focal point of the Church's attempt to convince the populace of the viability of religion. This place was Lourdes, the site of many miracle cures during the late nineteenth century and, in fact, up to our day.

The shrine of Lourdes, where many faith cures took place, was comparatively new in the late nineteenth century, dating from 1858, when Bernadette Soubirous, an illiterate and asthmatic peasant girl of fourteen, had visions of and conversations with the Blessed Virgin Mary on about eleven occasions. Her story, though wrapped in myth, is relatively simple.

Bernadette was born in 1844, the oldest child of an intensely religious Catholic family residing near the Pyrenees, cursed with hideous poverty. The Soubirous family lived in an old jailhouse belonging to some generous but distant relatives, because M. Soubirous was an incompetent businessman. Too softhearted with his customers, he could not get them to pay for the grain he milled. Of the nine children born to Mme. Soubirous only five would survive to the age of ten. Bernadette was stricken by cholera in 1855, suffered from chronic asthma and malnutrition, and deteriorated physically after reaching adolescence. Her delicate health compromised her physical activity.

In the middle of February 1858 Bernadette, one of her sisters, and a girl friend set off to find firewood in the countryside near Lourdes. Lagging behind because of her asthma, Bernadette heard the wind blowing even though the poplar trees in the vicinity were not swaying. She noticed the bending branches of a wild rose-bush near a grotto. Moving closer, she saw a wonderfully beautiful girl with an indescribable smile on her face, who was dressed in white and blue and had a rose pressed beneath each foot. She motioned to Bernadette to come closer. Blinking her eyes to make sure that she was not dreaming, Bernadette, overcome with reverence, knelt to say her rosary. When she finished, the beautiful girl disappeared.

Rumors of her vision spread all around the countryside, and the girl's mother forbade her to revisit the grotto. But Bernadette

was drawn back to the grotto by an inexplicable force. The vision
recurred, but this time the girl in white and blue spoke, and
Bernadette fell into an ecstasy. In this state she carried on conversations with the girl, who counseled penitence and prayer and
told a secret that Bernadette would never reveal. After having
many visions and conversations, the girl said that she was the
Immaculate Conception.

Soon a furor developed around Bernadette. The people of the
village and the surrounding countryside had been following her to
the grotto and watching her enter into trances; the authorities, both
religious and civil, were not sure what to make of all this. She was
interrogated by civil servants, castigated by priests, and slapped by
nuns, none of whom believed in the visions. Still, the girl in white
and blue returned, and the crowds, watching Bernadette in her
ecstasies, grew larger. A mass contagion was under way as nonbelievers were converted and newspapers recounted the story of
the visionary who saw what others could not. The weirdness of the
situation reached its culmination on February 5, 1858.

On that day Bernadette, in an ecstatic state, moved backward
on her knees out of the grotto, then forward on her feet searching
for something. In a trance state she bent down and scraped the
muddy soil with her hand. Reluctantly digging deeper, she soon
discovered some muddy water, which she drank. It seemed as
though the girl in white and blue had told her to drink the water
from a hidden spring, which Bernadette, in her ecstasy, had
quickly located. Some of her followers in the crowd soon dug
deeper. Seemingly miraculously, they discovered a gurgling spring,
whose water was soon bottled and drunk for its curative properties.

Before long, cures at Lourdes were reported and visionaries
multiplied. One girl plunged the paralyzed fingers of her right
hand into the spring and was cured. Five women carrying candles
passed into a crevice they saw in the grotto, searching for the girl
in white and blue. Emerging later, they claimed that they too
had seen her. The miraculous spring was channeled into a basin,
and soon pilgrims began coming to Lourdes seeking a cure for the
incurable.

Instructed by the Immaculate Conception to tell the Church
authorities of her desire to have the Lourdes grotto become a place

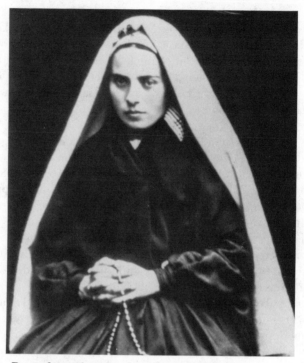

Bernadette shortly after the visions. (Studio Noël Viron, Lourdes)

of pilgrimage, Bernadette did just that. Then she slowly receded into the background, first to her parents' home, then to a nearby religious school, and finally, in 1866, to a nunnery at Nevers. Although believers and nonbelievers alike would flock there just to glimpse the visionary-saint, Bernadette hated being a celebrity and spent thirteen years as an invalid in her "white chapel," as she called her bed. Her asthma worsened; her appetite failed; she coughed up blood; she developed bed sores and became infected. In the spring of 1879, after a long agony, Bernadette died in an armchair beside her "white chapel," clutching a crucifix.

Though such doctors as Auguste Voisin at the Salpêtrière would call her a hallucinator and mentally ill, it was not the person of Bernadette on which medical attention centered from 1866 onward but rather Lourdes itself. By the 1890s Lourdes had become a massive shrine. Invalids flocked there by the trainload. The tiny little village in the Pyrenees became a religious tourist trap of the first order.

No one was surprised when the novelist Emile Zola was seen one fine August day in 1892 waiting in a queue to take the train to Lourdes. It was rumored that this naturalist author, this proclaimed enemy of religion, was collecting material for a new book entitled, simply, *Lourdes*. Zola intended his book as an antireligious polemic. He perceived Lourdes as a monument not to God but to the greed of the priests who ran it, and believed that the miracles performed there were only hoaxes.

Zola the good atheist was not moved after seeing one girl cured of pulmonary tuberculosis and another of ulcerated sores on her face, attributed to so-called trophic neurosis. Employing ghoulish naturalism, he described in *Lourdes* (1894) one of these cures, that of a paralyzed and disfigured woman named Marie Lemarchard. "At last the neckerchief fell aside. . . . Lupus [used here as a descriptive term meaning a discoloration or disfigurement of the face] had attacked the nose and mouth and gradually progressed there; an ulcer was slowly spreading under the crusts, eating into the mucous membrane. . . . The cartilages of the nose had been already eaten away, the mouth was inwards and twisted to the left by the swelling of the upper lip; and it resembled an oblique slit, repulsive and shapeless. And blood mixed with pus was oozing from the large, livid wound." Many doctors who examined Marie considered her to be suffering from a neurotic disorder, called a trophie neurosis. She had many of the Charcotian stigmata of hysteria, including paralysis and anesthesia as well as an unstable and overly emotional personality. Zola agreed with this diagnosis and especially stressed her emotionality. Following her from the train, Zola witnessed the paralyzed and disfigured girl surrounded by believing attendants, who lowered her into the miraculous body of water where the cures usually occurred. Marie soon leaped forth, her paralysis gone, and shouted, "I'm cured! I'm cured!" Moments later, her face was completely healthy save for some minuscule scars.

Zola sneered at the notion that she had been cured and called the whole event a hoax perpetrated by the priests from beginning to end. He argued that she was a hysteric who had lost her paralysis because of her suggestibility. He noted in his book that she became paralyzed again on the train ride back to Paris. Her face, however, remained healed.

Though the public really knew what to expect of Zola in his upcoming book, they still awaited *Lourdes* on pins and needles. Hence the *New Review*, a young literary journal in England, looked about for a prominent doctor to cast some light on the miracle of Lourdes on the eve of the publication. The journal found their man in Charcot, who took up the challenge in 1892.

In his article "Faith Healing" the aging Charcot admitted that he had seen numerous cases of faith healing. He wished to examine these cures as a scientist, so that he and other doctors might harness this faith healing for the sake of medicine. Basing his belief on his clinical observations, he dismissed the idea that the cures were hoaxes. Yet he also made it clear he thought that the miraculous-seeming phenomena were simply natural events. Supernatural explanation did not exist for Charcot. Perceiving scientific explanation as progressing year by year, he felt that the science of twenty years earlier—that is, 1870—was just beginning to investigate the influence of mind on the body. However, he believed that by 1890 science had thrown much light on the issue. He himself was beginning to see mind, or psyche, as distinct from spirit, and, therefore, psychology as separate from theology. With this separation in mind, he saw avenues of explanation that were scientific but not only materialistic.

In this article Charcot delineated a cluster of recurring conditions under which miracles have been known to occur. As he saw it, a miracle is a "natural phenomenon" produced "at all times, in the most different degrees of civilization and among the most various religions." Although he never broke away from his usual position that such miracles could occur only among hysterics, he nonetheless conceded that such miracles actually occurred.

When a hysteric is pronounced incurable, wrote Charcot, he nearly loses hope as the disease progresses. But then he hears vague and distant rumors of a shrine, a religious cult, or a miraculous tomb where miracles occur, where the lame are made to walk, and ulcers and cancers disappear in an instant. He begins to hope, and so he prepares for the journey. It is a long and arduous one. Money, food, companions are collected. Rumors of cures grow louder as he boards the train, the cart, or the coach bearing him toward the shrine.

The shrine itself proves a wondrous place. The sufferer falls in with others seeking cures. A cluster of doctor-priests, aided by a curious class of persons called intercessors, who are usually women, examine the sufferers. Usually looming in the shadows of the shrine is the figure of a beneficent being, a Saint Francis, a Saint Theresa, or a Saint Bernadette. A period of penance follows, of praying and waiting. The shrine is adorned with votive tablets, sculptured forms representing arms, legs, necks, and breasts, and the discarded crutches of those cured by past miracles. The faith in a cure grows stronger, becoming a force in its own right, a vital force, a fixed idea. Ultimately the sufferer is lowered into a body of water. The idea, nurtured on every side, incubating for days, for weeks, springs to life as the sufferer approaches the water, and the mind heals the body.

While spelling out this age-old outline of events leading to miracles and of circumstances surrounding the faith cure, Charcot continued to shout that they were due to hysteria and only hysteria. In fact he was defining more than just hysteria. The Master was doing an interesting bit of sociological and psychological work. He was approaching the idea of symbols and rituals. He is speaking of recurring patterns in human thought and behavior far beyond his notion of hysteria in the seventies and eighties. Specifically, he was making it clear that the strength, the energy, the vitality of the healing idea exists not in the mind of the doctor, not in his magnetic personality, his animal magnetism, or his brilliance, but rather in the mind, however humble, of the patient.

This concept was part of a magnificent progression on Charcot's part. He started with the Zeus myth, which located the etiological moment of neurosis in a shock in the environment—in the bolt of lightning that nearly struck the man walking toward Paris, or in M. C.'s rape of Louise, or in the shock of the railway on the patients' nerves—and then connected this shock with an idea of fright in the patient. This is what Charcot called autosuggestion: a terrifying idea of injury, of death, that grew in the mind and played a role in the development of the hysterical symptom.

In his analysis of faith healing Charcot progressed even further.

Mapping out the healing ambience, the crutches, the doctor-priests, the body of water, all the accouterments that helped incubate in the patient the idea of healing, Charcot attributed the sudden and miraculous-seeming cure to a second autosuggestion. As the sufferer was lowered into the water the idea of being cured coalesced and mind affected body.

Charcot saw in faith healing a mighty force that he wished doctors could somehow understand, without compromising themselves as scientists, and harness for humanity. He thus shifted his attention away from materialistic modes of explanation—the neurotic as hereditarily tainted in his brain—to more psychological levels of understanding—the neurotic as undergoing painful emotional experiences. Though he himself never lived to follow out the intellectual progression of this subtle but momentous shift announced in his faith-healing paper, younger medical men were quick to perceive the crucial nature of Charcot's elusive thinking and follow his lead.

One such doctor was William James. Having studied in many medical centers in Europe, including Paris, James grasped many of the tiny threads of Charcot's thought and moved forward in important new directions. Yet it is not only James the doctor and psychiatrist but James the nerve sufferer who played an important role in this progression. His own personal troubles became central to his psychological thinking. His confusion over his own career—painter, doctor, psychologist, or philosopher—epitomized the confusion of an individual trying to make sense of a world without order or purpose. *The Varieties of Religious Experience* makes his neurotic suffering universal.

Early in life James faced a painful dilemma. He possessed both scientific and artistic abilities and was in a dilemma over which career was better for him. While his father favored science, he originally favored art, and in 1858, aged eighteen, he joined an artist's studio. After a year and a half of painting—and indeed he showed talent—William developed eye weakness and indigestion. These symptoms, later diagnosed as neurasthenia, kept him from serving in the Civil War and forced him to give up painting as well. In 1861 he made the decision to take up a scientific career and so went off to Harvard.

He continued, however, to be plagued with eye weakness and

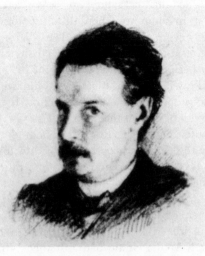

William James, doctor, psychologist,
nerve patient. Self-portrait. (From
F. O. Matthiessen, *The James Family*)

indigestion, as well as backaches, general weakness, and depression. In 1863 he enrolled at the Harvard medical school but interrupted his program in 1865 and again in 1867. Traveling to Europe, he frequented spas in Bohemia and France but also continued his medical studies, now in psychology and the nervous system, in Berlin.

In 1870 he seems to have undergone a kind of religious experience. While studying at the Salpêtrière in Paris he encountered a highly disturbing patient—a green-skinned idiot—with whom he apparently identified. He feared that very little separated him from becoming just like this man. Given the reigning Degenerate, Prometheus, and Onan myths, such a fear seemed well grounded. Alcohol, masturbation, overwork, so much in life seemed likely to touch off neurosis. As part of his personal upheaval and insight James reached the conclusion that the state of his mind very much influenced the state of his body. This elusive connection played a significant role in his later decision to become a psychologist. Only his own will seemed to hold him back from nervous dissolution, his own will to believe. He forged ahead with his career.

In 1871 he finished medical school and was given a teaching post at Harvard, first in anatomy, then in physiology, and later in psychology. He never really practiced medicine, but he read widely in the literature on neurosis. His conviction that mind influenced body became the underpinning of his growing interest in psychology. This idea contradicted the thinking of Lombroso, Nordau, and the proponents of the Degenerate myth, who stressed the inevitability of brain derangements. Though James the man continued to suffer nagging pains, emotional despondency, and lassitude, James the thinker progressed steadily toward a view of mind and body as equal and commingling in a pluralistic universe cluttered with meanings and uncertainties.

James had no love life until he was thirty-four years old. Then one day his father, while attending a club meeting, met a young woman named Alice Gibbens and was so taken by her that he came home to tell Will that he had just met Will's future wife. Once given parental permission to have a sensual life, James met and married Alice. He went on to father four sons and one daughter, and wrote highly successful books on philosophy, psychology, and religion.

However, James remained a nerve sufferer, with endless prostrations, depressions, and back and eye aches. These nagging symptoms, which were never cured by his many trips to the spas of Europe, pushed him in the direction of psychic studies. He had originally been interested in mediums and Christian Science healers, not only as a scientist but also as a patient seeking relief from his symptoms. Vibrant in the classroom, an innovative teacher, he remained hypochondriacal, neurotic, and depressed in private life, though he was given at least some relief by the faith healers.

Out of his own personal turmoil as well as from the growing intellectual struggle between agnostics, atheists, and materialists on the one hand and spiritualists and religious believers on the other, James began collecting a number of case studies of common men and women who had had psychic experiences. Automatic writing, séances, and religious experiences interested him most keenly. From these interests he spun *The Varieties*.

Arguing in a much more balanced manner than Lombroso or Nordau, Krafft-Ebing or Bourneville or even Charcot, James captured in *The Varieties* the two sides of the dilemma of religious experience, dispassionately and sympathetically extending the idea in more humanistic directions. Like his friends Pierre Janet and Frederic Myers, James was essentially a psychologist with very strong intellectual roots in philosophy as well as a religious life of his own. Hence he drew his more temperate picture of religious and emotional experiences as stemming not only from neurological upset but also from individual psychology.

Like all the medical and psychological writers of the day, James began his book with a chapter entitled "Religion and Neurology," in which he presented the familiar theory that religious figures such as Christ, Mohammed, and Buddha were all really neurotics, hereditarily determined religious geniuses. They suffered from an odd commingling of nervous instability and superior intellect. "Often," he wrote, "they have led a discordant inner life, and had been melancholy during a part of their career. They have . . . been liable to obsessions and fixed ideas; and frequently they have fallen into trances, heard voices, seen visions, and presented all sorts of peculiarities which are ordinarily classed as pathological." Up to this point James's argument does not vary from that of Moreau, Lombroso, Charcot, or any of the other medical materialists of the age.

However, James took his argument in a very different, in fact an opposite direction. He was willing to admit the reality of mental and nervous illness in "religious geniuses," to see many saints— notably ascetics—as very ill and even perverse individuals. But he took the offensive against Lombroso et al. by stating, "We are surely familiar in a general way with this method of discrediting states of mind for which we have an antipathy . . . medical materialism seems indeed a good appellation for the too simpleminded system of thought we are considering. Medical materialism finishes up St. Paul by calling his vision on the road to Damascus a discharging lesion of the occipital cortex, he being an epileptic. It snuffs out St. Theresa [of Avila] as an hysteric, St. Francis of Assisi as an hereditary degenerate." Once the medical materialists had labeled the religious figure, they usually felt they had won the day, that any religious experiences must necessarily derive from illness. Though James agreed that many of these figures were mentally ill, he still saw it as important, meaningful, critical to listen to what they were saying and take it seriously.

He suggested that the psychologist must "judge the religious life by its results exclusively, and I shall assume that the bugaboo of morbid origin will scandalize your piety no more."

James launched into the study of religious experience armed with a reverence for personal religion. The bulk of his book described the religious experiences of many men and women, some geniuses, some ordinary men. What characterized so many of these cases were moments of disembodiment, of hallucinatory experiences, of dreamy times when the religious individual verged on touching, seeing, or feeling God or some other power. As Krafft-Ebing did with homosexuality, James collected little confessions from various religious individuals. These he mingled with biographical sketches of famous persons. He set out to argue that the unseen world is real, that it is connected with the world of the subconscious or the subliminal (two words coined by James's two friends Janet and Myers, respectively), and finally that the experiences of religious conversion, sainthood, and mysticism are all part of this vast and very real world of the subconscious or subliminal, which is the domain of the medical psychologist.

James admitted that the person who has had religious experiences is probably in the minority. He described a cluster of movements in nineteenth-century America and Europe, to which he gave the glib name of the Religion of Healthy-Mindedness, as appealing to the vast segments of the Western world that see mental sickness in religious experience. Citing the ideas of social evolution and technological progress as the cornerstones of this healthy-minded religion, he spoke of the advance of liberalism as leading to the casting aside of the more morbid "old hell fire theology." He constructed an imaginary interview with one of these "coarse-meated," health-minded Philistine individuals, which reads like this:

Question: What does religion mean to you?
  Answer: It means nothing; and it seems so far as I can observe, useless to others . . . the God-idea was begotten in ignorance, fear and a general lack of any knowledge of Nature . . .
Question: What comes before your mind corresponding to the words God, Heaven, Angels, etc.?

    Answer: Nothing whatever. I am a man without religion.
These words mean so much mystic bosh.
    Question: Have you had any experiences which appear provi-
dential?
    Answer: None whatsoever . . . a little judicious observation as
well as knowledge of scientific law will convince anyone of that fact . . .

This healthy-minded individual represented not only most Philis-
tines but also most late-nineteenth-century Westerners.

Rather than looking at the world through the eyes of these
mentally healthy, modern individuals, James attempted to come
to grips with a more foreign, frightening, and "sick" view of the
world, in which the evil aspects are the very essence of our life and
"the world's meaning most comes home to us when we lay them
most at heart." James saw those who have religious experiences as
Sick Souls, constitutionally depressed and more sensitive to pain,
more acutely aware of misery. He argued that the "sanguine,
healthy-minded" individual lives on the "sunnyside of the misery
line," while the "depressed and melancholic," those prone to religious experiences, live beyond it, "in darkness and apprehension." His argument was essentially based on heredity, seeing the
healthy-minded person as born with "a bottle or two of champagne to his credit," while the depressive type is born stone sober.
Life's hard experiences could deplete our "animal toughness" and
lead to a "little irritable weakness and descent of the pain thresh-
old," which "brings the worm at the core of all of our usual springs
of delight into full view, and turns us into melancholy metaphy-
sicians."

James described two men as exemplifying the hereditarily
cursed modern man: his contemporary, Leo Tolstoi, and . . . himself! Although he disguised his own confession as that of a young
Frenchman, the biographers of both William and Alice James
suspect that the second Sick Soul is really the morbid Will James.

Tolstoi had long been tormented with painful melancholy.
"Behold me then," wrote the Russian, whom James quoted, "a
man happy and in good health, hiding the rope in order not to
hang myself to the rafters of my house where every night I went to
sleep alone; behold me no longer going shooting lest I should

yield to the too easy temptation of putting an end to myself with my gun."

James wrote of himself in the following manner:

> Whilst in this state of philosophical pessimism . . . I went one evening into a dressing room to procure some article . . . Simultaneously there arose in my mind the image of an epileptic patient whom I had seen in the asylum, a black haired youth with greenish skin, entirely idiotic, who used to sit all day on one of the benches . . . He sat there like a sort of sculptured Egyptian cat or Peruvian mummy, moving nothing but his black eyes and looking absolutely non-human. This image and my fear entered into a species of combination with each other. *That shape am I*, I felt, potentially.

Both religious sufferers—James and Tolstoi—struggled with melancholy, the sense of impossible-to-articulate wretchedness. Behind their every movement there crouched a mockery of their lives. Tolstoi represented well the civilized human being—surrounded by his material possessions, his wife, his properties, his modern conveniences—who lacked a larger purpose. The black-haired idiot with whom James identified left him trembling to the very core of his being, since so little separated him from this idiot in an asylum. The religious and philosophical doubts of these two men plunged them into deep despondency. They had to admit to themselves that more optimistic world views, based on either religious or scientific certainty, seemed challenged by the exigencies of the real world. Poverty, cruel illnesses, and utter despair were everywhere. Their souls were haunted by recriminations, dreads, morbid scruples, and irrational impulses. An utter night of the soul reigned.

What is remarkable about the Jamesian idea of religious experience is precisely how modern-sounding it is. In fact, the title of James's book, *The Varieties of Religious Experience*, is in many ways misleading. The book actually concerns a specific neurotic type in the Victorian period, the Religious Self-Tormentor, who parallels the person suffering from an identity crisis in the late twentieth century. The nineteenth-century neurosis was dressed in the garments of moral scruples, whereas the modern dress is more existential and philosophical. This neurosis mingled the age-old religious ideas of asceticism, purity, strength of soul, and charity. The Religious Self-Tormentor struggled to reform his religious and moral convictions on a higher plane. This was precisely the struggle that such men as George Beard, Max Nordau, and so many other doctors themselves underwent. Much of the struggle took place subliminally or subconsciously, James believed, and the act of religious conversion—when Saint Paul fell from the horse; when one troubled young Englishman felt another presence, supposedly God, in his bedroom and gained religious faith; when a tormented French Jew had a vision of the Blessed Virgin in a Catholic church—took place in a magical moment when the different levels of the self converged and broke through from the subconscious and a higher vision was apparently reached.

Although the more dramatic forms of this religious conversion experience occurred in the nervously unstable, the suggestible, the emotionally sensitive, James thought it had a more universal, less pathological significance. The experience of the religious genius, the nervously unstable person, was only a more dramatic form of a crisis that all truly sincere and serious men and women faced in their lives.

To be sure, James believed that the excesses and fanaticism of some "saints," notably the Catholic ones, were indeed morbid and pathological. "Francis of Assisi kisses his lepers," writes James. "Mary Margaret Alacoque, Francis Xavier, St. John of God, and others are said to have cleansed the sores and ulcers of their patients with their respective tongues; and the lives of such saints as Elizabeth of Hungary and Madame de Chantal are full of a sort of revelling in hospital prurience disagreeable to read of, and which makes us admire and shudder at the same time." James makes his readers admire and shudder when he tells of his near-contemporary Saint John Vianney, who imposed on himself the dicta that "he should never smell a flower, never drink when parched with thirst, never drive away a fly." Also, James described the "psychopathic" fourteenth-century German mystic Henry Suso, who "secretly caused an undergarment to be made for him . . . into which a hundred and fifty brass nails, pointed and filed sharp, were driven, and the points of the nails were always turned toward the flesh . . . Suso next tells of his penitences by means of striking [a cross placed against his chest in order to force] the nails deeper into his flesh." To James, the Catholic saint of medieval vintage, such as Bernadette or Louise Lateau, was no longer worthy of emulation, but was rather to be feared, since she was mentally sick.

"A strange moral transformation," he wrote, "has within the past century swept over our Western world . . . It is not expected of a man that he should either endure or inflict [physical pain], and to listen to the recital of cases of it makes our flesh creep morally as well as physically." Even the Catholic writers, wrote James, have to admit resignedly that times have changed and that self-flagellating sainthood in the fifteenth century is the masochism in the late nineteenth century. Krafft-Ebing and he would have to agree.

But James argued from a highly complicated and sometimes shifting point of view about religion. He constructed a richly embroidered and multidimensional world that included mental turmoil, an internal division of the self, and ultimately the great moment of religious conversion, when the turmoil mounted to a higher level. This was the experience of many common men and women of the nineteenth century, believed James. Reared in a simple world of religious certainty, the Victorians saw their convictions shattered by a pluralistic world of materialism, capitalism, and militarism. The scientific perspective seemed intellectually and emotionally satisfying only to a point. The Victorian neurotic, who still carried along his religious baggage, found himself mired in a spiritual crisis. Growing despondent, he might become neurasthenic, depressed, or at least morose, brooding. He passed into adulthood only when the religious conversion experience culminated in a new direction, religious or otherwise. Only then could he become whole again.

The religious convert could then move forward into a religious life, the capitalist into the marketplace, the Aspiring Aesthete into an artist's studio or a writer's garret, and the doctor into the world of scientific medicine. All of these career choices grew, James believed, out of a similar moral struggle. The conversion to scientific atheism, to Nietzscheism, to the muscular Christianity of people such as Dr. Livingstone and Robert Browning, were all results of this Victorian experience of religious conversion. While Lombroso saw religion in many ways as either an atavism or an anachronism, James saw the solemn and reverential nature of religion, the need for breathing room for the subjective experiences of the individual, as living concerns.

Probably more than any of the practicing doctors of "neurotic science" heretofore discussed, James presented the conversion experience and the world of nerves and nervous sufferers in a subtle, subjective, and dynamic manner. Yet despite his stature and persuasiveness, Lombroso, Bourneville, and many religiously doubting doctors remained adamant materialists. At least part of the materialists' strength lay in the observation that many of those who had religious conversion experiences did not act with more maturity afterward but in fact became embroiled in meaningless fanaticism. These rational doctors believed in the neurosis of Louise Lateau and Bernadette of Lourdes, seeing morbid religiosity in their ecstasies and weird visions. They also could not bring themselves to look very carefully at the experiences of religiously tormented persons, since these Saintly Fools seemed so sick. The subjective experiences of which James was speaking seemed to be just the end products of brain centers and reflexes, of electricity and biochemicals. Hence the value of all religious turmoil could be dismissed. The revolution of empathy was stymied. The movement in science and medicine away from religion left many intelligent Westerners progressively less able to believe in the old religious stystems and more prone to perceiving those who did as distasteful, ludicrous, even pitiful.

But a deeper respect was growing for the subjective, the personal, the psychological. Charcot's later work on faith healing and James's book represented this more psychological trend. Severed from the roots of any specific religion, this movement among doctors and in society at large tended to examine more diligently the scruples, the painful thoughts, the self-loathing of Religious Self-Tormentors, and the symbolism of the patron saint, the shrine, the prayer, for persons cured by faith. In placing less emphasis on the brain and giving new credence to personal emotions, ideas, and symbols, a few doctors inched toward a much more subtle comprehension of how to listen to human sufferers, how to feel compassion for their symptoms, how to confront their pain.

TWELVE

Private Lives

W*HEN* Victorian doctors did listen to their patients, they often heard about their love lives. Krafft-Ebing's homosexuals and Charcot's hysterics suffered from a slow and unsettling debate in their heart of hearts about their own sexual escapades. Many of Beard's neurasthenics were worried about their nocturnal emissions, their onanism, their masturbatory fantasies. Mitchell's and Playfair's invalids were worn down by childbirth and deserted by menfolk or were pining away in meaningless spinsterhood. Am I saint or sinner? Geneviève and Louise asked themselves and their doctors in the Salpêtrière. Am I sinner or neurotic? Krafft-Ebing's patients asked. Is my neurasthenia caused by my onanism? My sexual fantasies? Did this villain of a man bring about my hysterical pregnancies? Doctors hoped to answer these questions for their patients.

Sex and love in the late Victorian period possessed a rich complexity. On the one hand, high-minded and prudish attitudes toward sexuality really did prevail among the middle classes, the bourgeoisie. On the other hand, the Paris of Marcel Proust circa 1895, the London of Oscar Wilde, the Vienna of Krafft-Ebing were vibrant worlds in which promiscuity, sodomy, lesbianism, and prostitution seemed everyday affairs. Between these two worlds lay a balance the Victorians called moral health.

This was a delicate balance that could be tipped by a whisper.

Proust's father's book on neurasthenia counseled the parent to keep quiet about sexuality when dealing with the suggestible child. Krafft-Ebing and many other doctors attributed many of the problems of sexuality to popular literature, which implanted wicked ideas in the heads of young ones. Bernheim discussed Dr. X, an evil doctor who hypnotized a poor delicate woman into having an illicit affair with him. Many doctors seemed to counsel a steadying marriage and a solid career as a way of getting over self-doubt, sexual obsessions, and morbid thoughts. Anxiety about sexuality centered on the question of whether certain persons, notably women and children, should be exposed to it at all or whether it should be whispered about behind their backs. The conclusion often was that once the suggestible one was introduced to licentiousness and debauchery, he or she was only too ready to plummet into the pits of profligacy and remain there forever.

The struggle to prevent such a downfall was waged on many levels in late Victorian times. The Norse gods and mythical figures of Wagner's operas were victims of unbridled excess and immoral passions on the German stage, stimulating and intriguing the Aspiring Aesthetes. Such libido and aggression, Nordau feared, might suggest that the bonds of marriage could be broken very readily. Phaedre was overcome with passion for her husband's son on the Paris stage, and fathers such as Marcel's feared that a like idea, implanted in the sensitive heads of their offspring, could lead to passionate fantasies strong enough to ruin them. In the family the picture presented was that of strict parents versus demurely obedient or rebelliously defiant children. In the individual a battle ensued between the painful sense of duty to parents and to society and the desire to feel satisfied in life. The intense struggle of licentiousness versus morality, unbridled sexuality versus will power, played itself out in the private lives of many Victorians.

One entrée into the private lives of the Victorians, their love lives and their attitudes toward romance, can be found in the literature of the period. Madame Bovary, for instance, married a silly old apothecary for security, then chased vainly after happiness with dashing men. Her life ended in a desperate suicide. Tolstoi's Anna Karenina cast off her drab Russian husband and ran away to western Europe with a gallant viscount. Still, she was racked with confusion and desperation and finally flung herself in front of a train. This tension between love and romance on the one hand and duty and society on the other hand appears in many, many pieces of Victorian literature.

Though a study of Victorian literature is truly revealing of the prevailing ideas about love and sex, it is hard to separate the lives and attitudes of the authors from the travails of their troubled characters. Gustave Flaubert and Tolstoi possessed very strong, rather eccentric points of view, thereby making it difficult to generalize from their works. It seems less inherently confusing to describe the private lives of some flesh-and-blood Victorians. Women's lives seem especially apropos, since Victorian men often perceived them in a complex manner that led to painful conflicts concerning love. Love played a central part in women's vulnerability to "nerves," to the various Victorian neuroses. Men invariably saw women as weaker, more ignorant, childlike, but also as angelic, inspirational, asexual.

Sexuality and duty, societal mores and personal interests conflicted in the lives of a number of eminent Victorian women: George Sand, a shocking figure whose sexual promiscuity and cross-dressing—as well as her famous novels—won her the diagnosis of neurotic genius from Lombroso; Elizabeth Barrett Browning, the wife of Robert Browning, for many years a bed case, to use Mitchell's term, but also a Lombrosian genius; Elizabeth Siddal, the model and wife of Dante Gabriel Rossetti, a victim of anorexia, headaches, general depression, and suicide; George Eliot, a neurasthenic according to Beard, a genius according to Lombroso; and Alice James, the younger sister of Henry and William, another bed patient, unsuccessfully treated by a group of Victorian doctors. All five of these women were neurotics in one or more of the ways the Victorians used the term. Each struggled with her sense of duty to parents or society and the Victorian ideals of women as innocent, ignorant, and childlike.

Perhaps the most notorious woman in the nineteenth century was George Sand, who loomed as the perfect antithesis to Victorian womanhood. She was the sinner triumphant, the genius who broke the bonds of women's duty to home and hearth and never seemed to pay for it. Born in 1804 to a father who was an illegitimate member of an ancient noble family and a mother who was a camp follower and prostitute of the French Army of the

Revolution, George Sand was originally named Aurore Dupin. She inherited the pride and intellectual curiosity as well as the lust for experience of her forebears. She read avidly and loved to go hunting in men's garb from an early age. She was high-spirited and adventurous even as a child. After her father's sudden death and her mother's return to the life of a prostitute in Paris, little Aurore was left in the province of Berry with her noble grandmother. The elderly woman sent her to a convent, where she received her formal education. Though she contemplated becoming a nun, her grandmother yanked her back to Berry to be wed. Because she was a wealthy heiress, a great marriage seemed her only choice in life, aside from the nunnery or suicide.

As the years passed, the spirited young girl continued her wide reading and so came under the sway of the Romantics, notably Rousseau and Chateaubriand. She began to doubt her Catholicism. When her grandmother became very ill and lay dying, Aurore sat nursing her, reading Byron's *Lara* and Chateaubriand's *René*.

When her grandmother died, her hated mother reappeared and whisked her off to Paris. Soon, out of desperation but also—or so she believed at the time—motivated by a passionate, romantic love, she married a gentleman named Casimir Dudevant. Like a good Romantic, she wanted to share everything with him. Books, music, art, all that quickened her heart and sent her into reveries and ecstasies she bestowed on Casimir. But she found too late that all fell dead on the thick skull of her husband. He preferred drinking, riding to hounds, and playing card games. Within a year or so after her marriage, following the birth of a son, Maurice, Aurore grew despondent. Finding that her idea of love, culled from various romantic books, was unfulfilled in marriage, she began to experience headaches, palpitations, and a cough.

These neurotic symptoms seemed common to women in the nineteenth century who felt trapped in marriages or in families. The stories of such women frequently ended at this point. The bed patients lay suffering and moaning and aching for years and eventually died. However, there was something exceptional about this spirited French girl. Though for a while she believed herself to be a consumptive, and even went on a religious retreat at the suggestion of her confessor, she found a way out of her misery.

Shortly after her disillusionment with Casimir she met another man, Aurélien de Sèze, with whom she had a platonic relationship. Although Casimir was jealous and at first forbade this friendship, she convinced him of its importance, and she and Aurélien wrote letters and saw each other. Casimir soon retreated into the background, fornicating with a servant girl, with Aurore's approval. The young wife grew intellectually bolder during the next few years and became well known and well liked in artistic and literary circles in Berry.

Fond of dressing in men's clothes since childhood, Aurore continued this practice as her intellectual and personal spheres widened. Now in her middle twenties, she had loosened the ties to her drunken husband so thoroughly that when the Revolution of 1830 broke out she deserted him and fled to Paris to become involved in the upheaval. "Life," she wrote from Paris, "is as gay among bayonets, rioting and rabble as it would be in the piping days of peace."

In Paris she fell head over heels in love with Jules Sandeau, a frail and sensitive poet. They boldly lived openly as lovers in Paris and together began writing a novel, *Blanche and Rose*, about two women, one an artist, the other a nun. From then on, the life of George Sand—her pen name—is devoid of any physical nervous symptoms, except perhaps attacks of dyspepsia, which sometimes kept her in bed late in the morning. She had no more fear of consumption, headaches, or palpitations, no more fits of weeping, no more religious retreats. Lombroso, who pored over her autobiography looking for neurotic symptoms, was forced to admit that though she had been prone to bouts of melancholy, she was not nervous. Perceiving her own feelings and desires as the ultimate concern, she cared little about societal mores. As long as she was true to herself, she felt she possessed integrity. Jaunting around Paris in a top hat and a black coat, smoking cigars, George Sand was notorious from then on, ostracized by polite society, yet very important to the intellectual and artistic community of Paris.

She soon fell out of love with Sandeau, whom she found aimless and lazy. Though she suffered from a deep melancholy when she left him, she was soon having minor affairs, a veritable female Don Juan. By one lover, Stéphane de Grandsagne, an aging tubercular, she had a daughter, Solange. Between affairs she sometimes contemplated suicide or reconsidered going into a cloister, but she always found another lover around the corner.

Her greatest love after Sandeau was the dazzling and handsome romantic poet Alfred de Musset. Meeting in the spring of 1833 at a great literary dinner given by an editor, the two were immediately struck with each other's charms, physical and spiritual. Soon they were gallivanting around Paris, a notorious couple, envied and adulated. As their intimacy deepened, Musset found that the hidden side of the splashy Sand was a cold and priggish woman. At the same time, Sand realized that behind Alfred's suave élan there lay a frail, self-pitying and uncertain man. Nonetheless, in December 1833, the celebrated lovers decided to travel to romantic Venice, where Sand hoped to experience some secret revelation. Once there the ebullient poet was quickly beaten in a brawl and fell into a deranged state of mind caused by a brain fever (either mental illness or typhus). He was delirious and hallucinating. Sand summoned a doctor named Pagello, with whom she sat at Musset's bedside. Before long she had fallen in love with Pagello and had taken him to her bed. When Musset regained his wits, he saw what had happened and ran back to Paris alone.

Sand followed, leaving the doctor behind. She and Alfred were reunited for a while. Soon, however, she tumbled into bed with other men. Always believing herself true to her own feelings, she never was a victim of moral scruples, fears, obsessions, self-doubts of any depth. Though occasionally melancholic, she always regained her equilibrium by returning to her estate at Berry. There she could write, see her two children, Maurice and Solange, enjoy the beauty of the countryside, and feel self-assured. She wrote prolifically and carried on many minor affairs. The years 1834 to 1837 proved to be but a prelude to her most celebrated, most tumultuous, yet most enduring love, that for Frédéric Chopin.

The great composer and the woman of letters met in 1837. Introduced through mutual friends—Franz Liszt and Marie d'Agoult, two lovers whose affair was notorious (she had deserted her nobleman husband to run off with him)—Chopin and Sand soon were madly in love. She swooned and felt joyous palpitations whenever he played. She loved to crawl under his piano and lose her being in the resonating chords as he played. He, like so many other men, could not resist this beautiful rebel in men's clothes. Though Chopin still suffered from being scorned by a beautiful Catholic virgin back in his homeland, Poland, he tarried for years with the shocking Sand. They were so enthralled with each other that they decided to run off to Majorca. There a pattern threatened to repeat itself when Chopin fell desperately ill and Sand had to nurse him. Spitting up blood, temperamental, sensitive to the slightest noise, he was an insufferable invalid. However, instead of taking up with a doctor, Sand found great comfort in nursing him. Calling him her third child, she brought the consumptive composer back to Berry to live with her.

Though Chopin proved too delicate and weak for sexual intimacy, the two lived together for nearly a decade. Wintering in Paris, summering in Berry, he wrote brilliant musical scores and she fine pieces of fiction. Still, many things began to come between them. Their political perspectives were at loggerheads; he was an inveterate monarchist, she a republican and liberal. Also, he and she began to quarrel and intrigue with each other and with her children. Whereas George was encouraging her son Maurice in his romance with a penniless female cousin named Augustine, Chopin saw this attachment as shocking and ill-advised and so sided with her daughter Solange, who was herself just jealous of Augustine. Chopin also backed Solange in her desire to marry a local aristocrat, whom George judged to be tedious and boorish, another Casimir Dudevant. There also simmered a mutual jealousy between the two males in the life of Sand, Chopin and her son, Maurice. In 1846 Chopin departed from Berry on strained terms with Sand. They both seemed to want a reconciliation, but Chopin was never to see her again. His consumption worsened in London, and the lonely composer died in great misery many miles from his companion.

By now over forty, Sand settled down emotionally. Closely involved in the Revolution of 1848 and deeply disappointed by its outcome—the Second Empire—she remained connected intellectually, emotionally, or sexually with nearly everyone of any importance in artistic France until her death three decades later in 1878. She was an incredibly vivacious woman throughout her long and healthy life.

What is so astonishing about George Sand was her ability to

take the old ideas of what is masculine and what is feminine and turn them on their heads. All four of the important men in her life—Casimir, Sandeau, Musset, and Chopin—were inferior to her, either intellectually or physically. She came to see Casimir as a fraud, Sandeau as a lazy ne'er-do-well. She sadistically reversed roles with Musset by having an affair while he was sick. She treated Chopin like a child in the very years when her children were maturing. She led an adventurous life, casting off organized religion, social norms, and male-female stereotypes. Through this superhuman effort she could live essentially free of neurosis. She played out in real life the adventures of such fictional women as Anna Karenina and Madame Bovary. But instead of paying for her sins, she seemed to thrive, winning great influence and acclaim. Though she was a degenerate genius to Lombroso, her life was an attractive one.

Sand's life was clearly not open to most women. Elizabeth Barrett Browning, Elizabeth Siddal Rossetti, George Eliot, and especially Alice James all suffered debilitating nervosity. Even though they all possessed exceptional talents, they struggled to reconcile themselves with Victorian ideas of duty.

Elizabeth Barrett was a highly interesting invalid whose poetry illustrates the painful admixture of the desire to be rebellious and the need to remain a Victorian woman. Though sentimental, her poetry also possesses a serious moral fiber that is preeminently Victorian. Her epic poem *Aurora Leigh* was said to have been read by many blossoming British and American maidens under their bedclothes, but the rebellion of Aurora Leigh smacks of English duty and tradition, hardly warranting the term "rebellion" when compared with George Sand's deeds. In her *Sonnets from the Portuguese* the central figures are King Cophetua and the Beggar Maid, two stark Victorian figures from an Alfred Tennyson poem. The king idolizes the maid but still remains the one in charge. Elizabeth's life with Robert Browning in many ways embodied this poetic vision. Her romantic death of consumption only deepens the glamour of her life, maladies, and works.

Born in 1809 to Edward and Mary Moulton Barrett, Elizabeth, the oldest of eleven children, lived an exceedingly sheltered life. Her mother died in 1829, leaving Mr. Barrett a widower and Elizabeth seemingly destined to be a spinster who would care for

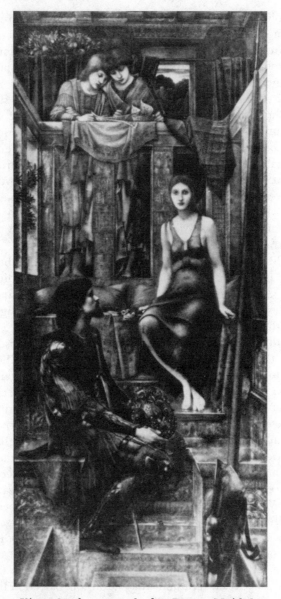

King Cophetua and the Beggar-Maid by
Edward Burne-Jones, or woman on a pedestal. (The Tate Gallery, London)

him forever. Her father proved to be an old-fashioned parent who chose to shelter his children from the cares of the world. For instance, even though he was nearly ruined in the 1830s when the slaves were freed in Jamaica, where he had sunk a fortune into sugar plantations, Mr. Barrett kept all his financial worries hidden from his children. He tried to create a pastoral retreat in a country house in the south of England. Here Elizabeth enjoyed an extended childhood, dreamily looking out at an immense garden through the stained-glass windows in her room. In exchange for this sequestered life her father demanded strict obedience. Obeying him as best she could, Elizabeth grew deeply involved in contemplation and reading.

She proved to be a child prodigy, learning Latin and Greek by the time she was eight, and publishing her first poem when she was fifteen. She also suffered from backaches. Ripening into a delicate woman with an appealing face and dark curls falling to her shoulders, she left her dream world when her family moved to London in 1835. Elizabeth was twenty-six when they settled on Wimpole Street. Though the shy and wan girl was introduced into London literary society because of her literary genius, her contacts were few, since her father seemed not to want his daughters to meet men or even have many friends, let alone marry. Soon Elizabeth sank into chronic invalidism and was told by consulting doctors to avoid all stimulation, including reading. She withdrew into her room, where she gave herself up to writing and dreaming.

In her mid-thirties, Elizabeth began to spit up blood, so her doctors recommended that she take a long rest by the sea. She went to Torquay, on the North Sea, to rest and recuperate. Here she whiled away three years waiting for her health to improve. The spitting of blood stopped, but the chronic weakness and back pain continued. She was ordered to stay in a room away from books. Aside from these prescriptions, there was no active treatment available in the 1840s. Her various family members, including her father and her favorite brother, Bro, came up at intervals from Wimpole Street.

One morning in 1841 Elizabeth quarreled with Bro, and he went off for a little sail. A storm sprang up; his boat was lost, and his corpse was washed up on the beach three days later. The "moral shock" of her dearest brother's death prostrated Elizabeth.

She was transported back to Wimpole Street on a stretcher suspended within a carriage by a thousand springs.

There she languished on her bed for another three years, too depressed and too weak to walk. It was during this time that she began to take the "medicant" morphine to kill her pain and to help her sleep. Secluded in her sickroom, getting no exercise, dreaming romantic dreams, she wrote poetry and received only a few visitors. One was Florence Nightingale, and another her dear father, with whom she would kneel at her bedside and pray every evening.

During those years, 1841–45, she continued to write poetry, notably "Lady Geraldine's Courtship." In this poem a servant reads to his lady the poetry of certain notable Victorian authors, including Wordsworth, Tennyson, and a young man named Robert Browning. Thus it happened that one day in 1845 the bedridden Elizabeth received a letter from the thankful Browning which threw her "into ecstasies." She answered in kind, and the letters of mutual poetic admiration flowed back and forth.

This young dandy (thirty-three to Elizabeth's thirty-eight) soon invited himself to an audience in her sickroom. There he found his hostess lying on a sofa with her dog, Flush, beside her. Browning and Elizabeth found much in common, and soon, oddly enough, her health and spirits rose, permitting her to go by coach to Regent's Park with him. The young poet's visits to that darkened room continued, and Elizabeth's father sometimes bumped into Browning on the stairway, but Barrett never grew jealous, since Elizabeth was an aging spinster.

That winter, despite her improved health, Elizabeth's doctors advised her to hurry south to avoid consumption. While Barrett resisted this counsel, Browning waited in anguish, as he had fallen madly in love with the poetess. Meanwhile Elizabeth found herself in a state of heightened emotional turmoil. To defy her father and go south seemed a terrible deed, an overstepping of filial piety. Yet she was deeply puzzled as to why her father would endanger her health. To make matters more perplexing, Browning proposed marriage. Though she loved him, she could not help wondering if she would be sacrificing his happiness on the altar of her infirmity if she accepted.

Ultimately she made her choice. In September of 1846 she and

Browning were secretly married and eloped to the Continent in the company of Flush and her maidservant, Wilson.

Her health rallied wonderfully during the next few years, relative to what it had been. Though she always remained frail, delicate, pale, and quite dependent on morphine, she no longer required Flush to polish off the last morsels on her plate. Pregnant in 1847, she had a miscarriage, and she tried again and again to have a child. Finally, in 1849, at the age of forty-one, she succeeded in giving birth to a healthy son.

Living in Italy in the British and American colony of the mid-Victorian period, she developed a fascination with both liberalism and séances. She admired George Sand and favored the movement of the Italians toward unification. Also, she attended many a séance and table-rapping session. With her love for Browning and her son, affectionately called Penini, and her poetry, these two enthusiasms seemed to sustain her somewhat.

Still, she languished. Her father never spoke to her again. He never wrote and always considered her as dead. He never acknowledged her son as his flesh and blood. He returned her letters unopened and refused to meet her on her visits to Britain. Although her literary fame grew, and her political liberalism as well as her dramatic elopement with Browning were seen as revolutionary, she wished for the love of her family. Indeed, her enthusiasm for séances may have been based on a desire to communicate with her dead mother. When her father died in 1857, her interest was heightened even more.

As the 1850s passed and her fame increased, her health worsened steadily. At the age of forty-three she suffered another miscarriage and hemorrhaged profusely, needing to be packed in ice to stop the blood flow. Later her doctors conjectured that this massive loss of blood may have played a role in her increased susceptibility to infections. Described as sensitive, high-strung and morphine-craving, she sustained a series of terrible "moral shocks" from 1857 on. Her father's death in 1857 was one, Louis Napoleon's sellout of the liberal Italians to the reactionary Hapsburgs in 1859 was another. News of the latter brought on violent palpitations and coughing fits. In 1860 one of her sisters, Henrietta, who, like herself, had been disowned by her father for marrying, died suddenly; the same year a good friend and famous medium admitted she was a fraud. These "shocks" seemed to Elizabeth's contemporaries to have played a major role in her marked deterioration by 1861. Though she spat up blood profusely, lost all appetite and became almost skeletal, her death that June, really a horrible one, none-theless seems a piece of poetry. As she lay coughing painfully one night, Browning came to her side. Lifting her up, he inquired tenderly, "How are you, my love?" "Beautiful," was her last word. She died, smiling, in his arms.

While Sand represented the female Degenerate at her most shocking, the Genius at its most sinful, Mrs. Browning embodied the Angelic Invalid myth at its most attractive, as well as the Genius myth at its least sinful. Sand had been freed from the strictures of her family at a young age and so strode recklessly into the wide world. Mrs. Browning's life was less flamboyant, less bo-hemian. She suffered like many Victorian women without a direc-tion in life or a romance. Sheltered by father and family, she was sustained by her poetry. As her body wasted, her mind secretly developed. When the young Browning appeared on the scene, the aging angel acted courageously and so emancipated herself from paternal tyranny. Her poetry blossomed. She gave birth to a son.

Still she tried desperately to reconcile with her father, who proved implacable. Rebuffed so cruelly, she sank slowly into in-validism and languished in Italy. The sad but attractive death of this Genius, this Angelic Invalid, seemed fated.

The story of Elizabeth Barrett Browning's life is in some ways similar to that of another memorable Victorian woman, Elizabeth Siddal. However, Mrs. Browning's life experiences represented the Victorian ideals of womanhood and manhood at their best. She and Browning were like a lady and lord. She was gentle, he was noble. She delicate in health, he sturdy. Elizabeth Siddal strove for the same ideal but never achieved it. Her miscarriages were tragic. Her lover, Dante Gabriel Rossetti, was no Browning. He was a rake.

Born in about 1835 to an artisan father and a mother of noble but poor ancestry, Elizabeth (Lizzie) got a job at a milliner's shop in London when she was sixteen. Here many a lovely shop girl could be seen through the large display windows. She was first noticed by a painter friend of Rossetti's, Walter Deverell, for whom she sat as a model. With her long pale hands, arms, and legs, and a full head of rich red hair, she was an astonishing vision to behold. Soon the young painter gentleman Gabriel Rossetti pirated her away from Deverell, an extraordinarily beautiful specimen himself, whose tragic death shortly thereafter left Lizzie haunted.

At that time, about 1850, Rossetti was in the midst of consolidating his own school of painting, which he and his two friends John Everett Millais and Holman Hunt came to call the Pre-Raphaelite Brotherhood. Backed by the art critic John Ruskin, these three men developed their own philosophy of art, which in fact influenced Rossetti's relationship with Siddal. Central to their creed was the notion that society was moving toward destruction and the artist must try to halt this headlong rush. The Pre-Raphaelites scorned the ideals of liberalism and progress, then so popular, and yearned for a return to a preindustrial culture. They embraced the Middle Ages as their ideal. Though the actual style of painting they adopted was quite in keeping with that of other painters in the mid-Victorian period—namely, a painstaking, greatly detailed naturalism—their subject matter was not only the common man experiencing his everyday joys, sorrows, and tedium, but also unreal characters stepping from the pages of Arthurian romance. They specialized in lovers such as Lancelot and Guinevere, Arthur and Morgan le Fay, Tristan and Isolde, as well as Dante and Beatrice.

Some of their subject matter was, of course, not out of keeping with the general middle-class Victorian sensibility. Mrs. Browning's *Sonnets from the Portuguese* and Alfred Tennyson's popular poem *The Idylls of the King* inspired as well as complemented the Pre-Raphaelites' rather sugary concept of courtly love and despair in love, of the lover's being jilted and pining away. In short, Rossetti, Hunt, and Millais were inhibited Victorians who felt uncomfortable with their own sexual natures.

Three specific types of sensitive women are discernible in their paintings, all of which are present in much other popular Victorian art. First, the Fallen Woman, a hybrid of the Angelic Invalid and the suggestible woman led astray by her lover and her own passion. Such Arthurian creatures as Guinevere and Isolde fascinated Rossetti and his colleagues, as did real-life prostitutes. A second favorite was the Woman on a Pedestal, an Angelic Invalid

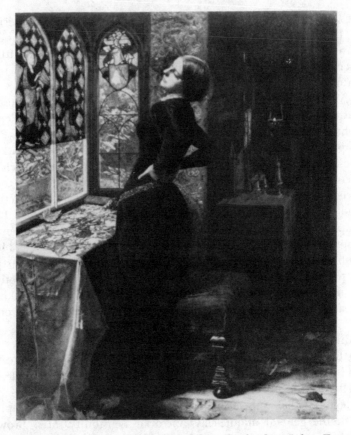

Tennyson's Mariana, or woman with a backache. John Everett
Millais, *Mariana*. (The Makins Collection, Washington, D.C.)

whom the man can revere from afar: Dante's Beartice or the
Beggar Maid in a painting by an early disciple, Edward Burne-
Jones, are good illustrations. The Beggar Maid literally sits on a
pedestal above King Cophetua. The final and perhaps most typical
figure was the Jilted Woman, the ingenuous creature whom the
rake leads on, then tosses aside most cruelly. Millais' painting
"Mariana," named after a Tennyson poem, shows a woman gazing
out of a stained-glass window and saying to herself "I am aweary
. . . He cometh not" as she strikes a modified arc-en-cercle and apparently develops a backache. Another Millais painting, "Ophelia,"

shows the woman jilted by Hamlet floating dead within a flower-spangled stream.

This fascination with sensitive women—fallen, on pedestals, or jilted—is mirrored in the relationships the Pre-Raphaelites had with women, especially their models. Their concerns also expressed a fear for the place of art and human sensibility in an industrialized liberal society. Art, feminine in nature, was being put on a pedestal, jilted, or prostituted in a masculine, striving, and aggressive society in which sensibility and fine perceptions and feelings seemed at worst passé, useless, and at best a private matter, guarded and nurtured in delicate-nerved wives and daughters and models.

The Pre-Raphaelites were all middle-class men, embarrassed around women. They tended to put women of their own class on pedestals—while looking to lower-class women for romance or sex. It was common among the painters of Rossetti's clique to mimic with their models King Cophetua's relationship to the Beggar Maid. The model was to be worshiped and adored, but she was also clearly a beggar, often a lower-class trollop. The artist still dominated; he could pull her down from her pedestal or jilt her at any minute. Rossetti's friend Hunt, for instance, kept a woman named Annie Miller, whom he not only painted but also tried to educate. He paid for lessons in elocution and deportment, training her to be his wife, and kept her waiting for years before finally dismissing her. Rossetti, who was a member of an Italian-English family struggling to be middle-class, wanted to see himself as artistically, intellectually, and socially superior to Lizzie Siddal. Since her father was only an artisan, it seemed natural for Rossetti to house Lizzie in an apartment and employ her as a model, while keeping her a secret from his family. Embarrassed to admit his own sexuality to his stern mamma and virginal sisters, he let years pass before introducing Lizzie to them and finally marrying her.

What attracted Rossetti to Siddal—the spelling was Siddall until Rossetti chose to drop the second *l*—was not only her magnificent hair, height, pallor but her growing talent as a painter in her own right. At the same time he was attracted by her morbid languor, which he captured on canvas time and again. She was prone to attacks of depression, to laconic, morose, even peevish periods, as well as having poor appetite and being generally weak.

Despite his fascination with these qualities, Rossetti had her taken by the wife of a fellow painter to see a famous physician, Dr. Garth Wilkinson, in the early fifties. Though it is unclear what he diagnosed, he recommended a change of scenery and sent the ailing model to Hastings by the sea for the air and the rest.

It seemed clear to many friends of Rossetti and "the Sid," as she was called, that her problem was a simple, if unspoken one: that she was yearning for him to propose marriage, not to mention a sexual relationship, which she refused to have with him until they were married. Another interpretation is that Lizzie herself was stalling, perhaps pining away for the very handsome though very dead Deverell. In either case, both she and Rossetti were sexually timid. Soon friends of the couple consulted and eventually persuaded two women, Barbara Leigh-Smith and Bessie "the Brick" Parkes, to supervise Lizzie in the pre-Mitchell rest cure prescribed by Wilkinson. These two women loathed the Pre-Raphaelite idea of a mentally and physically starved woman at the command of a medieval lord of the castle, a tightly corseted woman with a lined forehead and a head overloaded with hair and underloaded with brains. So they carried off the ailing painter-in-embryo to Hastings by the sea in an attempt to revitalize her and perhaps turn her against Rossetti.

The cure was only moderately successful, and Lizzie returned to London. She then tried to contact Deverell via séances, and began taking laudanum, an opiate. Thus the early 1850s passed with the artist and the model wrapped in a kind of paralysis, Rossetti enthralled with the weak but beautiful Lizzie, who still idealized Deverell.

In 1855 Holman Hunt set off for Palestine to paint, leaving his model and wife-in-training, Annie Miller, in London. Very quickly Annie and Rossetti grew closer and closer. Though the details are vague, it is clear that the two became lovers. When Lizzie discovered their liaison, her symptoms may have worsened. At least she had someone to blame for her incessant headaches, peevishness, and general weakness. Though she and Rossetti continued their painfully long engagement, he became familiar with London night life, perhaps an habitué of prostitutes. His friends came to marvel at his facility with ladies of easy virtue—street girls and trollops.

From 1855 on, Lizzie's life seemed to be in a sensitive balance. On the one hand, she had her own talent as a painter. Rossetti, at least to some degree, encouraged her to paint, and Ruskin, the art critic, even gave her an annual salary on which she could live and paint. On the other hand, Lizzie's health continued to deteriorate. Ruskin sent her off to Oxford to visit the Regius Professor of Medicine, Dr. Acland. With her long legs, hands, and neck, her dull eyes and her thick hair, she seemed an embodiment of the Victorian tubercular type. Happily, Acland found no signs of consumption but did diagnose "power long pent up and now overtaxed." He suggested rest and a vacation in the south. So, like Elizabeth Barrett Browning, she went to Paris in the winters of 1854 and 1855. Yet her enigmatic illness only deepened.

In 1857 Rossetti met and befriended William Morris and Edward Burne-Jones, two young Oxford undergraduates with whom he undertook the painting of a series of murals in Oxford. There the three met a new model, Jane Burden, daughter of a stable keeper, whom they immortalized in these murals as Guinevere. In the same year Lizzie grew sick and was sent to the country for a rest. Gabriel went to visit her but remained distracted by his work in Oxford. Also, in London he met a woman known as Fanny Cornforth, who was probably a prostitute. He dedicated much of his time to painting her as Mary Magdalene while they carried on an affair. Throughout the three years 1857–60 Lizzie and Gabriel remained engaged, unable to become sexually involved, to marry or to part.

In 1860, shortly after the marriage of Morris to Janey Burden, Gabriel wrote his mother to announce his marriage and then set off with Lizzie for Paris. Soon afterward Lizzie became pregnant. She got a cradle and baby garments and even became merry. It is just possible that Gabriel shared her mood and remained faithful to his young wife. But then she had a miscarriage. Lizzie took to her bed, never really rallying. Though she modeled occasionally in her apartment, she never painted again. She stayed in her room and received few visitors. Sleepless, with little appetite, she increased her laudanum dosage. Slowly she became fascinated with death.

At that time the little humpbacked, alcoholic poet Algernon Swinburne entered the lives of the Rossettis. Swiftly he fell head over heels in love with the fragile and beautiful Lizzie, and she may have used him to make Rossetti jealous. In the midst of this complication she probably became pregnant again, by Gabriel. Once more her hope of giving birth to a healthy child gave her new life, a new sense of purpose, and a few months of health. Then came the lamentable stillbirth of an infant girl. Lizzie was smitten and withdrew more and more into the would-be nursery, where she was seen by many friends rocking the empty cradle and singing.

One night in 1862, following a quarrel at a restaurant, the unhappily married couple returned home. Rossetti insisted on going out again. Many hours later he came home to find Lizzie dying, an empty laudanum bottle beside her. He reportedly found a note pinned to her chest: "My life is so miserable. I wish for it no more." A friend who rushed to her side seems to have snatched this note away to stifle the scandal of her suicide. Rossetti blamed himself for her death and buried the only manuscript of his best poetry with her.

He remained haunted by her image for the rest of his life. Gabriel swiftly moved into larger, more opulent quarters, in the company of Swinburne and his "house-keeper," Fanny Cornforth, but he wallowed in guilt for the next twenty years. He completed a portrait of Lizzie in 1864 called "Beata Beatrix," which shows her on the verge of death. Painting and repainting Lizzie, hoarding his pictures and sketches of her, the artist turned to drink and drugs and forsook the original Pre-Raphaelite manifesto of rebellion against industrialized society, to which he really had been only minimally committed. Selling his paintings for large sums, he exchanged his own talents for lucre. Six years after Lizzie's death Rossetti had the manuscript that he had buried with her secretly exhumed. He published it for profit. Then, eaten with deep remorse for defiling her grave, he turned to séances to contact her soul. Shortly thereafter he went mad. Hearing voices and believing that a conspiracy of critics was mounting against him, he suffered a slow, steady decline in his health. He withdrew more and more from all social contact and gradually saw his talent run dry. He died, very unhappy, in 1882.

Despite all this turmoil, in the closing two decades of his life Rossetti had created on canvas a new subtype of the Angelic In-

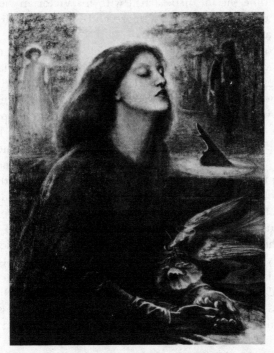

Dante's Beatrice in a trance, or Lizzie with a
headache. Dante Gabriel Rossetti, *Beata Beatrix*. (The Tate Gallery, London)

valid, a complex figure that can be called the Sensual Woman. She
is no longer an angel but rather a voluptuous creature, with thick
hair and appealing lips, who is absorbed in her own pain and
stares languorously, sorrowfully, inscrutably at the viewer.

Even more than his earlier works, Rossetti's paintings of the
Sensual Woman intrigued the *fin-de-siècle* audience. His vision
reflected a larger trouble haunting the Victorian age. Beyond the
widespread fear of machines, the popular press, and the spread of
alcoholism was a growing fascination with sexuality. The Sensual
Woman, the ultimate rendition of the Angelic Invalid, symbolized
the sensibility of society at large, growing plump and sexually
aware, succumbing to material progress and creature comforts. At

the same time the idealistic artist, with his Victorian view of sexuality as repugnant, withdrew more and more into self-absorbed escapism and worship of the past.

The Rossettis' tragic love and Gabriel's subsequent art present in some ways a darkened version of the Brownings' relationship. Both women were sensitive, delicate, chaste, and creative. Elizabeth Browning was more fulfilled in her poetry, in her intellectual life, and in her marriage; Elizabeth Rossetti was unhappily married, her painting unremembered, her intellectual liberation stillborn. While Mrs. Browning had a young Roland in her knightly husband, Lizzie had only a self-absorbed poet-painter who frequented prostitutes. The two women stand forth as two versions of Victorian womanhood sacrificed on the shoals of love, martyred by the cruelty of their men—one by her father, the other by her husband. A passion that burned ever so brightly in their delicate hearts consumed their frail forms. In the medical jargon of the day, the cares and woes, the slings and arrows of the world, had shocked their delicate constitutions and so prostrated and exhausted them. Stripped of the poetical language of the period, Mrs. Rossetti's miserable death and Mr. Rossetti's obsession with sensual and inscrutable women can clearly be understood as flights from reality, a movement into a personalized aestheticism in which love is unattainable and really becomes a prelude to death. With these more somber ideas Victorian medical thinkers had yet to come to grips.

George Eliot's story, by contrast, is not that of a Sensual Woman whose pain is unnameable. Hers is a tale of a "strong-minded woman," as Thomas Carlyle called her, who, for the sake of her relationship with a man, defied convention, yet could never entirely shrug it off. George Eliot suffered quietly for her rebellion, and out of her suffering she wrote great modern psychological novels.

She was born Mary Ann Evans in 1819, her father an artisan turned businessman, in Warwickshire, England. Shy and diffident, Mary Ann suffered from not being pretty—"magnificently ugly—deliciously hideous," wrote Henry James years later, after she had become famous, but merely ugly and hideous before her fame.

Her most beautiful attributes were her mind, her charitable spirit, her beautiful temperament. Her mind is what carried her for many years. Sent off to boarding school by her parents, she read deeply and learned many foreign languages, including Greek, Latin, Hebrew, German, and French. On the death of her mother in 1836 Mary Ann returned home to keep house for her father. Although she had gone through a phase of ardent evangelical Christianity in her youth, by the time her formal education ended she had read so much that she had developed grave religious doubts. Thus she refused for a while to attend Anglican church services with her father. After he threatened to throw her out for this rebelliousness, the two struck a compromise. She was to attend services regularly but could carry on her antireligious studies in private.

Remaining unmarried, Mary Ann managed her aging father's household for years. During this period her health became impaired for the first time. Headaches, faintness, and general weakness plagued her, though the application of leeches apparently offered some relief. Meanwhile she undertook the translation from German of the 1500-page *The Life of Christ*, by David Friedrich Strauss, a highly critical biography that, when published in English, deeply affected thinking in England about Christianity. Even after its publication in 1846, however, she didn't reveal that she had done the translation, and remained the spinster daughter to her religiously orthodox father until he died in 1849.

Immediately after his death the liberated young woman set off for the Continent with friends. During her stay in Switzerland her health improved markedly. Over the next few years she drifted back to England and became a ghost editor for an English periodical, *Westminster*. The chief editor, later a doctor, was John Chapman, who was involved in an interesting sexual entanglement, which grew more complicated once Mary Ann, now calling herself Marian, appeared on the scene. Much in the manner of Fielding's *Tom Jones*, Chapman had a splendid arrangement in old London. In his late twenties, he lived with his wealthy forty-three-year-old wife, their children, and a lovely governess, Elisabeth, who was his mistress—all in one household. Soon Marian came to live with this happy family.

Chapman loved her for her mind, and possibly her body, though the evidence for their liaison is sparse, since he discreetly cut out of his diary many of the entries for this period. George Eliot's biographer writes, however, "There can be little doubt that Marian was guilty of some indiscretion, probably more serious than holding hands."

While she was living with Chapman, Marian's health deteriorated. She endured headaches whenever she read and wrote. Her teeth decayed, and she suffered from agonizing toothaches from then on. These problems were aggravated by eyestrain. Gradually, however, she drifted into the intellectual circles of London, meeting some of the same people the Rossettis and the Brownings met. When her relationship with Chapman proved desperately unsatisfactory, she left the *ménage à quatre*, despondent.

Again she met a man she thought she could love—the evolutionary thinker Herbert Spencer, another notoriously ugly Victorian. During many long walks around London, Marian and Herbert developed warm mutual feelings. Marian was falling in love. Then Spencer unexpectedly developed nervous symptoms— insomnia and "an overstrained heart"—and the relationship cooled. Rejected by the man she loved, she grew deeply depressed. Her headaches worsened. She took to bed, complaining of rheumatism in her shoulder. As time passed, she slowly recovered.

Then things suddenly changed. A new man, regrettably married, entered her life. He was George Henry Lewes, an intellectual of the first order, just then working on a *Life of Goethe*. The two talked of German literature and philosophy. Her headaches lifted and her spirits brightened.

Soon Lewes was confiding his deep and most painful secret to her, the immorality of his wife, Agnes. Lewes, Agnes, and John Thornton—also married—were involved in a most curious relationship. Although Lewes and Agnes had three sons of their own, her next two children, though surnamed Lewes, had been fathered by Thornton. For a number of years Lewes had been willing to be cuckolded. He even treated Thornton's bastards as his own. But by the time Lewes met Marian Evans he was sick and tired of the whole mess. He spilled all his woes on Marian, who only loved him the more.

As the trust between Lewes and Marian deepened, their love grew. Eventually they saw no recourse but to act, even though they both knew that English mores preferred the hypocritical arrangement of Lewes, his wife, and Thornton to any open, if honest, defiance of the marriage contract. In 1854, when Marian was thirty-five years old, she and Lewes ran off to the Continent together.

This romantic, if homely, couple spent most of the next year on the Continent. While he finished his book on Goethe she began a translation of Spinoza. During the eight months they spent in Weimar and Berlin she found continental society more understanding of her arrangement with Lewes. They met another notorious couple, Liszt and his mistress, Princess Caroline Sayn-Wittgenstein, who had deserted her Russian husband in order to follow him to Weimar. Her husband had originally ignored this liaison but then decided to divorce her. Marian and Lewes became intimate friends with the princess and the composer and so felt encouraged to flout English mores. Still, their months on the Continent were marred by the news that many old friends in England were casting them off. It was clear that unpleasant rumors about their involvement were being bandied about in England, with Marian depicted as the Fallen Woman, even the temptress.

While crossing back into England, Marian suffered severe headaches that prostrated her for about three days after her arrival in Dover. She may have been suffering from tension headaches while she and Lewes waited in Dover to hear from the estranged Agnes, still in London. Agnes seemed willing to accept Lewes's arrangement with Marian, provided he continued to support her and her children. Lewes agreed to this plan.

The "marriage" of Lewes and Marian remained a solid one from then on, even though Marian was plagued with headaches, weakness, and social shyness for the rest of her life. Old friends remained cool to Lewes and his new "wife" for years to come. Her nervous symptoms usually grew worse when she and Lewes were in London, usually diminished when they sojourned in the English countryside, and invariably disappeared during continental vacations. Marian recognized a psychic element in her illness, but she also seemed to believe in a commonly accepted physical reason, the London air.

Then Lewes began to suffer from some nervous symptoms of his own, including ringing in his ears and headaches. Though he remained a garrulous and clever raconteur who never was at all shy, his symptoms were sometimes compatible and sometimes competitive with Marian's. Many of their jaunts into the English countryside and across the channel into Germany and Switzerland became visits to spas for their health. The two essentially developed a neurasthenia *à deux*.

In the 1860s Marian Evans started writing fiction. At first sorely lacking confidence, she plodded on, with the support and protection of Lewes. Her first few works, *Scenes of Clerical Life*, published in 1858 under the pseudonym George Eliot, proved successful. But revealing her true identity was a tricky matter, since Lewes was convinced, with good reason, that if the true author of *Scenes* became known, George Eliot would be judged harshly by the critics. Furthermore, Marian seemed sensitive to any negative criticism, and Lewes protected her by reading all newspapers, all letters, before she could see them, so he could dispose of any hurtful comments that might prostrate her.

Nonetheless George Eliot continued to write and was soon renowned as a great author, perhaps the greatest living English novelist. Queen Victoria herself deeply admired *Adam Bede*; Dickens, the poet laureate Tennyson, Browning, and the world at large were rapt in admiration and also puzzled. Who was George Eliot? Finally, in 1859, the world came to know who had written these masterpieces. Since others had come forward to pronounce themselves the author of *Adam Bede*, Lewes and Marian decided to drop the pseudonym. Though her publishers feared the effect that the announcement that Mrs. Lewes or Marian Evans or Marian Evans Lewes had written *Adam Bede* would have on the sales of the book, she could not resist writing to the *London Times* to denounce the impostors, and she also confided the truth to select friends, who then spread the news around England.

Over the years following this revelation the ostracized Marian became the world-renowned George Eliot. Although much of "polite society" still could not accept her, the literary world did. She remained essentially a recluse for the rest of her life, though she employed her husband as her ambassador to many social gatherings where she would have felt uncomfortable. While writing she would always suffer excruciating weakness, "bilious" headaches, and dyspepsia; London always rendered her sickly, and rest in the country would invariably be her medicine. Her major social outlet was her Sunday-morning open house, when such people as Browning, Tennyson, the Burne-Joneses, and Henry James would come to meet this genius, sip tea, and discuss art and society. Nonetheless, up to 1870 most polite women avoided her, and only emancipated women such as Barbara Leigh-Smith and Bessie "the Brick" Parkes, two early suffragettes, would-be saviors of Lizzie Siddal, became her women friends.

By the early seventies lords and ladies finally began calling on her, and in the late seventies she was even offered a special audience with two of Queen Victoria's daughters, the royal princesses. Society gradually came to overlook her "marriage" to Lewes. When he died in 1878, George Eliot suffered great despondence, losing much weight and experiencing fainting spells, headaches, and nausea. However, in 1880, after consulting Sir James Paget, a prominent British doctor who knew her well, she decided to accept the marriage proposal of John Cross, a man twenty years her junior. With this marriage came total social respectability. Even her brother Isaac, alienated from her because of Lewes, broke a long silence to write and wish his notorious and famous sister the greatest happiness. When George Eliot died in the same year she was a well married and socially accepted woman.

Yet this acceptance had an ironic posthumous twist. John Cross made an effort to have his wife buried in the Poet's Corner in Westminster Abbey, since her achievement seemed unparalleled in the history of womanhood. Though he found a few influential supporters, many British men of letters could not imagine a woman who had flouted the rules of Christian marriage being laid to rest in the Abbey. They turned a deaf ear to her husband's pleas, and George Eliot was ultimately denied a place among the august dead. Her "marriage" to Lewes and her sex haunted her even beyond her grave.

George Eliot was the model neurasthenic, according to no one less than Dr. Beard. She suffered from headaches, dyspepsia, and general nervous weakness, not to mention toothaches and eyestrain, because of too much brain work and too much social pressure. All of her symptoms were aggravated by the city. She was a female Prometheus who burned out too many light bulbs.

Yet such a theory of brain power and nerve force fell short in explaining her symptoms in any depth. From a more psychological point of view, it seems likely that her guilt-inducing arrangement with Lewes and, before that, her relationships with her father and

Chapman contributed to her despondency, her headaches and dyspepsia. Being near London may have set off her symptoms precisely because both Chapman and the real Mrs. Lewes dwelt there. Furthermore, her literary work may have catalyzed her symptoms, not because of the sheer amount of cerebral force she expended—as Beard's theory of neurasthenia or Lombroso's theory of genius would argue—but because of the characters and plots, moods and tones she called forth. The intricacies of her novels, in fact, reached much further into the realms of psychology than Beard's idea of nervous exhaustion. Characters such as Dorothea in *Middlemarch* and Dinah and Hetty in *Adam Bede* capture much of George Eliot's personal dilemma. Dorothea defied Victorian mores by refusing to remain a widow and marrying a young artist. Hetty fell head over heels in love with the dashing gentleman Arthur Donnithorne. Once impregnated by him, she was deemed a Fallen Woman and suffered miserably. Dinah courageously accepted her vocation as a charismatic preacher and spoke her mind openly to the world.

For every Lizzie Rossetti or George Eliot, however, there must have existed in Europe and America thousands of women who never escaped from the family hearth, who lived and died unknown. If Mitchell is to be believed, thousands lay languishing all over the West, reading *François le Champi* and *Sonnets from the Portuguese* under their bedclothes and never leaving their homes. Such a woman, it seems, was Alice James.

The James family is a celebrated one, not because of Alice but because of two of her brothers, Henry and William. Decidedly an eccentric family, it is well suited to a study of Victorian neurosis. All five of the James children led troubled lives. The two youngest sons, Robertson and Wilkinson, always lived, dissatisfied, in the shadows of their two brainy older brothers. Yet, having brains in the James family was a trial in its own right. Whereas Henry James, Sr., expected great things of his boys, especially William and Henry, he also instilled in all five children morbid fears and inhibitions that made it difficult for them to have a mature emotional life.

During the 1850s and 1860s the James family moved restlessly back and forth from Europe to America. From a Victorian perspective Henry James, Sr., seemed a peripatetic nerve patient looking for a cure. From a more modern point of view he appears, in part, to have been an emotionally troubled individual looking for satisfaction or purpose. In either case, because of their uprootedness, the family members found it difficult to form relationships outside of the family and so came to rely on one another too much. In addition, Henry James, Sr., had the idea that good character was founded on innocence, so he isolated the family from outside influences, especially popular culture. Though he titillated all his children with brief stays in such interesting places as Paris, London, and Switzerland, he invariably prevented them from knowing these teeming European cultures. This idea of innocence extended most especially in the direction of his only daughter, Alice, born in 1848.

Described as a "dear little creature and very sweet girl" during her childhood and adolescence, Alice had often been left behind when her older brothers set off into the great world of Europe and America—first because she was the youngest, later because she was a girl. Thus she whiled away the time, looking forward to a great future that never came. Postponing her happiness as the family moved from place to place, she felt strangled throughout her youth, as her needs, her education, and her friendships were considered secondary to those of her brothers. A serious, plain-looking adolescent, she looked older than her years with her hair pulled straight back and coiled in a braid and her conversation and clothing tending toward the severe and neutral.

In 1864 the family finally settled in Cambridge, Massachusetts, to be near William, who was studying at Harvard. Then sixteen years old, Alice had had no apparent nervous problem and had lived a cosmopolitan, though socially sheltered life. In Cambridge she finally began to develop close relationships outside the family, generally with women. In about 1866, however, Alice began to have nervous crises—her older brothers being too inhibited to describe them in any detail in any of their written works. She may have been struggling with her budding sexuality or the lure of forming close relationships outside the family. Her symptoms apparently included general fatigue, delicacy of health, and easy excitability—really nothing more than what any Angelic Invalid was expected to feel.

The family became worried, however, and elected to send her to

New York City for treatment by Charles Fayett Taylor, a doctor whose book *Movement Cures* reads like Beard's, but with a misogynistic twist. He believed that girls who were exposed to an over-abundance of emotional and intellectual stimulation, as Alice had been in Europe, overused their brains and so prevented the rest of their bodies from receiving proper nourishment. Nervous exhaustion was the outcome. He followed the therapeutic approaches of a Swedish massage and exercise specialist named Peter Ling, stressing stimulation of the muscles and rest for the mind. This insidious cure of letting the mind lie fallow was one that Mrs. Browning had received and rebelled against and which had likewise been prescribed for Elizabeth Siddal, though it had been applied only intermittently.

But Alice took Taylor's advice very seriously. Returning from New York in 1869, she convalesced, letting her mind lie fallow. Soon she relapsed. Her recurring "fits" might have warranted the diagnosis of grand hysteria. Her life of idling mixed with weight lifting and horseback riding had no direction. Always the relapses would occur, and she never developed a relationship with any male outside of her family. There was no Mr. Browning, no Chopin, no Rossetti.

During this same period, 1866 to the early 1870s, the only males in her life, her brothers, were undergoing neurotic crises of their own, especially Henry and William, the true "brain-workers." Henry eventually escaped to Europe and to art and novel writing, William into a marriage and a career as a psychologist, but Alice remained at home with her parents, resting and having fits, recovering and relapsing.

In 1872 she and Henry set off for the Continent, and her health rallied, only to relapse after her return home. No suitors arrived, and when William, the brother who had been the most flirtatious with her during her adolescence, married a girl named Alice in 1878, Alice James suffered a series of severe fits and may even have gone insane, though she was hidden from the view of society in the James home in Cambridge. Too ill to attend her brother's wedding, she found that the more her health worsened, the more tender and solicitous her parents became. She seemed to become a veritable Octopia Darnell, as depicted in Mitchell's *Roland Blake*.

A demanding, pesty, self-centered martyr, she wasted time and health and talent. Her health improved only in the late seventies, when she was befriended by a feminist named Katherine Loring Peabody, a spinster of tough fiber. Mrs. William James always hinted that this relationship was a homosexual one, and Henry James seems to have used it in his novel *The Bostonians*.

In the early eighties both her parents died, and Alice's health deteriorated. In 1883 she was placed in a Boston hospital for the nervous but not insane, and there she underwent a modified version of Mitchell's then popular rest cure, which involved supervised nutrition as well as hot air, vapor baths, massage, and galvanic and faradic treatment of muscles and nerves. She grew a little stronger but still remained debilitated. In 1884 she saw a Russian emigré physician who recommended exercise. Once again she was enthusiastic for a while but was soon disappointed. This remained her pattern with doctors and cures throughout her life, and as her biographer puts it, these doctors were probably the only males who touched her adult body.

In 1884 she decided to go to England with Katherine Peabody and Katherine's sister Louise, who was then dying of tuberculosis. Alice's brother Henry was bemused to observe Katherine running from one invalid to the other. As Louise spat up blood and coughed violently, Katherine would hurry to her, and then Alice would have a fit. The harassed Katherine would then hurry back to her. During the years in England, 1884 to 1892, Alice did little but read George Sand, George Eliot, and her brother Henry's works, though she also began a diary. She was treated with cannabis. She went to water resorts, notably the Royal Leamington Spa, where she lived in genteel debility. Later in life she was treated with hypnosis, which her brother William had been urging for years. It was especially helpful when Miss Peabody was the hypnotist. Alice greeted the diagnosis of her breast cancer in 1892 as a sweet release. This last malady at least was tangible. She died, ironically, on the same day and at the same hour as her mother had ten years earlier.

Alice James was the model bed patient, the well-to-do *malade imaginaire* whose life lacked purpose, who used her neurasthenia to mask deep emotional troubles, probably based on her inability to leave her family and develop mature emotional relationships. Her doctors applied many of the fashionable treatments of the day, such as electricity, rest, hypnosis, water, and travel. Each offered a flicker of hope but invariably failed.

In all of these Victorian vignettes, save that of Alice James, the theme of love is prominent. The lack of apparent love life for Alice may hide the strength of her loving feelings for her brother William or her father or her dear friend Miss Peabody. Love seemed so central to the life of a good Victorian. The romantic entanglements of George Sand shocked and fascinated the world. The romances of the Brownings and the Rossettis were the stock of Victorian literature. The plodding love between Marian Evans and George Lewes gave George Eliot both solace and pain. The Victorians could see that love and passion quickened the heart, put color in the cheeks. Love seemed intimately connected to the vital force itself, to the nervous energy that so many Victorian doctors saw as essential to the etiology of neurosis.

Yet love also led to heartache, sleeplessness, agonies at sunrise, conflicts with family, with duty, with reason, with religious beliefs. In the personal pain that love inflicted lay, many Victorian doctors admitted, the source of many cases of nerves. Few denied that the chagrin of the lover, the disillusionment of the rejected one, the shock of a telegram bearing the bad news of the death of a parent, a spouse, or lover were critical.

The question was how to theorize about and treat these cases, how to help the patient by talking about his loves. Electricity, massage, milk rest, sojourns at the sea, magnets, and hypnosis all revolved around physical, not emotional theories of disease and cure. Beard, Mitchell, Charcot, and the other doctors were speaking of rebuilding the body, revitalizing the nerves. Certainly in all their treatments a psychological component was at work, but Victorian medicine was still groping toward a theoretical understanding of the psyche.

The best efforts by 1890 had been made by Charcot and the Salpêtrists in their work on ideas and autosuggestion as causing and curing illness, by Bernheim and the Nancy school in their discussion of suggestibility, and by Krafft-Ebing and the early sexologists in their thinking about sadism, masochism, and other illicit sexual compulsions. The work of Lombroso and Nordau on the lives and works of certain artists and of James in the area of religious experience also showed the movement of medical thinking away from the purely physical into the realm of the psyche. Out of this intensely absorbing medical environment a few men developed theories of nervous illness in which psychology held an even more convincing place. The most notable of these were Charcot's disciple Pierre Janet (1859–1947) and Sigmund Freud (1856–1939), who not only studied under Charcot, Bernheim, and Oppenheim as a young man but also lived in Vienna when Krafft-Ebing was working and reworking his *Psychopathia Sexualis*.

We can see a momentous stride being taken toward a deeper understanding of "nervous illness" in the study of the narrative history of these men's patients and in the compassion and empathy that such study evokes. Like the Moderns, the Victorians were intrigued by personal histories in which an individual was seen in realistic surroundings, entering into emotional conflicts with his family, his enemies, his friends, his loves. Certain doctors, such as Janet and Freud, shared this widespread interest, and following the leads of Charcot, Bernheim, Krafft-Ebing, Nordau, and James, they spun out ever more complex descriptions and theories based on personal histories.

At this point Victorian doctors faced a parting of the ways. Certain medical men, such as Hughlings Jackson and some erstwhile followers of Charcot such as Pierre Marie, turned back toward medical research that modeled itself after the natural sciences and followed a rigorous scientific method which excluded the individual's subjective experience. In this type of approach, love had little place. Other medical men, such as Janet and Freud, grew intensely interested in individual, psychological, and more speculative means of explanation. In their studies, human passions could remain central. We can see a crucial separation in the study of nervousness and neurosis between the frankly neurological and the psychological. The first group of doctors was trying to delve more deeply into human anatomy and physiology. The second group developed psychological models that utilized personal histories. Though Janet continued to believe that weakness of the nerves underlay all mental maladies, and Freud in fact borrowed from thermodynamic and evolutionary language in explaining neuroses and never denied the importance of heredity, their approach to suffering and loving human beings was intensely personal.

THIRTEEN

Private Pain

AT the center of George Eliot's novel *Adam Bede* is a scene that captures the private pain of the Victorian in love. The gentleman/villain, Arthur Donnithorne, is anguished over his having succumbed to the charms of the little dairymaid, the lovely and sprightly Hetty, with whom he has made mad and illicit love in the woods on his estate. Arthur had led poor Hetty on by encouraging her to daydream of becoming a lady, the wife of a gentleman. The two had fallen prey to their emotions. He struggles to unburden himself of his pain while partaking of a good English breakfast with the country parson, Mr. Irwine. Mr. Irwine, a fine strapping fellow, more of a rider to hounds than a cleric, is eating with great relish.

Arthur too eats his eggs, ham, and cold fowl, all the while mulling over his resolution to tell the cleric of his faux pas, a typical one for a gentleman—having a tumble with a lower-class lovely. As he hesitates, Mr. Irwine discerns the turmoil in his young friend. He even considers asking Arthur to speak. But Mr. Irwine is too polite; his manners get in his way. Arthur's unburdening never occurs, poor Hetty is impregnated and later spends her days wandering the globe as an outcast; the novel moves on toward a sobering denouement.

This failure of the fictional clergyman to break through the veil of manners assumed by an English gentleman seems distant in time and space and world view from the painful but meticulous effort of a very real doctor in Vienna to understand the prickly and unspeakable sexual side of humanity. But the gulf between the two seems less difficult to span if one remembers the Victorian's fascination with love's complexity and centrality. What the English cleric lacked, Freud possessed, namely, an uncanny ear for the echoes of this tumult, a scientific commitment to inquiry, and the ability to tell his patients, despite convention, precisely what he thought they were really thinking.

How did he gain this insightfulness? Surely Freud can be seen as a genius in the Victorian sense: a man with a monomania, namely, seeing sexuality everywhere—in dreams, in slips of the tongue, in childhood, in everyday wishes and fears. Such an interpretation is, however, too glib, too superficial. As Freud and his followers were to do with their patients, we would do well to review the life history of the man, in order to appreciate the dimension of his genius.

Born in Moravia, a primitive province in the decaying Austro-Hungarian Empire, Freud had moved at an early age to the rapidly growing and richly cosmopolitan Vienna. Here he received an excellent education in all-male schools and then at the University of Vienna. Though he fantasized about becoming a great statesman, he decided at the age of seventeen to study medicine.

Once enrolled in medical school, Freud took an overly long time to graduate. Tarrying in the neurophysiology laboratory of Ernst Brücke, a colleague of Hermann von Helmholtz (who had first measured the speed of electrical current in nerve tissue), Freud did some original research on the nervous system of eels. After graduating in 1881 at the age of twenty-five, Freud received excellent training as a neurologist under Theodor Meynert, a renowned neuroanatomist and physiologist, as well as a neurologist and psychiatrist. By then Freud was steeped in the Victorian medical tradition of linking mind and brain together via anatomy and physiology. However, he grew interested in Charcot's work. Having received a fellowship to travel abroad, Freud went to Paris to study under Charcot, who was just then—in 1885—making his fascinating equation of hypnosis and traumatic neurosis. After about five months in Paris and a month in Berlin, where he studied under Oppenheim, Freud returned to Vienna and translated a few of Charcot's works into German.

In 1886, the year that *Psychopathia* was first published and two years before Krafft-Ebing assumed the professorship in Vienna from Meynert, Freud married and set up a private practice. Though originally a neurologist, Freud moved gradually in the direction of psychiatry. He remained intrigued with hysteria, as his visit to Nancy to see the work of Liébeault and Bernheim in 1889 attests.

Though conservative in many ways—politically and socially, ostensibly in his family life and habits—he lived in a city teeming with artists and intellectuals who were probing into the crevices of the mind and unleashing weird and phantasmagorical creations on the public. Undoubtedly these avant-garde artists stirred Freud's imagination. Also, as his interest in the psyche deepened, he found that many of his patients simply liked to tell him about their woes. One of the recurring themes of his patients, many of whom were upper-middle-class Jewish women, was their love lives and especially their secret sexual experiences. Freud did not avoid these delicate topics. During the 1890s a large number of his patients told him they had literally been sexually seduced as children by their parents, their nurses, or their siblings. When Freud presented to a Viennese medical gathering in 1896 his thesis that sexual seduction in childhood caused hysteria, he was coldly received. Krafft-Ebing himself is reported to have called the theory a "scientific fairy tale."

Though many authors have questioned the story of Freud's frosty reception, it does seem probable that his theory would appear unlikely to a medical world steeped in ideas of nervous degeneration, of brain power and exhaustion, of shocks and stresses caused by civilization. In such a world Freud's idea must have seemed simplistic.

In this decade of his life, roughly 1890–1900, Freud himself was quite neurotic, with serious symptoms including a train phobia and a superstitious preoccupation with numerology and dates, all relating to the date of his own demise. He also had a miserable period during his early thirties when he feared he was dying of a heart malady. Behind his neurotic sufferings was his long-standing addiction to nicotine. Freud's friend and physician by mail, Wilhelm Fliess, recommended in this period that the young Freud give up cigars, as they might be the cause of his palpitations and therefore of his fear. Freud struggled with his addiction, but he never succeeded in giving up nicotine, and eventually he parted ways with Fliess.

Though he rejected Fliess's theory of how his neurosis was born, Freud did delve into his own psychological makeup. By way of his own dreams he thought he had tapped into a stupendous and powerful part of his mind, in which he believed the roots of his own neurosis lay. During his self-analysis, as he called his dream study, he noticed that his own neurotic symptoms diminished, his mental pain dissolved, and he stumbled on a new idea of how a neurosis was born, which he later called the Oedipus complex, after the Greek myth in which Oedipus kills his own father and marries his mother. Freud concluded that his various hysterical patients had not always been literally seduced by their loved ones; rather, they wished to have been. This wish, which he thought came to life in the child's unconscious mind, was the kernel around which later symptoms developed. He believed these symptoms could be alleviated only by the analysis of dreams, which seemed to be the phantasmagoric creations of every neurotic and in which the illicit Oedipal wish could still be recognized in a disguised form, as in art.

Freud's concepts were powerful, but he was not alone in the eighties and nineties in concentrating on unconscious phenomena and on the pain of the individual as central to the breeding of a neurosis. Charcot's study of passionate attitudes and Bernheim's notion of suggestibility both rested on the idea that beneath the waking mind existed a sleeping subconscious mind, which displayed itself most dramatically in hypnotism. These men influenced Freud, his mentor in Vienna, Josef Breuer (1842–1925), and Janet, the young doctor in Charcot's Salpêtrière, all of whom then began to emphasize the mind and the realms beneath consciousness in their patients.

Janet and Breuer had difficulties with Freud's notion that the child's wish to kill one parent and marry the other was at the root of a neurosis. But both men had much in common with Freud. What united these three doctors was their emphasis on talking with their patients and unraveling the turmoil beneath the manners of society—the private passions, loves, fears.

Many have tried to identify the origins of Freud's thought, but as with any genius, it is impossible to reproduce those moments of creativity that were his while he was smoking his cigar. Yet one rather interesting aspect of his thought has often been neglected, namely, the origin of the very modern concept that patient and doctor together could tear aside the veil of manners and enter the psyche, the mind, the emotions, the private turmoil, and in so doing, effect a cure.

Patients had for ages been treated by private doctors, who charged fees and always kept their secrets. This was the approach of Mitchell, Krafft-Ebing and Liébeault, to mention a few of the more compassionate and perhaps charismatic doctors during the decades when Breuer, Janet, and Freud were on the scene. All of these doctors were intuitive psychologists, whether they knew it or not. Hypnotism, for example, offered a way in which the mind, with its passion and pain, could be approached in a ritualized and fairly safe manner. Its popularity in the eighties and nineties paved the way for a dazzling new inroad into the psyche.

In the early 1880s a startling case came to light in Vienna. What makes it especially striking is that it predated much of Charcot's work and all of Bernheim's. A pretty young woman, Bertha Pappenheim, from an exceedingly wealthy Jewish family, fell seriously ill in her home. In December 1880 a doctor was summoned: Breuer, a popular internist whose private practice had been growing by leaps and bounds, especially among the burgeoning Jewish population. In many ways a more optimistic, less neurotic man than his young friend Freud, Breuer found Bertha lying in her big bed, paralyzed and hallucinating. She spoke gibberish in four tongues.

Bertha's case may have paralleled that of Alice James. Though we know little about Alice's illness, whose specific symptoms are shrouded in Jamesian quiet, we know much more about the twenty-one-year-old Bertha, or, as she came to be known, Anna O., whose father then lay dying in the next room. Breuer found her "autohypnotized," as he described her condition, and he chose to listen to her utterances in four tongues. Visiting her every evening, he found her frequently in this peculiar talkative state, a second state as he called it. He simply let her speak and speak and speak. For a while she was unintelligible. Yet he remained at her bedside for months as her father deteriorated.

Breuer noted that Anna passed in and out of two essentially different states of mind. In the first, which occurred each morning, she was her usual self, though she felt sad that her father, whom she loved dearly, was dying of tuberculosis in the next room. In the second state—which followed a period of somnolence in the afternoon and continued after sunset—she would awake in a tormented and irritated frame of mind. She would throw pillows at her governess and enter into disputes of little import with her mother and attendants. She also complained to Breuer of seeing black snakes writhing in the room, a skull hanging in the air. Her language was garbled, and she frequently stopped speaking in the middle of a sentence. She even became mute for two weeks early in the treatment. This was the state Breuer called autohypnotic, following the ideas of many other doctors during this period who were beginning to think in terms of hypnosis when describing the subconscious mind.

After speaking in four languages in her delirium (or her period of passionate attitudes, as Charcot would have called it) Anna would talk coherently. But she also suffered complete paralysis, areas of anesthesia, and contractures of her right arm, partial paralysis of the other three limbs, a nervous cough, and had problems with hearing and vision. By the conventions of the 1880s she was decidedly a hysteric, and would be considered even more so in the nineties, when Breuer, familiar with Charcot's work, began to write up and publish the case. Breuer visited her almost nightly for a number of months. Her garbled language, her halting speech, her complaints of losing time continued unabated until March of 1881, when she finally spoke only in good English.

Breuer surmised that his patient had—in the jargon of the day —suffered a psychic shock secondary to her nursing her beloved father from July to December of 1880, when she had sat up at night knitting and keeping a vigil. Anna was a dutiful female, like the heroine of Mitchell's *Roland Blake*. She had seemingly brought on her hysteria by self-sacrifice. Breuer believed that her second state of mind, the one marked by visions of snakes and a skull and peculiarities of speech, had taken hold during those months of turmoil. He learned that she had in fact been suffering from somnambulism while nursing her father, but it was only in

December 1881, when the paralysis and contractures became generalized, that she had become a bed patient.

As the months passed, Anna seemed to benefit from simply talking to Breuer during the evening. She began to tell him little
stories, sad and pretty, in the style of Hans Christian Andersen's
fairy tales. They dealt with a girl filled with anxiety, sitting near a
dying loved one. Breuer found that telling these little stories gave
her comfort, and a missed day of storytelling left her restless and
irritable.

When she suffered a relapse at the time of her father's death in
April of 1881, the girl and her mother moved to the country, and
Breuer decided to make long trips to their country house two or
three times weekly. Always arriving in the evenings, always finding
her in the autohypnotic state of mind, he would listen to her
stories and would later learn that she had awakened the following
morning in a docile and cheerful state of mind. Her various hysterical symptoms were slowly disappearing, so doctor and patient
would take slow and pleasant walks through the garden as they
talked.

After a vacation Breuer returned to find Anna moody and irritable, her poetic vein exhausted. Her hallucinations had
worsened and began to improve only when she returned to the city
in the fall and Breuer came every evening as before. Then, in
December 1882, she relapsed markedly, and the two states of mind
took a peculiar turn. The hallucinatory state deepened and
lengthened, and what had been the first, clear state of mind took
on an ominous and eerie quality. She seemed awake and lucid, but
poor Anna still thought she was living in the house where her
father had died one year earlier, though the Pappenheims had
moved to different houses in Vienna, to get away from the memories of the dead father. She seemed uncannily to be reliving every
day of the past year, precisely one year later, as Breuer learned by
consulting Mrs. Pappenheim's diary.

This odd state of affairs continued into the following summer,
when a new symptom suddenly developed. In the midst of a heat
spell the girl refused to drink. One evening when she was in the
second state, Anna spoke of seeing her English governess allow her
dog to drink water out of a glass on the floor. She remembered

being disgusted and angry at the dog and the governess. Now, as she told the tale, to Breuer's amazement, her symptom of refusing to drink water suddenly vanished. She reached for a glass of water and drank thirstily. The symptom never returned after she unburdened her memory.

From then on, Breuer and Anna systematically approached each new symptom and all the old symptoms. Doubling his number of visits, he came in the morning, hypnotized her, got her to concentrate on all the traumas that in the past might have set off a particular symptom. Anna would relate numerous events, ultimately leading back to her experiences in the early part of 1880. When Breuer returned in the evenings to find her in her auto-hypnotized state, he would remind her of these traumatic memories. Anna would then vent her anger, fear, or sadness, and the symptoms would disappear.

The most intractable symptoms proved to be the paralysis in her right arm, her visions of snakes, and her visions of a skull. The first two were traced back to a terrifying experience in the summer of 1880, when the young Anna was waiting in her father's bedroom for a doctor to drain the serous fluid from his diseased lungs and thus give him some relief. Anna had drifted into a funny state of mind while keeping her vigil. She had been drowsing, leaning on her right arm, which had fallen asleep. She had been roused suddenly by the whistle of the train carrying the doctor to her father's rescue. She had apparently started up and seen a snake slithering toward her father, a vision born of the shadows of her dreams and the darkness of the room. As she reached out to save her father from the snake, she found her arm paralyzed, and so the later symptom of paralysis began. The next day, when she was gathering some sticks for firewood, she thought for an instant that one of the sticks was a snake, her hand recoiled in fear, and thus the symptoms deepened. Once Anna relived the terrors of these memories, the paralysis disappeared forever, as did the hallucinations.

As for the skull, she recalled an experience from the same year when she had risen in an exhausted state of mind, after a night of watching her father, and had gone to visit an aunt who lived nearby. Upon entering her aunt's house she had looked up, as the door opened abruptly, to see a face, her own, in a mirror. The face dissolved in her mind's eye and recomposed into her father's face and then suddenly into a skull. She screamed and fainted on the spot, and the vision returned time and again through the summer of 1880 and into the year 1882, until Anna told Breuer of her experience. Then this symptom too vanished.

With all her symptoms dissolving in catharsis, Breuer decided to fade out of the picture in the summer of 1882, satisfied with the results. He wrote later that Anna took a vacation from Vienna and after a time came to enjoy perfect health.

The true story grows murky, however, following these remarkable breakthroughs. In Breuer's conversations with Freud, and in Freud's with his biographer and disciple Ernest Jones, there remains room for doubt about what really happened. Breuer seems to have related to Freud that at the end of the treatment, when the old symptoms were gone, a new, frightening one suddenly appeared. On the very evening the internist said goodbye to his patient, a servant came running to his home summoning him back to the Pappenheim residence. There, to his amazement, he found the girl in the midst of a hysterical pregnancy, sweating profusely, writhing and clutching at her bloated and engorged abdomen, screaming that Breuer's child was about to be born. The good physician hypnotized the girl, reverting to suggestion in the manner of Bernheim and Liébeault. He apparently told her that she soon would get better. Then, uttering superficial condolences to Frau Pappenheim, he is said, by Jones, to have fled the house and sped off to Venice for a second honeymoon with his wife.

Regardless of what truly happened in the months following this first talking cure, patient and doctor never saw each other again. The years passed, and Bertha, according to Jones, relapsed and was placed in a sanatorium. Later still she moved to Frankfurt with her mother. There she became progressively interested in social causes and feminism. Though Freudians might make much of her special interest in reforming young Jewish prostitutes, she nonetheless did important pioneer work with orphans and children who were the victims of white slavery. Dying mercifully in 1936 before the Holocaust reached its peak, Bertha was commemorated in postwar Germany with a postage stamp bearing her portrait for her achievements in social work.

After Bertha left his care Breuer ruminated on the case, and he

told the hair-raising tale to Freud. Breuer admitted that he found
the treatment of Anna/Bertha too demanding, and his work and
interests moved in directions other than neurosis. His young
protegé, however, who had already been intrigued with hysteria
and hypnosis since his days with Charcot and Bernheim, began to
use hypnosis in his talking cure. By 1895 Breuer and Freud completed a book on the subject called *Studies on Hysteria*, in which
the Anna O. case was presented.

Meanwhile, in Paris, at the Salpêtrière, Janet was undertaking
some similar intimate studies with hysterical patients and was
making some parallel discoveries. He had been educated as a
philosopher before going into medicine. Always intensely interested in psychology, he had been weaned on Descartes, Rousseau,
Renan, Taine, and other great thinkers who had mingled the
search for philosophical truth with the search for understanding
the heart of human beings. He had a second education as a doctor
precisely so he could work as a medical psychologist. Sent off to Le
Havre for his training after medical school, he met a famous hysteric, Léonie, on whom he did telepathic experiments. These
extraordinary studies, the results of which he later thought false
because of the overzealousness of his assistants, nonetheless caught
the eye of Charcot. The Master invited the promising young man
to the Salpêtrière in 1889.

In the next few years Janet stumbled on his own talking-cure
technique, in which hypnosis played an important role. His cases
tended to lack the intensity of the Anna case, yet they became well
known in the 1890s. Perhaps the most famous was that of Mme. D.
If Breuer's Anna O. is tragic in tone, Janet's Mme. D. has a comic
cast.

In August 1891 Mme. D. was sitting at her sewing machine in
her little house in Calais, her husband was at work as a carpenter,
and her children were off at school. The daughter of an alcoholic
father and a slightly nervous mother, the thirty-four-year-old
Madame D. had always been afraid of snakes and spiders and
was easily frightened and prone to fainting. Hence her nervous
system seemed susceptible to the psychic schock she was about to
experience. As she sat sewing, a stranger, an anonymous villain,
appeared at her doorstep. This was no melodramatic nightmare,
although it reads like one. Turning to greet him, Mme. D. heard

him say, "Madame, prepare a bed. Your dead husband will be brought to you." Mme. D. lowered her head onto her sewing machine, growing paralyzed with shock. Then the stranger placed his hand on her shoulder and continued, "Do not cry so much. Go and prepare a bed." In a twinkling he was gone and was never heard from again.

The devastated woman sat paralyzed and weeping, and her cries attracted her neighbors, who came crowding around her. A messenger was sent to fetch her hard-working husband. As he approached his home, still very much alive, someone shouted, "Here he is!" Mme. D., imagining his cadaver, was overcome by an attack of hysteria.

While her husband and family watched and suffered along with her, she was delirious for three days, reliving her traumatic encounter with the stranger, seeing the body of her husband, crying out for pity for her orphaned children. For brief spells during this period of passionate attitudes she became conscious and seemed better. Then the delirium would recur and the visions and fears would overcome her. She would twist and turn in her bed, shouting and screaming. Finally she awoke from her delirium and discovered that her husband was alive. She was overjoyed and embraced him wildly, and friends and family all hoped she was better.

Soon, however, it was noticed that she suffered from a peculiar form of amnesia, resembling that of inveterate alcoholics or individuals who had suffered concussions after being thrown from horses or after train accidents. Like a concussion victim, she had forgotten not only the incident with the blackguard who had announced her husband's death but also the six weeks prior to the event, back into July of 1891. Like an alcoholic, she could remember nothing that anyone said to her, nothing that she did in the course of a day, nothing that she was supposed to do, from the day of her awakening forward. So she had to keep a notebook in an apron pocket and record everything. She would go to the market carrying her shopping bag. Consulting her notebook, she would buy a dozen eggs, reconsult her notebook, move on, buy beefsteaks. Confused as to where the bakery might be, she would consult her notebook again and follow the directions as if reading a treasure map. Not remembering what she wanted when she got there, she would look at her notebook and realize that she needed not only croissants but also three sticks of bread.

So things remained for three months. In late October of 1891 she was bitten by a mad dog and later could not even remember the experience. The poor woman was taken to Paris for the Pasteur's rabies cure, which proved successful. She and her husband then made the rounds of the Eiffel Tower, the Tuilleries, the Arc de Triomphe. To M. D. it was a great occasion, his first trip to the capital. Yet always, at every turn, he was being questioned by his amnesic wife: "Where are we?" His staccato reply: "Paris." Her surprise: "Really?" Nothing seemed to stay in her mind, of Paris, of Pasteur, of anything.

The exasperated and long-suffering husband, acting on the advice of a Dr. J. of Calais, brought his wife to the Salpêtrière to see Charcot in October 1891. The doctors searched her body for areas of anesthesia, for hysterogenic zones, for paralysis and contractures, and came up empty-handed. Yet the three-day fit seemed hysterical enough, and she still had brief recurrences of the symptoms. Hence the diagnosis of an atypical hysteria was soon made.

Placed in a ward in the Salpêtrière, Mme. D. was torn away from her husband, who must have been relieved to return to Calais without this sieve of a wife. Appointing two of her bedmates to eavesdrop on Mme. D., Charcot awaited reports of her state of mind. The hysterical bedmates gained her confidence. Though Mme. D. undertook a cure of electricity, rest, and massage, she failed to improve. But Charcot learned from his agents that she talked in her sleep. What did she say? She spoke of the incident with the mysterious man, of the incidents of the day just passed, all supposedly lost from her mind.

Charcot included her in one of his presentations and questioned her about all the events in her life up to July 1891. She had a prodigious memory but remembered nothing after July 16, 1891. She could not even recall anything about the very Tuesday when she stood before Charcot and his august group of doctors. Nothing at all. She could not remember what she had had for breakfast. She could not remember what she had had for lunch. She was taken from the auditorium to be hypnotized, and when she returned she told all. She recalled when the mysterious man said to her, "Madame, prepare a bed. Your dead husband will be brought to you." She remembered the bite by the rabid dog, the journey to Pasteur in Paris, the Eiffel Tower, the Arc de Triomphe, the Salpêtrière, the names of her two bedmates, what she had had for breakfast and lunch on that very day.

Then she was awakened, and she forgot all. Her memory melted away like a bad dream. Recent memories were once again lost to her. Charcot had her hypnotized again and made a posthypnotic suggestion that she hold certain memories in her mind after she awoke. He awakened her, and she remembered a few items. Quickly, though, a shroud covered these memories, and within a few days she forgot them all again. At this point Charcot threw up his hands and turned the woman over to Janet.

Janet quickly grew curious about the fact that his new patient remembered many things in her dreams, as her ever vigilant bedmates continued to testify. He assumed that the lost memories were all hidden somewhere in Mme. D.'s subconscious and that they might be set free through some manipulation. He then made an intriguing new departure in treating her. He took over the idea of automatic writing, a technique fairly widespread just at that time, then pushed it in a new direction, changing it into automatic talking. This was carried out not under hypnosis but during distraction. He had an assistant involve her in a very animated discussion. (Unfortunately we never learn precisely what the content of this discussion was.) While she was distracted—that is, while she was consciously elsewhere—he would sneak up on her and whisper in her ear various questions, and he would receive answers. "What is the name of your intern?" "Monsieur Lavey." "How did you cut your left hand?" "With a piece of glass." Janet had found that he could communicate with her subconscious through his technique. This was a revelation. The part of her mind in which her memory was theoretically held captive now lay open.

Janet then used a technique that he had already employed on a few patients, which he called the cathartic technique of hypnosis. His hypothesis was that the evil memory of her experience with the stranger, a fixed idea, as he called it, had created her memory problem. In her dreams Mme. D. replayed the scene of August 1891 night after night. She frequently had serious difficulties falling asleep, fearful of this recurring dream. "In a word," wrote Janet, ". . . the terrifying events of August 28 have not disappeared from the mind of Mme. D."

Janet had gotten to know this woman far better than Charcot had. He had watched and observed and interacted with her carefully, taking copious notes on everything that she said, and he had concluded that her *idée fixe* was the central pathological agent. He contended that it had dissolved her ability to synthesize new data in her consciousness. Hypnotizing her, he spoke to her in her trance. Rather than ordering her to forget the incident—the technique that would have been used by Bernheim—he had her describe all the details that her subconscious mind could remember about the incident of August 28.

Janet perceived the pathological memory of the past traumatic experience as a plastic phenomenon that could be altered in the present by suggesting slight but significant alterations in the memory. First he changed her memory of the man. Over time, after many hypnotic suggestions, he transformed the trickster into none other than Pierre Janet himself. Then he changed the very words Mme. D. heard on August 28, 1891. Instead of the terrifying message about her husband, Mme. D. began to remember hearing, "Madame, prepare a bed. I would like to stay at your house in Calais."

As these subtle suggestions began to work their magic on the fixed idea, which Janet saw as a parasite in the mind of the hereditarily susceptible Mme. D., her memory began to reappear. Freudians might argue that Janet had intuitively stumbled on the idea that the psychotherapist represented at once the violator of the patient's home, her husband, and even her father. Also they might say that he was intuitively working on her sexuality by suggesting the idea that she prepare a bed for him. Regardless of the validity of these arguments, Janet began to see a return of Mme. D.'s memory concerning July of 1891, then August, and even the months before and during her hospitalization at the Salpêtrière. Janet reported that she literally grasped her head and complained of severe headaches and dizziness as the memories flooded back.

This treatment of assaulting the *idée fixe* and transforming it lasted for a little more than two years, from about January of 1892 until April of 1894. Her memory slowly and surely began to return. Never, unfortunately for M. D. and their children, never did it completely catch up. As her life advanced, she would always remember what had happened three weeks earlier, but nothing after. On September 21, 1895, she could remember what had happened up to the first of September, and so on. She remained difficult to live with, forgetting everything her husband or Janet had just said to her. Nevertheless she was discharged from the Salpêtrière and returned to Calais to live relatively happily ever after.

What is always so dissatisfying to us about Janet's work with this woman and other patients is his failure to go behind the incident, to look deeply at the psychic shock. For instance, he always believed that the mysterious visitor actually existed, never entertaining the idea of his being a fantasy for Mme. D., a strange male interrupting her boring life to announce the death of her uninteresting if hardworking husband. Perhaps she had just read *Madame Bovary* and was waiting for a dashing young cavalier to free her from her carpenter husband. Janet never even considered that she might find some pleasure in the notoriety she received in her town and at the Salpêtrière for her hysterical performance.

In this respect the case history of Mme. D., as reported by Janet, is a cartoon, a caricature of a Freudian talking cure. Mme. D. and her husband are never fleshed out as characters. If Mme. D. shrieked on hearing the trumped-up news of her husband's death and fell in a faint, then to Janet she was surely a degenerate, an overly susceptible woman, born to an alcoholic father and a nervous, fainting mother. He never made anything at all of the fact that her parents were separated because of her father's alcoholism and philandering. Mme. D.'s mother's silence on these issues when Mme. D. was a girl seemed only natural to Janet. With such material—from which Freud would soon weave the idea of early childhood trauma, within which a neurosis would ripen—Janet did nothing. Yet he cannot be faulted for what he did not know or, more correctly, did not believe was important. He did some interesting and highly innovative work with Mme. D. that was worth while in its own right.

Meanwhile Freud was directing his efforts and ideas into the area of hypnosis and hysteria. He pursued his studies single-mindedly in the late 1880s and early 1890s and was becoming a great expert. He had met Bernheim in Nancy in 1889, and he became his German translator.

Freud's own contributions to *Studies on Hysteria* are extensive. His four cases include a governess named Lucy, who developed a hallucination of burning pudding and was cured once she admitted she was in love with her employer, and Katherina, a nice country girl he met while he was vacationing in the Alps. She told him of her hysterical problems, which developed after she was raped by her father. The pathology of all four of these cases of hysteria and his next great case, himself, centered on a sexual event and perhaps a forbidden wish. One of his contributions to *Studies* was theoretical, namely the idea that in hysteria the patient suffered from a sexual wish that had to be repressed and then led to hysterical symptoms. Another was therapeutic, namely, the notion that in the treatment of hysteria a new technique, usually called free association, was more useful and practical than hypnosis.

As the next few years passed, Freud became progressively more isolated from Breuer. The internist was never comfortable with the idea of a repressed sexual wish, and Freud became more and more involved in examining his own psychological makeup. His study culminated in his *Interpretation of Dreams* of 1899–1900. While he was writing this great work Freud was employing free association and the theory of sexual wishes on many patients referred to him from colleagues in Vienna. One case, that of Dora/Rosa Bauer, was in many ways his greatest work.

Dora/Rosa was an eighteen-year-old girl who came to see Freud in the autumn of 1900. Freud had successfully treated her father for syphilis four years previously and had met Dora two years earlier. She was handed over to Freud by her father, who said, "Bring her to reason." Freud began to see her many times every week. He learned that she and her parents were all on bad terms with one another. Dora's father admitted to Freud that he was "getting nothing" from his wife. Meanwhile Dora's mother was trying to involve her in housework, while Dora wanted to attend lectures for women in Vienna. On one occasion Herr and Frau Bauer found a suicide note on Dora's desk, and later, when her father was quarreling with her, she suddenly fainted. "The attack was, I believe," wrote Freud, "accompanied by convulsions and delirious states." Her somatic symptoms increased: "Dyspnea, *tussis nervosa,* aphonia, and possibly migraines, together with depression, hysterical unsociability and tedium vitae which was probably not entirely genuine." We can see that Freud had his own ideas about trickery in hysterics.

He went on to say:

> More interesting cases of hysteria have no doubt been published, and they have very often been more carefully described [the cases of the Salpêtrists' Louise and Geneviève], for nothing will be found in the following pages on the subject of stigmata of cutaneous sensibility, limitation of visual fields or similar matters . . . I may venture to remark, however, that all such collections of strange and wonderful phenomena of hysteria have but slightly advanced our knowledge of the disease which still remains as great a puzzle as ever.

Freud noted that Dora had been treated with hydrotherapy and electricity without success and had come to him as a last resort. He saw his sexual-wish idea as the avenue of attack on her hysterical symptoms. And this avenue would be lined with the patient's dreams, which he could best interpret by asking her to make free associations.

He then laid out Dora's life history. Her father was a wealthy man who had suffered from a spate of infectious illnesses including tuberculosis, syphilis, and probably gonorrhea. Her mother was clean to the point of suffering from a "housewife's psychosis." Dora had lived within a resort town since her sixth birthday. Here the family met the K.'s, husband and wife, who became entangled in their home life. Frau K. became the friend of both Dora and her father, and Herr K. took a special interest in Dora, to whom he began to give little tokens of his friendship. Never fond of her mother, Dora was attached to her father and the K.'s through much of her young life.

Roughly four years before her treatment began, when Dora was with Herr K. at his place of business, he had grabbed her and kissed her on the lips. She had fled in disgust. Two years later she had been walking by a lake in the Alps when Herr K. asked her to sleep with him. Soon she realized that her father and Frau K. had been having a sexual liaison for years and that he might

have been hoping for her to become sexually involved with Herr
K. to keep him satisfied.

All of this Dora related to Freud in their first meetings. If her
father had wanted Freud to talk her out of being upset over his
liaison (reminiscent of the relationship of George Lewes, his wife,
and her lover), then Dora seemed to want Freud to side with her
and help her tell her father that he was a lecherous man.

Freud did neither.

He decided to approach the whole problem through Dora's
dreams. Fresh from writing the dream book, he attacked Dora's
dreams with great verve. In so doing he may have, as later psychoanalysts believe, made Dora think he was interested in sexually
violating her. Dreams are so personal; pursuing them vigorously
might have seemed comparable to penetrating her. In any event,
Dora complied and told her dreams.

Her first recorded dream goes thus: "A house was on fire. My
father was standing beside my bed and woke me up. I dressed
myself quickly. Mother wanted to stop and save her jewel box; but
Father said: 'I refuse to let myself and my two children be burnt
for the sake of your jewel case.' We hurried downstairs, and as
soon as I was outside I woke up."

Freud learned that this was a recurring dream that she first had
had after Herr K. had made advances to her in the Alps, and
further that Herr K. had once given Dora a jewel case as a gift.
"Then a return present," Freud said to Dora, "would have been
very appropriate. Perhaps you did not know that 'jewel-case' is a
favorite expression for . . . the female genitals, I mean."

"I knew you would say that," replied Dora. In the course of the
next three weeks Freud made a number of statements to this
adolescent that would be shocking at any time, let alone in the
Victorian age. He suggested that Dora really wanted a sexual
relationship, not only with Herr K. but also with her father. He
also emphasized the fact that in childhood Dora was not only a
bed wetter but a masturbator. Furthermore, in the text of the case
history, he suggested that Dora's hysteria was essentially a perversion of her sexuality, as she had somehow taken a "natural" feeling of sexual excitement toward Herr K.—who could in reality,
Freud thought, have divorced his wife and married Dora—and

converted this sexual energy into her various hysterical symptoms. Dora could not swallow the whole list of imputations.

In the closing days of the analysis Dora related a second dream:

> I was walking about in a town which I did not know. I saw streets and squares which were strange to me. Then I came into the house [away from home] where I lived, went to my room, and found a letter from Mother lying there. She wrote saying that as I had left home without my parents' knowledge she had not wished to write to me to say that Father was ill. "Now he is dead, and if you like, you can come." I then went to the station and asked about 100 times: "Where is the station?" and I always got the answer: "Five minutes." I then saw a thick wood before me which I went into, and there I asked a man whom I met. He said to me: "Two and a half hours more." He offered to accompany me. But I refused and went alone. I saw the station in front of me and could not reach it. At the same time I had the usual feeling of anxiety that one has in days when one cannot move forward. Then I was at home. I must have been traveling in the meantime, but I knew nothing about it. I walked into the porter's lodge, and inquired for our flat. The maidservant opened the door to me and replied that Mother and the others were already at the cemetery.

While Freud hammered home more and more sexual interpretations, Dora began to grow anxious. It is easy to make fun of Freud's interpretation of "train station" (*Bahnhof*) and "cemetery" (*Friedhof*) as related to an anatomical term for the region of the female genitals (*Vorhof*). This association may have been Freud's, but it was not necessarily Dora's. Also, Freud made much of her meeting the man in the woods and her questioning him, of her being away from home without her parents' knowledge (that is, perhaps, her running off with Herr K.), and so on. Freud's sexual monomania frightened the girl, and it is not surprising that she let him know on December 31, 1900, that she would stop coming to see him.

Returning a number of months later to let Freud know that she had told both the K.'s and her father that she knew of their sexual entanglements, she said goodbye to Freud under ambiguous circumstances, and they never met again. She soon married and moved away from Vienna.

Years later she was treated briefly by one of Freud's disciples, who described her as house-bound and chronically ill. She subsequently moved to New York. Developing many of the qualities of her mother, such as a mania for cleanliness, she died in the twenties of bowel cancer. A Freudian who knew her described her as "one of the most repulsive of hysterics, her death a blessing to those who were close to her."

The cases of Anna, Mme. D., and Dora in many ways represent three of the most intensive treatments of neurosis by psychological means as the nineteenth century gave way to the twentieth and as a physiological explanation of neuroses gave ground to psychological theories. The theories of Breuer, Janet, and Freud can be placed on a spectrum, ranging from the physiological to a mixture of the physiological and the psychological to the essentially psychological.

To Breuer, the power of autosuggestion depended on an aberrant state of the brain. He posited that Anna was in a "hypnoid" state when her various hysterical symptoms appeared. He argued that she was predisposed to hysteria, since her family tree was riddled with mental illness. But he saw the real source of the pathology as her nightly vigils at her father's bedside, when she was in a state of constant fright and fatigue and was susceptible to passing into the second state of mind, the hypnoid or autohypnotic one. In this state her nervous energy would move, not toward consciousness but toward the development of hysterical symptoms.

Arguing by analogy to an electrical system, he spoke of how the organ of mind in the "normal, conscious man" is connected to the organ of feelings and passions. An idea mixes readily with a proper feeling and is expressed through a proper outflow of passion—tears or an outburst of anger. Not so in the hysteric, who, through a combination of hereditary predisposition and a period of fright and exhaustion, can undergo a faulty neurological process. As Anna sat at her father's bedside in a hypnoid state, various nerve centers in the brain that played a part in circulation and digestion were called into play. When feelings such as anger or sadness were not properly expressed, the nervous energy was trapped below consciousness and converted into hysterical symptoms having to do with circulation and digestion. The nervous energy passed along paths that eventually became permanent. Through the cathartic approach the energy was redirected, and the idea was reconnected with the proper feeling. The emotion could then be expressed and the hysterical symptoms could disappear.

Janet's theory was less physiological but also less oriented toward emotions. His thinking centered around the fixed idea, namely, some experience of an individual that gets caught in the subconscious. The experience is so shocking or frightening that it upsets the synthetic faculty of the mind, which Janet associated with the higher brain centers. Mme. D.'s hereditary predisposition to superstitions and fears left her susceptible to the mysterious stranger. The horrid experience with him upset her ability to think straight, to remember. Also, the fixed idea got caught in her subconscious, the automatic part of her brain, and obstructed her ability to attend to and remember anything new thereafter. In his treatment Janet concentrated on reshaping this fixed idea into an innocuous idea that could be remembered without pain. This technique invigorated the synthetic functioning of the mind, weakening the power of the devastating idea to distract the person.

Though Janet's technique was also called the cathartic approach, it differed markedly from Breuer's, since emotions or affect played a less important role than ideas. Furthermore, Breuer simply expected his patient to remember the unhappy experience and to connect it with the dreadful feeling and passion. Janet actually went over and over the experience and tried to reshape it.

Freud moved far beyond both of these cathartic approaches and theories with his ideas of wish fulfillment and free association. His theory required evil wishes on the part of the hysteric, such as a desire to have sex with one's father or to be seduced by a married man, along with a great sexual curiosity and a tendency toward masturbation and even homosexuality (which Freud believed Dora had in her feelings toward Frau K.).

Freud's theory—at least at this point in his writings—was a clear and simple one based on "defense" and "repression," as he calls these phenomena. Young women such as Dora, Katherina, and

Lucy the governess—one cannot help wondering what would have happened if he had treated Mme. D. and Anna O.—all suffered from illicit sexual wishes that had leaped into their consciousness but were so aberrant, even perverse, that they had to be repressed —that is, unthought, pushed into the unconscious. From there these wishes connected to the various body parts, such as the throat, in the case of Dora's cough, or the right leg, in the case of her limp, and so forth. These symptoms revealed a symbolic connection, not an energy connection, as Breuer was positing. Dora's cough was connected to Herr K.'s kiss, her limp to her feeling that she had taken a "false step" in wanting to be seduced by Herr K. Freud's theory made the hysteric not a victim, as in the cases of both Anna O. and Mme. D., but an active agent in her own illness.

The major difference between the theories of Breuer and Janet on the one hand, and Freud on the other, is this new emphasis on the active role of the neurotic. Anna O. was a long-suffering Victorian Angelic Invalid whose self-sacrifice was her undoing. Janet's Mme. D. was a Degenerate whose tainted heredity was catalyzed into hysteria by a Charcotian shock. To be sure, both women were passionate Victorians whose loves for father and husband were central in the breeding of the neuroses. Nonetheless both were victimized by heredity and environment. The doctor used hypnosis, talking, compassion, and personal closeness to save them.

Meanwhile Freud made a brilliant departure in developing his own myth about neurosis. Oedipus may have fallen into the trap of killing his father and marrying his mother and then blinding himself after recognizing what he had done. But Dora, if Freud could have helped it, would not have suffered, since she would have recognized her evil wishes through free association and dream analysis, and in so doing she would have been freed from her symptoms. In helping her reach this recognition he expected the symptoms to vanish. His theory was very definitely not one of brain but of mind. Though he never denied the importance of heredity and environment in the breeding of neurosis, his neurotics were able to shape their own minds. Furthermore, the realm of symbols and archetypes looms large in Freud's work. For Freud the patient's wishes hold center stage. Electricity, spas, rest, even hypnosis—all of the Victorian instruments for fighting neurosis—

fall by the wayside. Sexuality and dreams, really just wishes escaping in disguise, are at the core of the theory. Talking, associating, analyzing are the tools of cure.

Freud believed that he was uncovering time and again the startling fact that there existed a split between what the Victorians, and all humans, wanted to think and what actually existed in the mind. In their heart of hearts, men and women were not simply good and delicate and sweet and fair or lecherous and hideous and ugly. Everyone was capable of murder, lust, perversion, and incest, as well as of love and compassion. Even the good little girl virtuously minding a dying relative, the good housewife sitting at her sewing machine, the innocent adolescent setting forth into the wide world already possessed a nature at war with itself.

Freud was, of course, not the first to recognize this split. He acknowledged that many great artists such as Dostoevski, Zola, Rossetti, and Wagner were excruciatingly aware of this inner struggle. Other thinkers, such as Nietzsche and Marx, were working with similar ideas. Nor was Freud really the first doctor to outline this struggle. Krafft-Ebing and his followers, the sexologists, were quite involved in studying it. But Freud, unlike all other medical thinkers, saw not only sexuality but illicit sexual wishes as so ingrained in every human being, in every minute of his waking life, that to deny them, to thrust them aside via an act of the will, like the adolescent who eschews masturbation, was no answer to the problem. Rather, the human being must admit his own centrally sexual nature and strive to channel it into creative directions.

FOURTEEN

Angels and Oedipus

REUD himself was a victim of a Victorian neurosis, his addiction to nicotine. Seeing it as related to the "primary addiction," masturbation, Freud used the drug to stimulate his nerves, his mind. Nicotine probably played a crucial part in the progress of his intense intellectual life, his spinning out a skein of books, articles, and monographs between 1900 and his death in 1939. His ideas of free association, childhood sexuality, defenses, unconscious conflict appealed to many in the West, and he gradually attracted many disciples.

As the years passed, Freud developed painful sores in his mouth. They festered and drove him to an otolaryngologist in the 1920s—his first ear, nose, and throat doctor since his old friend Wilhelm Fliess. The doctor diagnosed cancer. After a bloody operation he warned Freud to avoid cigars, to kick the habit, since smoke irritated the mucous membranes, thus heightening the possibility of a recurrence of the cancer. As he did with Fliess's prescription in 1889, Freud ignored the doctor's advice. Hence he suffered recurrence after recurrence of the cancer, operation following bloody operation. He stoically underwent this pain, this self-induced torture. He smoked cigars until his death at the age of eighty-three.

With Freud we have arrived in the modern world. We have left the land of picturesque Victorian invalids waiting for their heroes to arrive, mysterious victims of moral shock, convalescing and idling. We have entered a world of painful admissions of our own amoral desires. After the Freudians, neurotics could no longer be seen as passive victims of delicate nerves, of shocks, or of heredity. Instead, the neurotic becomes an active agent in his own demise. The various myths—Onan, Zeus, the Degenerate, the Angelic Invalid—seem less compelling. The roots of health, Freudians believe, are uncovered in the center of a maze. All of the unpleasant wishes, dreads, and desires the patient must lay bare in his heart of hearts. The drama of modern neurosis is fought within our minds. Health is within our own grasp if only we can capture those fleeting wishes, memories, fears—if only we want to be cured.

Freud depicted himself as fighting against the hypocritical attitudes of his time, the tendency to dress up sex as love, death as heroism, dreams as dreaminess. Like Emile Zola, he strove to lay bare in his prose much of what was unappealing in Western society, much that was hypocritical, in need of reform. Freud was bent on exposing to his patients and his society their embarrassing underbellies.

Though some of Freud's biographers question this picture of the Viennese doctor as a toppler of Victorian sensibility, there is much truth in the characterization. To be sure, sex was more commonly discussed than Freud would have us think. Krafft-Ebing's book on sexual perversion was widely read. But it is also true that it was seen as potentially corrupting its readers. The open, unbridled passion of the Wagnerian gods and mythical personages may have appealed to many on the stage, but Max Nordau saw such interest in open passion as prurient. The father of the James family, the parents of Marcel Proust forbade their nervous offspring to attend the theater out of fear of overexcitation and moral corruption. *Aurora Leigh* had to be read under the bedclothes by many Victorian girls, since doctors warned their parents that popular literature might well cause nervous collapse in their daughters. Sexuality was decidedly widespread in the arts and the popular press, but many individuals feared them for that very reason. Through suggestibility, imitation, and nervous weakness a delicate young person could be rendered a sexual pervert, a murderer, a rapist par excellence. Such fears linger into our century, but because of Freud's theories much of the whispering about the human drives toward sexual satisfaction and destruction has ended, and these drives have been accepted as essentially human.

However, though Freud's ideas of Oedipus, the id, resistance, the unconscious, gained momentum and disciples, many doctors in official medicine were not impressed. They did not give up the old theories but refined the old myths and continued their thinking, research, and clinical practices along the old lines of natural science. In so doing they made significant new discoveries that have given the old myths a new scientific character.

By listening to a patient's intensely personal narrative such a doctor could picture hereditarily diseased nervous tissue, unbalanced environmental forces, and individual psychic stresses and struggles as all playing a significant role in neurosis. The doctor's therapeutic responses could be at any of these levels. He could refine his theory from year to year to take account of developments in psychology, sociology, physiology, anatomy, immunology, laboratory techniques, and so forth. Though the growth of such an all-encompassing theory would be slow and undramatic, the medical thinker could continue to model his theory and research on both the natural sciences and the social sciences. The help he could give his patients by way of medications, social interventions, and psychological insights remained uncertain but boundless.

Such a medical thinker was Janet. Although he never collected round himself a group of disciples in the manner of Freud, he onetheless did serious work that to this day permeates French psychiatry especially. His eclectic mix of the physiological and psychological appears less brilliant than Freud's entrancing ideas about dreams, illicit wishes, childhood sexuality. Yet Janet's attempt to locate in the brain the functions of the mind is really the heart of modern psychiatry. His thought seems solidly mainstream, quintessentially post-Freudian, and very modern.

Though Breuer gave up his interest in hypnotism and hysteria after the publication of *Studies on Hysteria* in 1895, and many of the Salpêtrists, following Charcot's death in 1893, returned to studying straightforward neurological disorders, Janet in Paris and Freud in Vienna continued their work with psychological approaches to mental illness. Both made significant contributions to psychiatry. Janet's Madeleine and Freud's Wolf-man were cases that in many respects marked the culmination of their clinical work. In these cases they express some of their most deeply held convictions about neurosis and human nature. Freud found the penultimate traumatic moment, a hallmark of his theory: the primal scene. Janet found a restatement of the old theories of nervous tension and nervous exhaustion.

The two cases have little in common. Janet's Madeleine was essentially a Parisian bag lady, whereas Freud's Wolf-man was the heir of a huge estate in southern Russia. What the two share, however, aside from an interest in drawing and painting, is the label of neurotics in the Victorian sense.

Even this is a complicated characterization. Janet did call Madeleine, the heroine of his last great book, *The Anguish and the Ecstasy* (1926), a neurotic, but he also called her a neuropath and a psychasthenic, both dated terms, as well as a psychotic and a schizophrenic. Freud, meanwhile, defined the Wolf-man as an obsessive neurotic. Later analysts who read this case have suggested a much more disturbing diagnosis, such as a paranoid or "borderline" condition. Regardless of the subtleties of diagnosis, what one sees developing here is a two-tiered psychiatry—of the "haves" from a monetary point of view, the neurotics, who can afford an expensive treatment, and the financial "have-nots," the psychotics, who often cannot. Janet treated the indigent and very disturbed Madeleine within the confines of a decrepit ward of the crumbling Salpêtrière, while Freud treated the depressed but still very elegantly booted Sergei the Wolf-man at high fees in his office on the Berggasse in old Vienna. Though it is probable that the Wolf-man, like Madeleine, suffered from elements of a hereditary nervous problem, his condition was less disastrous, and his thinking and style of living never became so profoundly impaired that he had no recourse but an asylum in which to meet his end.

Despite this difference in clientele and theoretical stance the two great analysts both developed a profound and undying relationship with their patients. Their capacity for empathy may in fact have been the source of their cures.

At first glance Madeleine's case seems almost surreal. What originally attracted Janet to her in the late 1890s were her bizarre symptoms: incessant walking on her toes and saying that she would fly away. Looking over her case history, he fastened on the fact that her mother had died of a brain hemorrhage when Madeleine was a small child. Janet's starting point was hereditary taint and nervous weakness. So it seemed particularly significant that

Madeleine began to walk late and had weak legs, poor balance, and difficulty running and climbing stairs. Because of this weakness and a general debility—persistent coughing and occasional vomiting—she received her education at home. Janet also noted that she was impressionable and prone to violent trembling: "The sound of shoes, the grating of a saw, the grazing of a needle passing through wool caused her to tremble and could lead to fainting. Her morbid fear of storms, railways and automobiles brought about since childhood little nervous crises and periods of catalepsy." In short, Janet believed that her later tiptoeing and her almost religious ecstasies could be attributed to faulty nerves.

Madeleine proved to be an articulate woman. During her treatment she wrote Janet long letters daily. Indeed, after her discharge in 1902 she continued to write him weekly up until 1918, when she died from a heart ailment at the age of sixty-three. Though her ecstasies and tiptoeing first attracted Janet, it was her way of thinking, her interest in communicating with him that kept him involved. Also, the content of her conversation and correspondence piqued Janet's interest. This professor of the Collège de France loved the logical, theological, and philosophical discussions he had with the little Parisian bag lady. These intriguing talks may have been salutary, since it was through them that she developed a deep and abiding relationship with the great psychologist.

She told Janet that she believed walking on her toes was a sign of her being loved by God. She related it, first, to the fact that Christ's legs twisted in the same manner when he suffered on the cross and, second, to the Catholic notion that the Virgin Mary, the Mother of God, had been assumed body and soul into heaven. To Madeleine, walking on tiptoe meant that she too was on the verge of being assumed into heaven.

Janet proclaimed in *The Anguish and the Ecstasy* that there was an ecstatic living in the Salpêtrière. Constantly he compared her to Catholic saints prone to ecstasies, notably Saint Theresa of Avila, Saint John Vianney, Louise Lateau, and others. Most of these ecstatics lived under the protection of the Church. But Madeleine, Janet felt, was a saintly ecstatic who had fallen into the hands of a rationalistic scientist who could study her.

Madeleine's fantastic interpretations of her own symptoms were clearly psychotic by modern standards. Today her thinking would be called delusional. Yet a delusion by definition is a way of thinking that is considered alien to the majority of the community. Since most Frenchmen circa 1900 were Catholics, and in many ways superstitious ones, Madeleine's thinking was not that farfetched. In fact, at the time of her discharge from the Salpêtrière in 1902, she was approached by many priests and religious devotees to provide ammunition against many of Janet's antireligious statements.

Madeleine's life was filled with "singular adventure." Although sickly and nervously sensitive, she had contemplated becoming a schoolteacher. At the time of her first Communion, however, she

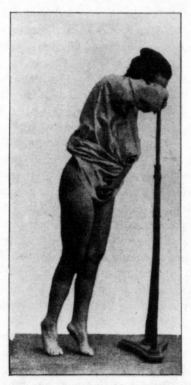

Madeleine, the angel on tiptoe.
(From Pierre Janet, *De l'Angoisse à l'Extase*)

considered giving herself totally to God. Starting at the age of eleven, she began to experience long periods—literally hours—in which she would remain absolutely immobile, lost in deep and peaceful reveries. She was afflicted by tormenting thoughts, veritable obsessions concerning her own sinfulness, her fear of pregnancy, of damnation. At age fourteen she became infatuated with a boy. While he was away at school, she waited impatiently for his return. Upon his homecoming she was devastated to learn that he had forgotten her completely. In a gesture reminiscent of Geneviève's long delirium after the death of Camille, Madeleine then renounced all thoughts of human love; indeed, she found sinful anything hinting of adolescent love. She began to perceive all worldly pleasures as devilish. If she loved dancing, she had to forsake it, and she did. If she enjoyed good food, she had to feed herself only bread and water, and even those she had to consume hurriedly so as not to enjoy them. Similarly with music, clothing, any pleasure in life.

She came to idealize misery, mortification, and the idea of sacrificing her life to the poor. She found her family too worldly, so she left home at the age of eighteen and went to Paris "to lead the life of a worker in one of the poorest quarters in Paris," as she later wrote Janet. Rejecting her real name and taking the name Madeleine, after Mary Magdalene, she cut almost all ties to her family and never divulged her real name to anyone in Paris. She was unjustly arrested for vagrancy and vagabondage and imprisoned for swindling, begging and prostitution. Using the last name of Le Bouc (a name by which she designated herself as both an "emissary" and a "scapegoat"), she devoted herself selflessly to the care of sick, dying, and impoverished women in the ghettos of Paris. Her moods and attitudes alternated between excessive soul-searching and exhilarating love of her life of self-sacrifice. The years rolled by, she grew older, poorer, a habituée of the slums of Paris.

By Christmas 1896 her legs began to ache, to burn like charcoal, and she noticed that she was beginning to walk on her tiptoes. She found that she tired easily, that her malady was undermining her life as an itinerant helper of the poor. She took herself to a hospital. She was examined there by doctors who thought she was suffering from an inflammation of the nerves secondary to either alcoholism or aborted pregnancy. There she was transferred to another hospital, where the diagnosis was hysterical contractures and the treatment was hydrotherapy and magnets. This treatment lasted about a year, but when she failed to improve, she was transferred to the Salpêtrière, where she soon caught the eye of Janet.

Since he knew how to talk to such patients, he soon got her to confide to him her fantasies involving crucifixion and assumption. Indeed, Janet began to notice her tendency to strike the crucifixion pose while asleep in bed and to enter into long and motionless periods of reverie and ecstasy lasting days, even weeks. She also manifested slight wounds in her feet and hands, veritable stigmata similar to those of Saint Francis of Assisi, and she passed into and out of extended reveries and ecstasies, as well as periods of self-torture and self-doubt. In short, her symptoms were comparable to those of Geneviève or Louise Lateau. So Janet's proclamation that he had a Victorian saint in the Salpêtrière had some truth to it.

Madeleine's ecstasies were wondrous to behold. While walking across the ward she would suddenly stand transfixed and remain motionless for up to twenty-four hours on end, not eating, not sleeping, not performing her bodily functions, while Janet himself observed for hours on end. She would not respond to questions, would not follow simple orders, except when Janet prefixed his commands with the words, "Ask God if he will permit you to . . ." Only then would she listen and act accordingly. At first Janet wondered whether she were simply paralyzed, in a coma, but he found that when he whispered various things in her ear during her ecstasies and then asked her later what he had said, she could always remember.

Janet made it clear to Madeleine that he was at best an agnostic, if not an out-and-out atheist, and doctor and patient became involved in a long and amusing series of debates, before, during, and after her ecstasies. Madeleine wrote him daily, gave him her paintings—which depicted her ecstatic visions—and came to describe her states of mind during these ecstasies in much detail. She admitted that sometimes she was in a state of forgetfulness, like sleep, but that even that state involved "delicious drunkenness, in which all my being plunges into a happiness of which I can say nothing. It is a kind of a material death . . . ," she wrote. "I am like a baby in the arms of her mother who from time to time opens

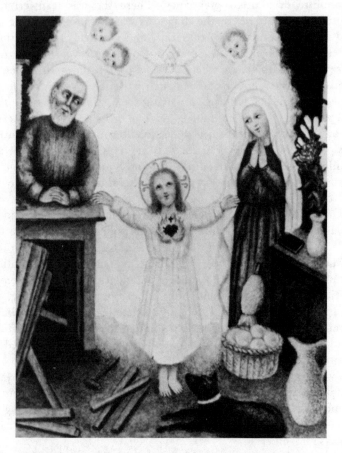

Madeleine's vision of the Holy Family. (From Janet,
De l'Angoisse à l'Extase)

her eyes and tastes the joy of being rocked and who then falls
asleep again."

Her ecstasies involved a drama about a loving couple, God and
Madeleine. Janet thought he had caught Madeleine in a heresy,
since in her ecstasies Madeleine had sex with God. In fact, she was
speaking in terms of a transcendental fusion of opposites, body
and soul. She swung rapidly back and forth between imagining
herself consumed in a pure union with God and seeing herself

entwined in a sexual liaison with the God-man Christ. She confided to Janet: "My being is drunk with divine kisses. Ah, if I
could communicate to you what I have experienced . . . I have just
passed a night of love and madness. Yes, it is true, God has made
me mad with love . . . cascades of tenderness which drown me. Do
not let me think that I only dream. I feel that I truly love God in
all manners . . . I could say to God: Lord, you wish to make me die
of love. My heart is too weak for the torrents which you spill
here." Yet she also wrote: "Virginity is a treasure which takes part
in the spiritual goodness of the Church, the principal virtue of the
holy person is in the purity of his body parts just as the strength of
Samson resided in his hair."

Her ecstasies transported her back to great moments in Christian history and transmuted her into great personages. In various
trances she was present at the crucifixion and at the Nativity. She
took on the role of Christ in the womb of Mary, and then she was
the Virgin Mary herself, pregnant with God. Then she was Jesus
born in the manger, Mary holding the child. Back and forth—
God, woman, lover, sufferer—the ecstasies flowed from moment to
moment.

Her most extraordinary ecstasies involved flying. "I seem to be
careening through the air, traversing space with the swiftness of the
wind . . . I climb to the top of precipices in moments, I descend
into valleys, then upward again. There are no more obstacles for
me. I pass through all places, narrow or inconvenient, with rapidity. I penetrate all that is in my way, like a shadow, like a spirit . . .
What ineluctable voluptuousness, I travel without touching my
feet on the ground. I am like a bird in the air, like a fish in the
water, everything obeys my lightest caprice."

This fantasy of flying, for all its modern sexual connotations,
explained to Madeleine's satisfaction her walking on her toes. She
was verging on flying away.

Like Anna O.'s private theater drawn from Andersen's fairy
tales, Madeleine's fantasies were based on the Gospel story of
Mary, Jesus, and Joseph, with Janet, interestingly, playing the
part of Joseph. Like Breuer with Anna, Janet was at times spell-
bound by Madeleine. She proclaimed that her joy was so great
that she never wanted to get better. Indeed, she described how, in
ecstasy, her mouth experienced a fresh and sweet savor, her nose

was filled with the odors of satiny perfumes, every part of her body was enraptured with voluptuous pleasure beyond the realm of words. She saw new worlds, new suns, opening before her. She saw the apocalypse, aghast at worlds annihilated, a planet unredeemable. She was a voyager in a world of psychedelic pleasures and pains beyond the realms of rational men.

However, Janet called her back, beckoned her to return from the land of joyous and painful madness where she sojourned one day so delightfully, the next so wretchedly. He tried logic, which did not seem to go very far with Madeleine. He tried to convince her she was ill. She sometimes listened, but usually turned a deaf ear. In time, however, he helped her to trust him. She saw him more and more as her spiritual director, who could give her comfort and sweet advice.

Like a good scientist, Janet divided her states of mind into a number of basic parts. Obviously her ecstasies were the central events, but leading up to and following them were the periods of torture, of melancholy, of soul-searching and self-doubt. These were the times when Madeleine was sunk in unrivaled pain. She suspected, during these stages, that her ecstasies were really the devil's tricks, that her marriage with Jesus was really a liaison with Mephisto. She believed that she was damned, that God hated her, that all her sweet ecstasies were chimerical—indeed, all but mad.

Janet seemed to capitalize on her doubts by pointing out heresies inherent in her religious visions. Also, whenever she wrote letters to various French officials to warn them that a dire apocalypse was at hand, Janet never hesitated to underscore the fact that her predictions never came to pass: that the anarchist never blew up the bridge, that the streets of Paris never grew slippery with blood, that this or that official was never assassinated. Janet taught Madeleine his sense of reality, his agnosticism, his religious doubts.

Though in her moments of ecstasy she continued to laugh at his logic, his rationalism, his belief that a good God could not exist in an evil world, her ecstasies and agonies grew less frequent as the years passed, and Madeleine lived more and more in a "state of equilibrium," as Janet called it. She remained a fervent Catholic, to be sure, but she was ultimately discharged from the Salpêtrière in 1904, to live with her sister. Janet had won the battle, and his theory that her religious ecstasies were a product of a faulty nervous system, or of nerve tissue firing awry, seemed supported.

Madeleine lived on through the catastrophes of the Great War, World War I, writing weekly to the aging psychologist-philosopher. Her letters lacked the great poetical passages of rapture, of delight, of pain that had been hers during her madness, when she predicted the end of the world, the destruction of France, and the Second Coming. Janet was surprised that Madeleine, now with support for her dire predictions—World War I, the greatest catastrophe in recorded history—never used it to confirm her apocalyptic point of view.

Janet classified Madeleine as a psychasthenic: literally, a sufferer with a loss of psychic strength. Her illness left her prone to losing control over her reason and descending—like a primitive Bushman, a child, or a drunkard—into periods of nervous weakness, when a lower, less rational side of her mind controlled her whole being. He suspected that her chronic cardiac and gastrointestinal diseases, both discovered at the Salpêtrière, might have contributed to her nervous weakness by preventing adequate nutrition and circulation in her brain. He saw her mad love for Christ as little more than an erotomania and compared her madness to that of other patients of his who believed that Colonel X or Abbé Y was in love with them or had impregnated them or was persecuting them. Thus Janet secularized this would-be saint. He had rationalized her glamour, taken away her wings, and in so doing placed us all in the gray humdrum of the modern world.

Janet's treatment of Madeleine was a marvelous event in medical history. He was one of the first in a growing tradition of mind healers who believed they could talk the madman out of his madness. It required a great hubris, a conviction that his beliefs were truer than Madeleine's, that his logic was more compelling than her transcendental visions. Yet by exercising such pride in his therapy, Janet performed an act of great heroism in seemingly curing a psychotic.

In his descriptions of Madeleine, Janet occasionally mentioned Freud. However, he generally dismissed the Freudians' approach as ludicrous, especially when he imagined them trying to interpret Madeleine's sexual ecstasies in terms of her desire to kill her mother and marry her father. Nonetheless Janet saw Madeleine's weird fantasies of becoming Christ in the womb of Mary as an amazing

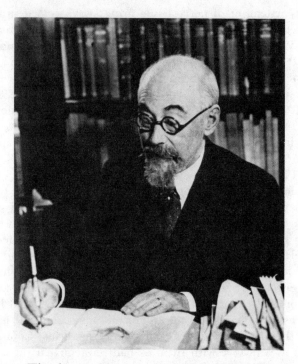

The doctor, Pierre Janet. (Studios Janet-Le Caisne, Paris)

piece of symbolism. The use of symbols was central to Freud's way of thinking, and in the case of the Wolf-man, Freud showed virtuosity in manipulating one of his patient's dreams to explain much of his neurosis. One dream image represented to Freud—and the Wolf-man concurred in this interpretation—the great primal scene, the moment when the child saw his parents in the midst of the sexual act.

The Wolf-man was a great character, one of the most celebrated in the Viennese psychoanalytic community of the 1920s. He was a living testament to the validity of psychoanalysis, and he wrote his memoirs to enrich the psychoanalytic literature.

Born in 1886 in southern Russia into a family of great landowners, Sergei the Wolf-man lived a sad existence almost from the time of his birth. His family was hereditarily tainted in the Vic-

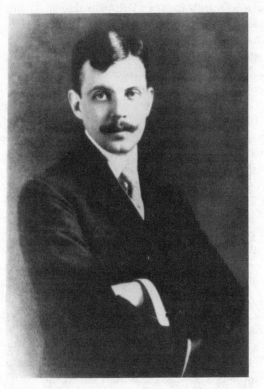

The patient, Sergei, the Wolf-man. (From Muriel Gardiner, *The Wolf-man: The Double Story of Freud's Most Famous Case*)

torian and post-Freudian sense. One paternal uncle, Peter, went mad when Sergei was a boy, and Sergei's father spent a good part of his adult life in various sanatoriums because of manic-depressive illness. Deep depression and suicide stalked the family.

Sergei clearly became a neurotic in his late teens. In 1906 his sister Anna went on a visit and—with little more than a hint to anyone—committed suicide. Sergei wrote in his memoirs that at this point he passed into a deep and dark depression. Freud took as a starting point for the Wolf-man's woes his contracting gonorrhea from a servant girl at the age of eighteen. Regardless of which version identifies the beginning, the years of deep unhappiness began to unroll for the Wolf-man. He gave up all plans for his future and joined the class of idle Russian rich, like a character from a Chekhov play, lacking a direction or purpose. By 1908, when he was twenty-two, his condition became so painful that he went to St. Petersburg to see a Professor B.

The professor made the usual diagnosis, neurasthenia, and recommended the usual treatment, hypnosis. "After greeting me, Professor B. made me sit down," wrote Sergei, "and said in a firm and persuasive voice: 'You will wake up tomorrow morning feeling fit and healthy. Your depression will completely disappear, gloomy and sad thoughts will stop, and you will see everything in a new and different light.' " All well and good; if a more extended hypnotherapy had followed, Professor B. might have been partially successful and Sergei may never have become the Wolf-man. The good professor, however, said during hypnosis, "As you know, your parents plan to donate a large sum of money for the foundation of a neurological hospital. It happens that just now the construction of a neurological institute is about to be started in St. Petersburg. . . . The realization of these goals is so important and worthwhile you should endeavor to persuade them to donate their funds to the neurological institute." The Wolf-man was so shaken by this bit of persuasion mixed with healing that he abandoned treatment by the unscrupulous professor. He elected to go to Germany for the Rest Cure. He went to Munich in the spring of 1908 to see Professor Emil Kraepelin, the greatest German psychiatrist then living, who diagnosed him as manic-depressive, like his father, and sent him to a sanatorium in the Bavarian countryside.

The night of his arrival there was probably the most momentous in his adult life. A fancy-dress ball was under way and he glimpsed an extraordinarily beautiful woman who was dressed as a Turkish concubine. With her blue-black hair parted in the middle and her chiseled features, she seemed to Sergei an apparition from the pages of the *Arabian Nights*. Within a few days he was head over heels in love with the intriguing demoiselle.

In fact, this apparition was a nurse named Therese, who worked at the sanatorium, a divorcée with a child named Else. These forbidding facts did not discourage the Russian invalid, who "now embraced life fully. And . . . [life] seemed to me highly rewarding, but only on condition that Thérèse be willing to enter

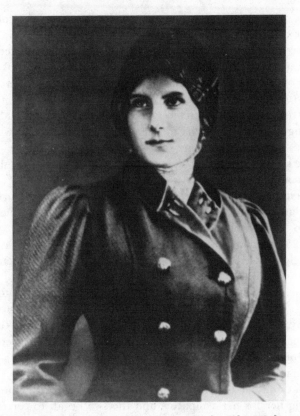

Therese, Sergei's czarina. (From Gardiner, *The Wolf-man:
The Double Story of Freud's Most Famous Case*)

into a love affair with me." Sergei was decidedly not a Victorian
prude; by this time he had had much experience making love to
servants and peasant girls. With reckless and passionate Russian
abandon, he pursued the lovely princess-nurse to her room a few
days later, burst into her quarters, and insisted on a rendezvous.
Though she gave him a time and place, she never appeared. Since
his happiness hinged on the favors of this fair woman, he asked
again for a rendezvous, which she never kept, and then another.

Meanwhile taking all the baths, massages, and other therapy
prescribed by the doctors, he noticed that his health was improving by leaps and bounds. Though rebuffed time and again by

Therese, who pleaded that love was not for her, that her profession and her child were her great passions, Sergei vowed that he would be successful. His moods swung wildly as Therese flirted with him, then gave him the cold shoulder. Eventually he spoke with his doctors about his love. They counseled forgetting Therese. He grew wretched, tormented, empty-feeling. Acting against the advice of the doctors, he left the sanatorium and moved to Munich. Awaiting the arrival of his mother from Russia, Sergei wrote to Therese, asking her to come to his hotel and say goodbye. To his surprise she complied, and they made love all night. Then she said a sad goodbye at daybreak.

His mother arrived soon afterward, and the two sojourned in Switzerland, where he poured out his torments to her. Then they went to Paris, where his Uncle Basel, like Krafft-Ebing, recommended a regimen of one-night stands with prostitutes as a cure for the lovelorn Russian. Sergei partook of this medicine plentifully but unsuccessfully.

In the summer of 1908 he and his mother returned to their estate. Then, as in a Shakespearean tragedy where misfortunes multiply, mother and son received a telegram informing them of the father's premature death—by suicide. The family went into deep mourning. The weeks crawled past and the brooding of the Wolf-man increased.

Then came a letter of condolence from Therese. He wrote back, thanking her for her sympathy, and the two began to correspond. He tried to find relief from his aching heart by throwing himself into his pastime of painting. That autumn he traveled back to Munich to consult Dr. Kraepelin again and, he admitted later, to see Therese. Sergei and Therese met one night, made furious love, and parted with the understanding that they would write.

Sent off to various sanatoriums by Kraepelin and other doctors, he refused to stay for very long in any one place and often traveled to Munich to see Therese. Sergei's moods varied greatly—joy, bliss, depression—as did Therese's. At times she was hopeful that they could be happy together, then doubtful, then forlorn because Sergei did not propose marriage to her. Sergei's mother and all of his doctors were adamantly against it. His mother seemed to consider it an out-and-out misalliance: a Russian gentleman heir and a Bavarian nurse divorcée. The doctors probably used a similar rationale but also did not hesitate to argue that, despite Therese's apparent stability as a nurse and mother, she was really a fickle and unpredictable hysteric, a divorcée.

Sergei began to note that his feelings for her were cooling. In the summer of 1909 he set off to meet Therese in Berlin, intending to sever the relationship. Once he saw her, however, he felt pulled in two directions. In a tempestuous scene in their hotel room she raged and screamed. She scoffed at his noncommittal attitude. One minute she spoke of leaving him, the next she pleaded for marriage. Then she began to pack her bags. The Russian remained lukewarm, and her hysterics passed. They "turned out the lights." That night was a sleepless one for Sergei, and the next day he left Therese without a word. He wrote her of his decision to break with her. Soon he was reproaching himself for writing this letter, yet he did not venture to undo it.

As the weeks on his estate lengthened into months, his grim despondency returned with all its nagging force, and his mother urged him to get in touch with a young psychiatrist in Odessa, Dr. D. "With his gold-rimmed spectacles and his square trimmed reddish beard," Dr. D. seems to have been a long-distance student of Sigmund Freud's. He explained to Sergei that emotional suffering could not be cured by baths, diet, or massage and that a talking cure and analysis was the only solution. Dr. D. had barely a clue as to how to go about this, but he was willing to give it a try. After a few weeks in the summer of 1909 Dr. D. finally admitted that he really could not do psychoanalysis, and he suggested that the noble invalid go to Vienna to undergo treatment with the master himself. Dr. D. even suggested that he go as Sergei's chaperone, his expenses to be paid by Sergei of course. Sergei consented.

Arriving in Vienna in January 1910, Sergei went to Freud and was much impressed with his personality. "Of course, I told Professor Freud of my stormy relationship with Therese in Munich," wrote Sergei, "and of Therese's visit to Berlin which had such an unexpected and fateful end. Freud's judgment on the former was a positive one, but he called the latter a 'flight from the woman,' and in accordance with this he answered my question of whether I should return to Therese with a 'yes,' with the condition that this would take place only after several months of analysis." The Wolfman's decision to remain with Freud seems grounded in the fact that Freud did not dissuade him from his relationship with Therese as the other Victorian doctors and his mother had, and may have encouraged it as a healthy development.

Dr. D., incidentally, continued to serve as companion to the rich invalid, appearing in the "role of maître de plaisir, the one who would decide how and where we would spend our evenings," only leaving Sergei in the autumn of 1910. Therese reentered the picture in late winter of 1911. Sergei, discovering that she had left her nursing job, had hired detectives to track her down. Now the owner of a small pension in Munich, she was visited by her lover one March day. "When I saw her," writes the Wolf-man, "I was deeply moved. She looked terribly rundown and her no longer fashionable dress hung about her body which had become so thin that it was scarcely more than a skeleton. . . . At this moment I determined never again to leave the woman whom I had caused to suffer so terribly."

Therese resolved to sell her pension and move to Vienna with Sergei. Freud had a rule that his patients shouldn't marry during analysis, and so the two lived together, unmarried, with the little girl Else. The curtain of this little drama goes down at this point, with Sergei silent about his treatment with Freud, which lasted from 1910 until the outbreak of World War I in 1914. At this point we must turn to Freud's case history to piece together the analysis itself.

Freud's case study began in about the fourth year of treatment. He explained a little about the adult neurotic conflict of the Wolf-man, namely, that he suffered from chronic constipation, which Freud attributed to anal eroticism. Also, the Wolf-man told Freud that he wished to defecate on him and have Freud perform anal intercourse with him. Freud said that the Wolf-man was not very depressed during all four years of treatment, so he discarded Kraepelin's diagnosis of manic-depression and suggested obsessive neurosis instead. This was really a major departure. Kraepelin was the doyen of German organic psychiatry, and Freud's rejection of his diagnosis and treatment was a turning point away from organic and toward psychological therapy.

The Wolf-man history, "From the History of an Infantile Neurosis," is an interpretation of Sergei's memories, half memories, and nearly remembered memories, as well as one highly

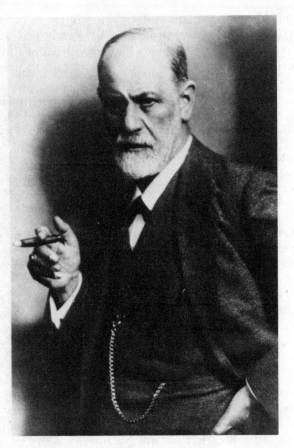

The doctor, Sigmund Freud.
(Mary Evans Picture Library of London)

riveting dream. Freud contended that adult neurosis was caused by distressing childhood experiences. Therefore an uncovering in analysis of an earlier problem could cure the adult illness. He was continuing to think along lines already elucidated in the Dora case, namely, that sexual wishes in childhood and sexually traumatic events set off neurosis. Pursuing his patient's memories back in time, back to early childhood, Freud developed Breuer's idea that a horrible memory and, as in the case of Dora, a despicable wish were at the bottom of every neurosis.

The ultimate memory and subsequent wish in the case of the Wolf-man he connected with the primal scene, which was transmuted into the well remembered childhood dream of this well-to-do Russian invalid. The dream went like this:

> I dreamt that it was night and that I was lying in bed. (My bed stood with its foot towards the window; in front of the window there was a row of old walnut trees. I knew it was winter when I had the dream, and nighttime.) Suddenly the window of its own accord opened, and I was terrified to see some white wolves were sitting on the big walnut tree in front of the window. There were six or seven of them. The wolves were quite white, and looked more like foxes and sheep dogs. They had big tails like foxes and had their ears pricked like dogs when they pay attention to something. In great terror evidently of being eaten by the wolves, I screamed and woke up.

Sergei recounted this dream early in the four-year analysis, and he recollected having dreamed it at about the age of four. Beginning with a series of associations the Wolf-man made to various fairy tales he had heard in childhood, Freud established that the Wolf-man's birthday was on Christmas day—that is, in winter—and that the Wolf-man had been involved in mutual physical exploration with his sister a short time before the winter of his fourth birthday. From this material and a series of other memories both clear and vague the psychoanalyst distilled and mixed the ingredients of this dream and the Wolf-man's adult symptom of constipation and his anal eroticism.

Freud built his case description around the dream, seeing the Wolf-man's adult neurosis as stemming from it and the ensuing anxiety. His idea was that the little boy had been involved in sexual investigations for a few years already, that his governess, his nanny, his sister, and his parents had all played little roles in his confused theories as to what the purpose of the penis was, as well as the anus and the woman's "wound," her vagina. He had fantasies about passive and active sexual contact with his sister, his father, and others. He had been stimulated to fantasize further after seeing various animals—dogs and sheep—copulating on his father's estate. All this, felt Freud, was incubating in the little boy's

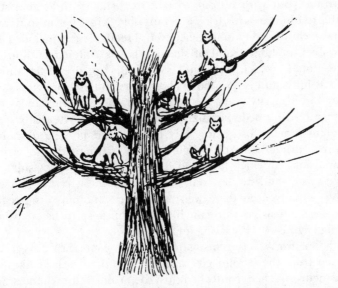

Sergei's sketch of his anxiety dream. (From Gardiner, *The Wolf-man: The Double Story of Freud's Most Famous Case*)

fantasies as he lay sleeping and dreaming one Christmas Eve waiting for his door to swing open and to see his presents hanging on a Christmas tree. The night, of course, ended instead in desolation, in fear, in the nightmare that needed explaining.

Freud concluded that it symbolized an earlier memory. One summer, at the age of one and a half or two and a half, the Wolf-man had awakened from a nap in the middle of the afternoon to see his parents copulating, his mother hunched over like a beast and his father looming over her like a wolf on his hind legs. Seeing this primal scene, thought Freud, he cried out and then defecated.

For many years Freud hovered on the point of believing that his neurotic patients had stored in their memories such primal scenes, such childhood traumas. He thought that if an analysis were carried out correctly, the proper memory or proper dream would be retrieved, would spring out, flashing like a hallucination before the inner eye of the patient. Armed with such a memory, Freud and his patient could begin to unravel the Oedipus complex, both heterosexual and homosexual, and the riddle of the neurosis would be solved. But with no one to talk to then, no child analyst on whom to unburden his fears and fantasies, Sergei began to develop various childhood phobias, believed Freud. These included fear of wolves, of horses, and of sheep. Also he suffered outbursts of aggression in which he would sadistically torture little animals such as birds and caterpillars. These fears and evil practices disappeared in his early years. His religious training at the hands of his mother transformed the anxiety neurosis into a ritualistic quasi-religious practice of kissing holy pictures and praying obsessively before bedtime, and this religiosity was transmuted into weirder compulsions in which he found it necessary to say "God-shit" and "God-swine" and similar contradictory phrases at certain odd moments. Finally even these weird neurotic symptoms disappeared, and the neurosis lay dormant like a syphilitic spirochete, an incubating engine of evil waiting for its moment.

The neurosis was reinstigated by the gonorrhea Sergei contracted from the servant girl, and later by the death of his sister. The neurosis then controlled his life, ruined his chances with women, even directed his love toward "persons who serve others," those of the servant class, peasants, a nurse. Because of his all-powerful neurosis the man could have no life of his own until he entered analysis and recovered his lost memories and then worked to reestablish all the lost associations of his memories to his present symptoms: his passivity, his indecision, his constipation, and his obsessions with defecating on Freud and having anal intercourse with him.

Just as many Victorian doctors who had treated Sergei considered his marriage to Therese to be a misalliance, so do many modern-day analysts regard Sergei's relationship with Freud to have been a misalliance. Freud appears to have committed some tactical mistakes in the analysis. For instance, at one point he took from the Wolf-man a sketch the patient drew of the primal scene. Later he met Therese socially and approvingly commented to the Wolf-man that she looked like a czarina. Modern-day psychoanalytic practice does not allow such interactions between patients and doctors.

Freud's theory in the case history is fraught with odd twistings and turnings, with *jeux de mots*, distillations, and far-fetched contortions. His treatment was nonetheless salutary for the beleaguered Wolf-man, who set off for Russia on the eve of the Great War to make arrangements for his marriage. Despite the outbreak of hostilities between Germany and Russia in August 1914, Therese came to Sergei in Russia, and the two were married in 1915. The war and the Russian Revolution of course destroyed the Wolf-man's wealth. Also, Sergei's mother and Therese disliked each other intensely. Despite these miseries, when the war ended, the Wolf-man and Therese set off for Vienna, where for four months Freud reanalyzed his returned symptom of constipation. The Wolf-man, now nearly penniless, got a job as an insurance agent.

Following the death of her daughter Else of tuberculosis, Therese grew uninterested in sexual contact with Sergei, since it seemed she could not have any more children. She became chronically depressed. Also, the Wolf-man never found any satisfaction in his insurance work. When Freud became ill with his mouth cancer, Sergei developed the delusion that his own nose had a hole in it. He required a brief reanalysis by a disciple of Freud's. In this analysis the Wolf-man spoke of his belief that many people were out to hurt him. When his new analyst interpreted this belief as due to homosexual wishes vis-à-vis Freud, somehow things fell together for the Wolf-man. He was seemingly cured.

Life seemed to be going pretty well till the Nazis came streaming into Vienna. Poor Therese, during an epidemic of suicide, took her own life in 1939. Beside himself with grief, Sergei ran crazy for a while, not able to find any respite until after a brief treatment by his second analyst in the summer of that year. His story goes on unendingly. The Wolf-man barely held himself together. He was decidedly a chronic bed patient who had to get out of bed to earn a living. There was probably a hereditary element to his illness, perhaps manic-depression, handed down from his father. Also, Sergei lived through the greatest catastrophes in Europe, World War I and World War II, and horrendous personal tragedies, namely, the suicides of his sister, his father, and his wife.

It is amazing that Sergei did as well as he did. Later psychoanalysts and psychiatrists have argued that the case is one of a far deeper disturbance than any neurosis, that castration anxiety, primal scenes, and homosexual wishes had little to do with this man's problems; that he really suffered from a genetic predisposition, a true mood disorder like Kraepelin's manic-depression; or at least that his childhood problem was pre-Oedipal, that the problem had more to do with a failure of mother-child attachment than with the vicissitudes of the sexual drive.

Regardless of these later theories, in the case of the Wolf-man, Freud puts forth the theory of a central moment, the primal scene, in the life of the neurotic. This idea was truly imaginative. The rapid growth of psychoanalysis, especially in America, from the 1920s until the 1960s, was the outcome of this compelling theory. Freud's ideas will always remain incredible to the uninitiated, unprovable to the philosopher and psychologist. Yet they will always remain fascinating, just as love, sex, and dreams themselves are eternally with us, yet forever elusive. In our age the word "neurosis" remains ultimately bound to human sexuality.

Meanwhile Janet's books gather dust. In his psychasthenic idea he reverted to the old notion of overexcitation and exhaustion of the mind, an idea as old as Cullen's lax and tense nerves, Cheyne's Angelic Invalid myth. But it is an idea that is forever new and intriguing to medical thinkers. Janet believed that a hereditary imbalance in the brain tissue ignited Madeleine's illness. He believed she suffered, not from the elusive illness we today would call neurosis but from a more organic mental illness, in which there was a biochemical imbalance in her brain tissue. Her ecstasies, her fantasies of being assumed into heaven fell to earth and again became the stuff of twisted nerve tissue. Alongside Freud's truly ingenious idea of the primal scene, that primitive moment when the child sees his parents writhing like demons, Janet's ideas seem too gray, too lifeless for the popular imagination, too stolidly scientific, perhaps too true for us to want to believe.

AFTERWORD

The old theories and myths about neurosis are not dead. Sunk though many may be beneath the flood of the years, in modern times at least a piece of every one of them has surfaced again. Though the psychoanalytic movement flourished, especially in America, in the forties and fifties, and will perennially attract devotees, international psychiatry is truly a polyglot congress in which physiology, psychology, and sociology blend and enrich one another. Psychiatrists have never forgotten and never will forget heredity and environment, the core materials in many of the myths. Attention to disturbed forebears, to cataclysmic events in life, to drug addictions, and to chronic medical conditions remain very much the substance of psychiatric diagnosis and treatment.

America's optimism, its affluence, its opportunities for the individual made this country the natural home of psychoanalysis. The denial of heredity, the apparently boundless plasticity of the environment, and the emphasis on the self seem central American postulates. All these factors, together with a large ambitious middle class, render America a fertile territory for a treatment in which the individual delves into his fantasies, his night and day dreams, and so reshapes the effects of his heredity, his environs, his life-style. This depth psychology, psychoanalysis, remains very much the treatment for Prometheus and the Genius. A person of the upper middle classes with the time, brains, and funds to undertake such an exclusive approach often turns to psychoanalysis. In many instances analysis makes the ambitious and ingenious person more able to be creative and capable. This is how many sophisticated Americans use the wisdom of analysis.

Most European and many American psychiatrists, meanwhile, have ignored or discarded much of Freud in favor of an organic psychiatry. Although small psychoanalytic communities do flourish in all American and European metropolises, many psychiatrists necessarily wear an eclectic garb. They still assume the existence of brain lesions—still undiscovered—in major psychiatric disturbances, psychotic and otherwise. Although psychiatrists no longer hail the Degenerate myth in its pure form, its notions of constitution, physiologic fault, and underlying lesion live on. Most psychiatrists are sure that schizophrenia, manic-depressive illness, and depression have underlying biochemical imbalances. In fact, the newest research posits that very specific biochemical deficiencies or excesses related to the adrenalin of the sympathetic nervous system, and even more subtle substances, are at work in these psychiatric disorders. This is a new biochemicalized version of the old nervous-exhaustion and overexcitation ideas.

Some theorists have even reactivated the old Degenerate myth. Substituting the more modern chronic schizophrenic for the Victorian idiot dying in an asylum, many meticulous theorists stress the interplay of heredity and family environment in the birth of this psychotic illness. Though a few celebrated psychiatrists have spoken of the schizophrenic as a misunderstood seer, other theorists posit that the ancestors of the schizophrenic are slightly disturbed and that organic predisposition and the inevitable peculiarities of language and parental communication interact to breed schizophrenia in the offspring. Though such a theory may be unpopular, too suggestive of inevitability and the individual's inability to help himself, many clever psychiatrists treat these patients with antipsychotic drugs and employ family therapy to reshape the odd languages, the "schizophrenic" communications.

But unlike infectious diseases such as typhus and yellow fever, many mental disorders—neurotic, psychotic, and the states between, the so-called "borderline" conditions—cannot be stopped like menacing foreigners at the border. Nor can they be cured by the patient's remembering a traumatic event in childhood. Nor have any modern wonder drugs wiped them from the face of the earth. Just as insulin controls diabetes or digitalis strengthens but does not restore the failing heart, medications and talking therapies merely contain the serious psychiatric conditions. The patients are doomed to chronic semi-invalidism. Many are exasperating in their failure to adhere to treatment regimens. Even those who take their medications and come to therapy often seem to be lacking an entire part of themselves, the ability to synthesize experience.

More minor psychiatric disorders are troublesome because of their apparent ubiquity. Psychiatric conditions have multiplied before the eyes of the psychiatrist. He can see pathologic interactions on street corners, on television. The Angelic Invalid myth has been democratized: most human beings are very sensitive creatures who feel anxiety and sadness, strong urges and nearly uncontrollable wishes, stemming from minuscule causes. In this respect we are all neurotic. Even with a very sensitive and perceptive psychiatrist who has undergone arduous training, the results of treating many widespread disorders are often ambiguous and difficult to quantify.

Though the treatment for minor psychiatric disorders might stress talking to get to the bottom of a problem—the substance of depth psychology—some very effective approaches have little to do with symbols and psychoanalysis. Effective treatments of phobias and impotence are a good example. The specific fears or the impotence may have a hereditary or constitutional component or they may be sexually related to early traumatic experiences. However, probably the best treatments are behavioristic. Though no psychiatrist believes that masturbation causes nerve weakness, phobias, impotence, or any other sexual dysfunctions, the new theories of faulty learning posit malfunctions quite akin to the faulty reflex-arc idea of the Onan myth. The reflex needs to be unlearned.

As for the Zeus and Noble Savage myths, which stressed environmental factors, many thinkers in psychiatry still underscore the importance of shocks and stresses in the formation of infections, ulcers, heart disease, and cancer. The interplay between stress, mental pain, and physical symptoms now seems richly complex. In cancer, for instance, psychiatric thinkers emphasize how psychological stress and slight immunological and endocrinal changes can join to undermine an organism's normal ability to destroy precancerous cells. Such insights into the interaction of mind and body by way of nerves and hormones can lead an individual to seek treatment through relaxation. Stresses and strains are always with us, always gnawing at our tissues, and only through basic means such as rest and relaxation are we to be freed from them.

Within psychoanalysis itself a new myth has largely replaced the Oedipus myth. Much emphasis is now put, not on the original triad, the child and his parents, but rather on the primal dyad, the mother and the child, or the primal Other and the Self. Problems with Self and with the relationship of the Self to others now stand as central in the theorizing of many depth psychologists. Nordau's and James's intimations about the Self placed the prototypical sufferer among specialized classes—those obsessed with a self-absorbed art, such as the Sinful Genius, and those weighed down with religious scruples, such as the Religious Self-Tormentor. In the past few decades the modern artist's fascination with the Self and the religious concern over goodness and badness seem to have become universal. The contemporary neurotic may still be obsessed with sex, but even sex is part of his problem with Self. By way of sex the Self recurs through procreation, and in intense sexual relationships the Other is always at hand. Is the Self and the Other good or bad, or some mixture? the neurotic asks. Enveloped in the Narcissus myth of neurosis, struggling in a vast expressionist landscape, he searches endlessly for himself, a Self lost somewhere in the past—a past in which the personal, the social, and the biological still remain curiously interwoven.

NOTES

Chapter 2. Founding Nervous Fathers

PAGE

32 "nervous . . . low livers": George Cheyne, *An Essay on Regimen* (London, C. Rivington, 1740), preface.

32 "the young gentry and free livers": see J. F. Payne, "George Cheyne," *Dictionary of National Biography* (London: Oxford Univ. Press, 1917), pp. 217–218.

32 "holiday companions": ibid., p. 218.

32 "All nervous distempers whatsoever": George Cheyne, *The English Malady* (London: Strahan & Leake, 1733), p. 14.

32 "a Relaxation or Weakness": ibid., p. 15.

33 "tender and delicate Constitution . . . too strong and high Food": ibid., p. 284.

33 "of an Honorable and Opulent Family . . . for want of due Care": ibid., p. 286.

33 "Since our wealth has increased": ibid., pp. 49–50.

34 "sense and motion injured": William Cullen, *A Synopsis of Nosology* (Philadelphia: Dobson, 1816), p. 51.

35 "a sympathy of the nerves": Robert Whytt, *Works* (Edinburgh: Balfour, Auld, & Smellie, 1768), pp. 489–496.

35 "the smell of grateful food": ibid., p. 496.

35 "irritation of the windpipe": ibid., p. 497.

35 "A too great delicacy and sensibility": ibid., p. 537.

36 "We are told of a lady": ibid., p. 539.

36 "by sudden terror, delicate women": ibid., p. 580.

37 "For her spirits . . . still continued very high": Jane Austen, *Sense and Sensibility* (New York: Nelson Doubleday, n.d.), p. 115.

37   "She could say no more": ibid., p. 171.

37   "two delightful twilight walks": ibid., p. 220.

37   "Hour after hour passed away": ibid., p. 225.

37   "her thoughts wandering": ibid., p. 226.

38   "Anatomists have discovered": Thomas Trotter, *A View of the Nervous Temperment* (Newcastle: Edward Walker, 1807), pp. 204–205; "The human stomach": ibid., p. 203.

39   *"The nervous system"*: ibid., p. 25.

39   "it is to be supposed": ibid., p. 39.

39   "frequent surfeits from high seasoned food": ibid., p. 45.

39   "I have known instances": ibid., p. 79.

40   "amidst the great effeminacy": ibid., p. 153.

40   The older of these two schools: Cecilia Mettler, *History of Medicine* (Philadelphia: Blakiston and Co., 1947), pp. 561–571.

41   "let us hope": Philippe Pinel and Isidore Bricheteau, "Névrose." *Dictionnaire des Sciences Médicales* (Paris: Panckoucke, 1819), Vol. 35, p. 565.

42   He describes one young woman: ibid., pp. 566–567.

42   "violent chagrin": ibid., p. 367.

42   "a great organic delicateness": ibid., p. 568.

42   "violent chagrin": ibid., p. 574.

42   "strong means of nourishing": ibid., p. 569.

42   "So many causes": ibid., p. 571.

42   "a celebrated actress": ibid., p. 581.

43   Somewhere in the mythical past: Jean-Jacques Rousseau, *Discours sur l'Origine de L'Inégalité (extraits)* (Paris: Larousse, n.d.), pp. 39–43.

43   His temptation: ibid., pp. 71–80.

43   He does not find greater happiness: ibid., p. 78.

43   Soon he is burdened: ibid., p. 43.

44   In all neuroses: Mettler, *History of Medicine.*

44   A product of this way of thinking: see Alfred Luton, "Névrose." *Nouveau Dictionnaire de Médecine et de Chirurgie*, Vol. 23 (Paris: J. B. Baillière, 1877), pp. 803–859.

46   "nervous spirits": Johannes Müller, *Elements of Physiology* (Philadelphia: Lea & Blanchard, 1843), p. 513.

46   "many physiologists and men of science": ibid.

46   "(1) That the vital actions": ibid., p. 515.

46   "Life . . . is not simply": ibid., p. 35.

46   "an onion taken from the hand of an Egyptian mummy": ibid., p. 36.

46   "branches of plants": ibid., p. 27.

46   It is almost disappointing: Fielding Garrison, *History of Neurology* (Springfield, Ill.: Charles Thomas, 1969), p. 206.

47   Another follower of Müller's: Moritz Heinrich Romberg, *A Manual of the Nervous Diseases of Man* (London: Sydenham Society, 1853), pp. 1–5, 275–278.

49   He believed that the various races: B. A. Morel, *Traité des Dégénérescences* (Paris: J. B. Baillière, 1857), p. 5.

49 "join in themselves the pugnaciousness": ibid., p. 37.
49 "the degenerate being . . . idiot or demented": ibid., p. 46.
49 "the existence of dangerous and unsafe occupations": ibid., p. 50.
50 lesions in the central nervous system: ibid., p. 53.
50 "the germ": ibid., p. 58.
50 "vicious organic disposition": ibid., p. 62.
50 "degenerates par excellence": ibid., p. 72.
52 "disequilibrium in the blood and nerves": Emile Zola, *La Fortune des Rougon* (Paris: Livre de Poche, 1978), p. 63.
52 "nervous crises": ibid.
52 "terrible convulsions": ibid.
53 "vital modifications, dynamic troubles": J. J. Moreau (de Tours), *La Psychologie Morbide* (Paris: Victor Masson, 1859), p. 32.
54 "gay delirium": ibid., p. 51.
54 "born and developed": ibid., p. 53.
54 "idiosyncratic hereditary nervous states": ibid.
55 "These children . . . are remarkable": ibid., pp. 71–72.
56 "the morbid principle of idiocy": ibid., p. 75.
56 "breaking of the cogs": ibid.
56 Reduced to a state: Fyodor Dostoevski, *The Idiot* (New York: Signet Classic, 1969), pp. 26–27.
56 The complicated workings of his mind: ibid., pp. 556–572.
57 The story ends: ibid., pp. 628–632.
57 "the virtue and the vices": Moreau, *La Psychologie Morbide*, p. 109.
57 "the grand social commotion": ibid., p. 118.
57 "Does the writer, the poet": ibid., p. 129.

Chapter 3. Medical Imagination in an Age of Empire

PAGE

61 Many medical illnesses won: Notable nineteenth-century neurologists with various disorders named after them include Charcot, Jackson, Guillaume Duchenne, Charles Edouard Brown-Séquard, Georges Gilles de la Tourette, Wilhelm Erb, Carl Wernicke, Albert Pitres, Pierre Marie, James Parkinson, Charles Bell, and George Huntington. See Fielding Garrison, *History of Neurology*, rev. and enl. by Lawrence McHenry (Springfield, Ill.: Charles Thomas, 1969).

61 These two titans: The British were there too, having militarily occupied Egypt in 1882, and the French were busy to the east, digging the Suez Canal. See James Morris, *Heaven's Command* (New York: Harvest/Harcourt Brace Jovanovich, 1980), and David Knight, *Robert Koch, Father of Bacteriology* (New York: F. Watts, 1961), pp. 96–98.

62 A renowned textbook: William Osler, *Principles and Practice of Medicine* (New York: Appleton, 1892), pp. 1–39.

63 Each . . . had an illness . . . named after him: Osler-Weber-Rendu

disease; Clostridium Welchii; and the Kelly and Halsted surgical clamps.

65 Then the great Pasteur arrived: René Dubos, *Louis Pasteur, Freelance of Science* (New York: Scribners, 1950), pp. 335–336.

67 Even Alfred Wallace: Loren Eisley, *Darwin's Century* (Garden City, N.Y.: Anchor Books, 1961), pp. 285–325.

67 In the 1830s: Marshall Hall, *Memoirs on the Nervous System* (London: Sherwood, Gilbert & Piper, 1837), and Johannes Müller, *Textbook of Physiology* (Philadelphia: Henry C. Lea, 1843), pp. 22–24, 67–70, 513–615, 548–560.

67 Ultimately, in 1891: Garrison, *History of Neurology*, pp. 165–166.

68 "It is a patient!": ibid., p. 219.

70 Darwin wrote that he stumbled: Charles Darwin, *Autobiography* (New York: Norton, 1958), p. 120.

70 Another economist, Karl Marx: Stanley Hyman, *The Tangled Bank: Darwin, Marx, Frazer and Freud as Imaginative Writers* (New York: Atheneum, 1962), pp. 121–123.

70 the German scientist Ernst Haeckel: Ernst Haeckel, *The Riddle of the Universe* (New York: Hargen Bros., 1900), pp. 109–123.

72 "My ancestors, idiots or maniacs": Alex de Jonge, *Baudelaire, Prince of Clouds* (New York: Paddington Press, 1976), p. 11.

Chapter 4. A Tale of Two Neuroses

PAGE

76 "My resources do not afford": A. Souques, "Charcot Intime," *La Presse Médicale*, May 27, 1925, p. 693.

77 He is said to have brought Nicholai and Gambetta together: Georges Guillain, *J.-M. Charcot: His Life—His Work* (New York: Paul Hoeber, 1959), p. 26, and Souques, "Charcot Intime," p. 696.

77 One day he was on his way: Souques, "Charcot Intime," p. 694.

78 "he held that by exemption from overteaching": Jonathan Hutchinson, "The Late Dr. Hughlings Jackson: Recollections of a Life-Long Friendship," *British Medical Journal*, Dec. 9, 1911, p. 1551.

79 just as Adam named the animals: Sigmund Freud, *The Standard Edition of the Complete Psychological Works* (London: Hogarth Press, 1955), Vol. 3, p. 13.

80 The biographical sketches: see especially Pierre Marie, "Eloge a J.-M. Charcot," *Revue Neurologique*, Vol. 1, No. 6 (1925), pp. 739–740.

81 His classification divided hysteria: J.-M. Charcot, *Oeuvres Complètes* (Paris: Progrès Médical, 1866), Vol. 1, pp. 320–333, 427–434, 436–439.

84 Jackson arrived in London in 1859: see Arthur Lassek, *The Unique Legacy of Dr. Hughlings Jackson* (Springfield, Ill.: Charles Thomas, 1970), and Sir William Hale-White, *Great Doctors of the Nineteenth Century* (London: Edward Arnold, 1935), and many articles by other authors.

86 "march": J. Hughlings Jackson, *Selected Writings of John Hughlings Jackson* (London: Hodder & Stroughton, 1931–32), Vol. 1, pp. 424, 427, 434 ff.

86 "organ of mind": ibid., Vol. 1, pp. 414, 417; Vol. 2, pp. 78, 84, 98.

86 "dissolution of the nervous system": ibid., Vol. 2, pp. 45–118.

87 "discharging lesion": ibid., Vol. 1, pp. 121, 141, 208, 209, 214, et passim.

88 One eyewitness: Occasional Correspondent, "Hypnotism in Paris," *Lancet*, July 29, 1882, p. 163.

88 "I seldom failed to attend": Axel Munthe, *The Story of San Michele* (London: John Murray, 1929), p. 296.

88 "a multi-colored audience": ibid., p. 296.

89 "art for art's sake": J.-M. Charcot, *Diseases of the Nervous System* (London: New Sydenham, 1889), Vol. 3, pp. 42, 94.

89 Charcot's female patients: Henri F. Ellenberger, *The Discovery of the Unconscious* (New York: Basic Books, 1970), pp. 98–101.

90 Munthe tells of meeting: Munthe, *The Story of San Michele*, pp. 302–313.

90 "morbid curiosity": ibid.

91 In London she makes the acquaintance of Sir Luke Strett: Henry James, *The Wings of the Dove* (New York: Penguin Classics, 1978), pp. 150–161.

91 Then, feeling extremely guilty: Theodor Fontane, *Effi Briest* (Baltimore: Penguin Books, 1967), p. 182.

91 There a Dr. Rummschuttel: ibid., pp. 183–185.

92 Thus he would lecture on a hysterical symptom: see, e.g., J.-M. Charcot, *Leçons du Mardi à la Salpêtrière* (Paris: Progrès Médical, 1889–92).

92 Geneviève: Désiré Bourneville and Paul Regnard, *Iconographie Photographique de la Salpêtrière* (Paris: Progrès Médical, 1877–80), Vol. 1, pp. 50–90.

93 "cerebral fever": ibid., Vol. 1, p. 51.

94 "sister" Louise Lateau: ibid., Vol. 1, p. 72.

94 "Monsieur et cher maître": ibid., Vol. 1, p. 73.

94 "I suffer . . . I have had enough": ibid., Vol. 1, p. 76.

94 "I am not a sordid woman": ibid., Vol. 1, p. 80.

95 "I love M. X": ibid., Vol. 1, p. 81.

96 Louise: ibid., Vol. 2, pp. 123–167 and Vol. 3, pp. 187–199.

101 Porcz: J.-M. Charcot, *Diseases of the Nervous System*, Vol. 3, pp. 261–273.

101 Pin: ibid., pp. 284–288.

103 a particularly valuable and timely case: J. Hughlings Jackson, *Selected Writings, op cit.*, Vol. 1, pp. 400–405.

104 "mental automatism": ibid., Vol. 1, p. 123.

105 "instability": ibid., Vol. 1, p. 179.

105 "exhaustion": ibid., Vol. 1, pp. 440–443.

105 "insanity": ibid., Vol. 1, pp. 198–199, 323, 366–384.

105 "In every insanity": ibid., Vol. 2, p. 411.

106 "the psychology of the nervous system," "the physiology of the mind": ibid., Vol. 1, pp. 86, 417, et passim.

106 "Our concern as medical men": J. Hughlings Jackson, *Remarks on Evolution and Dissolution of the Nervous System* (London: H. Wolff, 1833), p. 15.

106 "dynamic lesion": J.-M. Charcot, *Diseases of the Nervous System*, Vol. 1, pp. 278, 281, 284, et passim.

Chapter 5. The Railway God

PAGE

108 In the 1890s a little known Viennese neurologist: Sigmund Freud, *The Standard Edition of the Complete Psychological Works* (London: Hogarth Press, 1955), Vol. 1, p. 262.

108 "between the ages of 2 and 2½": ibid.

109 railway neuroses were a common phenomenon: see especially Esther Fischer-Homberger, "Die Buchse der Pandora: Der Mythische Hintergrund der Eisenbahn-Krankheiten des 19 Jahrhunderts," *Sudhoff's Archive* (1972), pp. 297–310.

109 Gioacchino Rossini: Cesare Lombroso, *Man of Genius* (London: Walter Scott, 1891), p. 18.

109 "I have several times had occasion to treat persons with fear of railways and travelling": Hermann Oppenheim, *Textbook of Nervous Diseases* (Edinburgh: T. N. Foulis, 1911), Vol. 2, p. 1149.

109 The American neurologist Philip Knapp: see F. X. Dercum, ed., *Nervous Diseases by American Authors* (Philadelphia: Henry C. Lea, 1895), pp. 135–170.

109 Charcot and Gilles de la Tourette: see, e.g., J.-M. Charcot, *Leçons du Mardi à la Salpêtrière* (Paris: Progrès Médical, 1887–89), Vol. 1, 121–125, 131–139, 527–535, and Georges Gilles de la Tourette, *Leçons de Clinique Thérapeutique sur les Maladies du Système Nerveux* (Paris: Plon, 1898), pp. 121–127.

109 It may be difficult now to picture: Fischer-Homberger, "Die Buchse der Pandora," pp. 292–315.

111 "I have heard strange noises": Axel Munthe, *The Story of San Michele* (London: John Murray, 1929), pp. 150–151.

113 In his book he cites more than two hundred cases: Herbert Page, *Injuries of the Spine and Spinal Cord and Nervous Shock* (Philadelphia: Blakiston, 1885), pp. 158–245.

113 "that of an apparently strong and healthy girl": ibid., p. 185.

115 "Our invalid was walking on foot": Charcot, *Leçons du Mardi*, Vol. 2, p. 438.

115 "It was three or four in the afternoon": ibid.

115 "You saw the lightning near you?": ibid.

115 "It gave me the idea": ibid.

117 Starting in 1888: see especially Hermann Oppenheim, *Die Trauma-tische Neurosen* (Berlin, August Hirschwald, 1889).

118 "psychic shock": Hermann Oppenheim, *Diseases of the Nervous System* (Philadelphia: Lippincott, 1900), p. 740.

118 "We assume that in the functional disorders": ibid.

118 "evoke molecular alterations": ibid., p. 741.

119 "auto-suggestion": ibid.

119 "was by the jar of the collision": *Kentucky Reports*, Louisville Southern Railroad Company v. Minogue (90:1890), p. 373.

120 "The defendant company ran one train": *Pennsylvania Reports*, Ewing et ux., Appellants, v. Pittsburgh, Cincinnati and St. Louis Railway Company (147:1892), p. 41.

120 "a horse car of the defendant": *New York Reports*, Anne Mitchell, Respondent, v. Rochester Railway Company, Appellant (151:1896), p. 108.

120 conductor who acted with carelessness: *Massachusetts Reports*, Margaret C. Spade v. Lynn and Boston Elevated Railway Company (168:1897), p. 285.

120 "It seemed as though I had turned to solid ice": ibid., p. 286.

121 In yet another case . . . In still another . . . In most cases: see, e.g., *Appellate Court of Indiana*, Kalen v. Terre Haute and Indianapolis Railroad Company (18:1897), pp. 202–213; *South Carolina Reports*, S. S. Mack v. South Bound Railroad Company (52:1897), pp. 323–344; and *Southern Reporter*, Lapleine v. Morgan's L&T R&SS Company (4:1888), pp. 875–878.

121 "To turn now . . . to nervous disability": Sir Clifford Allbutt, "Nervous Diseases and Modern Life," *Contemporary Review* (67:1895), pp. 214–215.

Chapter 6. The Mind in Splinters

PAGE

123 On May 6, 1877, a plump . . . blond girl: Désiré Bourneville and Paul Regnard, *Iconographie Photographique de la Salpêtrière* (Progrès Médical, 1877–80), Vol. 3, pp. 4–39.

123 "nervous crises": ibid., Vol. 3, p. 6.

125 Dr. Lambalt: J.-M. Charcot, *Oeuvres Complètes* (Paris: Progrès Médical, 1886–90), Vol. 9, pp. 225–227.

125 Dr. Burq: ibid., Vol. 9, pp. 213–224, and Occasional Correspondent, "Hypnotism in Paris," *Lancet*, May 20, 1882, pp. 842–843.

125 Vigouroux: Charcot, *Oeuvres Complètes*, Vol. 9, pp. 218, 483–501.

125 Marceline: Bourneville and Regnard, *Iconographie Photographique*, not just magnets, metals, and electricity: ibid., Vol. 9, pp. 213–277. Vol. 1, pp. 110–141.

127 Franz Anton Mesmer: see Robert Darnton, *Mesmerism and the End*

of the Enlightenment (Cambridge: Harvard Univ. Press, 1968), and James Wyckoff, *Franz Anton Mesmer: Between God and Devil* (Englewood Cliffs, N.J.: Prentice-Hall, 1975).

130 "A circular oaken case": Alfred Binet and Charles Féré, *Animal Magnetism* (New York: Appleton, 1889), pp. 8–9.

130 "when the agitation exceeds certain limits": ibid., p. 10.

132 "employed his leisure": ibid., p. 27.

133 "his friend Walker": ibid., p. 69.

134 "Provoked Hysterical Somnambulism and Catalepsy": Charcot, *Oeuvres Complètes*, Vol. 9, pp. 253–264.

135 catalepsy: ibid., pp. 300–301, 398–405.

135 The second stage, lethargy: ibid., pp. 301–302, 309–398.

138 The third hypnotic phase, somnambulism: ibid., pp. 302–304.

138 Liébeault was one of those general practitioners: see A. A. Liébeault, "La Confession d'un Médecin Hypnotiseur," *Revue de l'Hypnotisme* (1:1886), pp. 105–110, 143–48, and A. W. van Renterghem, "Liébeault et son Ecole," *Zeitschrift für Hypnotismus* (4), pp. 333–375, 1896.

139 "a process which exposed me": Liébeault, *La Confession*, p. 106.

139 "If you want me to cure you": van Renterghem, "Liébeault et son Ecole," p. 336.

141 "Sleep, sleep": ibid., p. 35.

142 One case was that of a man: ibid., pp. 349–365.

142 A handsome small man: Joseph Delboeuf, *Le Magnétisme Animal* (Paris: Alcan, 1889), pp. 48–79.

143 One story shows the laxness: Van Renterghem, *Liébeault et son Ecole*, pp. 366–369.

144 "weak-nerved, weak-brained, hysterical or women": Hippolyte Bernheim, *Suggestive Therapeutics* (New York, Putnam's, 1889), p. 5.

144 "common people, those of gentle disposition": ibid.

144 "very intelligent people": ibid.

144 Bernheim defined hypnosis: ibid., p. 15.

145 "a suggestion given during sleep": ibid., p. 38.

145 "There is one thing certain": ibid., p. 137.

145 *"effects the unconscious transformation"*: ibid.

145 the celebrated Battle of the Schools: see Robert G. Hillman, "A Scientific Study of Mystery: The Role of the Medical and Popular Press in the Nancy-Salpêtrière Controversy on Hypnotism," *Bulletin of the History of Medicine* (39:1965), pp. 163–182, and Henri F. Ellenberger, *The Discovery of the Unconscious* (New York: Basic Books, 1970), pp. 749–754.

147 "full of contentment and pleasure": J.-M. Charcot, *Clinique des Maladies du Système Nerveux* (Paris: Progrès Médical, 1892–93), Vol. 2, pp. 22–26.

147 In the summer of 1893, Charcot: see Georges Guinon, "Charcot Intime," *Paris Médical*, May 23, 1925, pp. 511–516, and A. Souques, "Charcot Intime," *La Presse Médical*, May 27, 1925, pp. 693–698.

150 "when the time had passed": A. Baudouin, "Quelques Souvenirs de la Salpêtrière," *Paris Médical*, May 23, 1925, p. 519.
150 "abominable cancer": ibid.
150 "There is no truth": ibid., p. 520.

Chapter 7. *A Proliferation of Perversion, an Epidemic of Murder*

PAGE

152 In 1861 the actress Sarah Bernhardt: see Paul Aubry, *La Contagion du Meurtre* (Paris: Alcan, 1894), p. 8.
152 *"peculiar attribute for transforming"*: Bernheim, *Suggestive Therapeutics* (New York: Putnam's, 1889), p. 137.
153 "common people . . . old soldiers . . . very intelligent people belonging to the highest grades of society": ibid., p. 5.
153 "carries out everything according to my command": ibid., p. 57.
154 Dr. X: Hippolyte Bernheim, *Hypnotisme, Suggestion, Psychothérapie, Nouvelles Etudes* (Paris: 1891), p. 157.
154 Eyraud and Gabrielle Bompard: ibid., pp. 148–149.
155 An excellent example of this widespread notion: Other examples are A. Vigouroux and P. Juquelier, *La Contagion Mentale* (Paris: Doin, 1905), and Paul Moreau (de Tours), *De l'Homicide Commis par les Enfants* (Paris: J. B. Baillière, 1888).
155 "our immortal Pasteur," "penetration of a morbid element": Aubry, *La Contagion du Meurtre*, p. 2.
156 "infected": ibid., p. 3.
157 For example, a Madame Lombardi: ibid., pp. 86–87.
157 Another example was a fifteen-year-old F. Lemaître: ibid., pp. 90–91.
157 "Menesclou poisoned me": ibid., p. 90.
159 Cesare Lombroso was a richly eccentric personality: see especially Gina Lombroso Ferrero, *Cesare Lombroso: Storia della vita e delle opere* (Turin: Fratelli Bocca, 1915), and Hans Kurella, *Cesare Lombroso: A Modern Man of Science* (New York: Robinson Co., 1910).
160 "This man . . . possessed": Cesare Lombroso, Introd. to Gina Lombroso Ferrero, *Criminal Man According to the Classification of Cesare Lombroso* (New York: Putnam's, 1911), p. xiv. Page nos. from here to citation of another work refer to this book.
160 "this was not merely an idea, but a revelation": pp. xiv–xv.
161 one-third of all criminals were born to be criminals: p. 8.
161 "as in chimpanzees": Ferrero, *Criminal Man*, p. 14.
161 "is frequently twisted, upturned": p. 15.
162 "fleshy, swollen and protruding as in Negroes": p. 16.
162 "an atavistic character common to animals": p. 18.
162 "an ape-like character": p. 19.
162 "the foot is often flat, as in Negroes": p. 21.
162 "there is a prevalence of large, pyramidal and polymorphous cells": p. 22.

162 "the number of nervous cells is noticeably below the average": ibid.

162 "To give up stealing would be ceasing to exist": p. 38.

163 "my chief pleasure is beheading": p. 39.

163 "fallen into disuse among the higher classes": p. 46.

163 Rizz: p. 54.

163 Rav: p. 55.

163 "Habitual resignation leads one to suspect an obtuseness in sensitivity": Cesare Lombroso and William Ferrero, *La Femme Criminelle et la Prostituée* (Paris: Alcan, 1896), p. 63.

163 "women feel less because they think less": ibid.

163 "develops between an inferior being . . . and a superior being": ibid., p. 115.

164 "Religious faith . . . is nothing other than suggestion": ibid., p. 127.

165 "true sisters of marble": ibid., p. 379.

165 "suffer from a milder form of the disease": Ferrero, *Criminal Man*, p. 101.

165 Charlotta, "hysterical and disequilibriated, but with an extraordinary culture": Lombroso and Ferrero, *La Femme Criminelle*, p. 415.

166 "after driving about the streets of Lyon with Gabrielle": Ferrero, *Criminal Man*, p. 113.

166 "of one hundred young girls": Lombroso and Ferrero, *La Femme Criminelle*, pp. 531–532.

167 "the dog . . . left to run wild": Ferrero, *Criminal Man*, pp. 135–136.

167 "This tendency to alter under special conditions": ibid., p. 136.

169 "sympathetic nature, penetrating eyes, and a persuasive voice": J. Wagner von Jauregg, "Richard von Krafft-Ebing," *Wiener Medizinische Wochenschrift* (42:1908), p. 2310.

173 *Venus in Furs* centers on the character of a young masochist: Leopold von Sacher-Masoch, *Venus in Furs*, in Gilles Deleuze, *Sacher-Masoch* (London: Faber & Faber, 1971).

174 "raising women to social equality with men": Richard von Krafft-Ebing, *Psychopathia Sexualis*, 7th ed. (Philadelphia: F. A. Davis, 1894), p. 4. Page nos. from here until the end of the chap. refer to this work.

174 "in that pure love from which springs": p. 5.

174 "effeminacy, sensuality and luxury": p. 6.

174 "large cities as the breeding places of nervousness": p. 7.

175 "degenerate Caesars": p. 58.

175 "that modern monster Marshalls Gilles de Rays": ibid.

175 "I opened her breast with a knife": p. 62.

175 "I am fond of women": ibid.

176 "The story of a prelate by Taxil": pp. 68–69.

176 "high boots and short jackets (Hungarian fashion)": p. 97.

176 "being whipped by handsome young persons": p. 102.

176 "[who] was accustomed to call": p. 116.

177 "neuropathic eyes": pp. 98, 103, 254, et passim.

177 two ways of becoming a homosexual: pp. 225–226.

178 "The hereditary factor . . . a transmission to descendants becomes possible": p. 228.
178 "Nothing is so prone to contaminate": p. 188.
179 "I took three or four times the usual dose": pp. 207–208.
179 "butchers, fakirs, drivers": p. 297.
180 "a certain Eliza Edwards": p. 302.
180 "had to discontinue treatment, owing to business": p. 344.
181 "after 6 months as a happy bridegroom": p. 352.

Chapter 8. Prometheus the Democrat

PAGE
186 The son of a New England fundamentalist minister: see Alphonso Rockwell, *Rambling Recollections: An Autobiography* (New York: Paul B. Holbin, 1920), pp. 180–232, and Charles Dana, "Dr. George M. Beard," *Archives of Neurology and Psychiatry* (10:1923), pp. 428–435.
189 These symptoms included tenderness of the scalp, headaches: George Beard, *A Practical Treatise on Nervous Exhaustion (Neurasthenia)* (New York: William Wood, 1880), pp. 34–117.
190 "higher orders": George Beard, *American Nervousness* (New York: Putnam's, 1881), p. 31.
190 "brain workers": ibid., pp. 193, 195, et passim.
190 Beard tells a ridiculous anecdote: ibid., p. 190.
191 Beard borrowed some of his thinking: see George Beard, "The Newly-Discovered Force," *Archives of Electrology and Neurology* (Vol. 1, No. 2, 1874), pp. 209–216.
191 "new principles until now buried": see Mathew Josephson, *Edison* (New York: McGraw-Hill, 1959), p. 129.
191 Another elusive link . . . Herbert Spencer: see George Beard, *Herbert Spencer on American Nervousness: A Scientific Coincidence* (New York: Putnam's, 1882).
192 "steam power, the periodical press": Beard, *American Nervousness,* p. 96.
193 fine organization: ibid., p. 26.
193 "who could not hold more than one bottle": ibid., p. 34.
194 "palaces": Beard, *Nervous Exhaustion,* p. 32.
196 "lights": Beard, *American Nervousness,* pp. 98–99.
197 Silas Weir Mitchell: see especially Ernest Earnest, *Silas Weir Mitchell, Novelist and Physician* (Philadelphia: Univ. of Pennsylvania Press, 1950), and Anna Robeson Burr, *Silas Weir Mitchell* (New York: Duffield & Co., 1929).
198 "powerful, strange head": Burr, *Silas Weir Mitchell,* p. 156.
199 One woman who pleaded paralysis: ibid., p. 184.
199 With another woman who refused to get out of bed: ibid.
199 "a lady of ample means": Silas Weir Mitchell, "The Evolution of the

Rest Cure," *Journal of Nervous and Mental Diseases* (1904), p. 369.
199 "passed through the hands": ibid.
200 "In two months": ibid., p. 372.
201 "our ancestors called . . . the vapors": Silas Weir Mitchell, *Lectures on Diseases of the Nervous System, Especially in Women* (Philadelphia: Henry L. Lea, 1881), p. 1. Page nos. from here to citation of another work refer to this book.
201 "women of the upper classes": p. 14.
201 "the daily fret and worrisomeness": ibid.
202 "change in social circumstances, love affairs": p. 218.
202 "the pests of many households": ibid.
202 "by ill luck the writing": p. 17.
203 "support herself by giving lessons in music": p. 23.
203 "a slow, steady, hopeful training": p. 29.
203 "half-conscious . . . a morbid birth gift . . . tea or coffee": p. 52.
203 "I confess that I too": p. 114.
204 "dotted with black marks": p. 85.
204 "I carried on a sort of starvation process": p. 88.
205 "every hysterical woman is liable": p. 180.
206 "embittered by losses of property": p. 186.
207 "a slow moral, molecular disintegration": Silas Weir Mitchell, *Roland Blake* (New York: Century Co., 1913), p. 246.
207 "whom she could drag": ibid., p. 191.
207 "on the verge of a denial": ibid., p. 45.

Chapter 9. Prometheus Goes to Europe

PAGE
215 "intellectual work is accompanied": Fernand Levillain, *La Neurasthénie: Maladie de Beard* (Paris: A. Maloine, 1891), p. 61.
215 Two other medical researchers: see Gilbert Ballet, *Neurasthenia*, trans. P. Campbell Smith (London: Henry Kimpton, 1911), pp. 49–50, 133–135.
216 The true, or shock, neurasthenic type: Georges Gilles de la Tourette, *Leçons de Clinique Thérapeutique sur les Maladies du Système Nerveux* (Paris: Plon, 1898), pp. 78–80.
Tourette described a degenerate, or hereditarily neurasthenic, young man: ibid., pp. 87–92.
218 "this weakness is inborn . . . poorly branched projections": Rudolf Arndt, *Die Neurasthenie* (Vienna and Leipzig: Urban & Schwarzenberg, 1885), p. 110.
218 "To wish to distinguish the neurasthenic": ibid., p. 124.
218 "atomic and molecular process": ibid., p. 131.
219 "Modern man . . . tries to hold up": Levillain, *La Neurasthénie*, p. 26.
219 "Always and everywhere . . . the sounds": ibid., p. 31.

219 Likewise, Krafft-Ebing preached against the vices: Richard von Krafft-Ebing, *Nervosität und Neurasthenische Zustände* (Vienna: Alfred Hölder, 1900), pp. 9–18.

220 "on a couch slung from the roof": William S. Playfair, *The Systematic Treatment of Nervous Prostration and Hysteria* (Philadelphia: Henry C. Lea, 1883), p. 41.

221 "reclining at length on a long couch": ibid., p. 102.

221 "I am sure that I could": ibid.

224 Through a series of spinning wheels: see Franz Carl Müller, ed., *Das Handbuch der Neurasthenie* (Leipzig: F.C.W. Vogel, 1893), pp. 495–505.

224 One Frenchman named Boisseau du Rocher: ibid., pp. 501–502.

224 Massage was another technique: ibid., pp. 260–303.

225 Dieting was another major treatment: ibid., pp. 330–354.

225 Sea baths were luxuriantly described: ibid., pp. 355–376.

225 The European doctors devoted chapter upon chapter: ibid., pp. 400–461.

228 "prepared for me . . . by Messrs. Brady and Martin": Julius Althaus, *The Failure of Brain Power (Encephalasthenia)* (London: Longmans, Green, 1898), p. 257.

228 "You will hardly believe me": ibid., p. 258.

229 The doctors were at least dimly aware: Müller, *Das Handbuch der Neurasthenie*, pp. 514–584.

229 Bernheim showed that of 30 cases: ibid., p. 580.

229 Baron Albert von Schrenck-Notzing hypnotized 40 people: ibid.

229 One French doctor named Auguste Voisin: ibid., p. 576.

231 Adrien Proust was a professor of medicine: see Robert LeMasle, *Le Professeur Adrien Proust* (Paris: Lipschutz, 1936).

231 Marcel Proust: see Robert Soupault, *Marcel Proust de Côté de la Médecine* (Paris: Plon, 1967); Georges Rivane, *Influence de l'Asthme sur l'Oeuvre de Marcel Proust* (Paris: Nouvelle Edition, 1945); and George Painter, *Marcel Proust*, 2 vols. (New York: Vintage Books, 1978).

232 The authors specifically speak of the neuroarthritic tendency: Adrian Proust and Gilbert Ballet, *Hygiène du Neurasthénique* (Paris: Victor Masson, 1897), pp. 17–18.

232 "safeguard the future of the children": ibid., p. 126.

232 "It is necessary to habituate the child": ibid., p. 148.

233 "at the approach of puberty": ibid., p. 154.

Chapter 10. Mephisto

239 Richard Wagner: see Robert Gutman, *Richard Wagner: The Man, His Mind and His Music* (New York: Harcourt Brace Jovanovich, 1974).

241 Paul Verlaine . . . Arthur Rimbaud: see Pierre Petitfils, *Verlaine* (Paris: Julliard, 1981), and Enid Starkie, *Arthur Rimbaud* (New York: New Directions, 1961).

243 Max Nordau: see Anna and Maxa Nordau, *Max Nordau: A Biography* (New York: Nordau Committee, 1943), and Meir Ben-Horin, *Max Nordau, Philosopher of Human Solidarity* (New York: Conference of Jewish Social Studies, 1956).

244 In his *Paradoxes*: see Max Nordau, *Paradoxes* (Chicago: L. Schick, 1886), pp. 116–202.

246 "Just as giants": Cesare Lombroso, *Man of Genius*, trans. from the Italian (London: Walter Scott, 1891), p. vi. Page nos. from here to citation of another work refer to this volume.

246 "genius is a neurosis": p. vii.

247 "promised land": pp. 336–352.

247 "motor epilepsy" . . . "psychic equivalent": pp. 337–338.

248 "the mirage of omnipotence": p. 343.

248 "Never . . . even among the Borgias": pp. 344–345.

248 "Napoleon wept not on account of true and deep feeling": p. 345.

248 "unpleasant witticisms . . . they granted him": p. 346.

248 "Taine has here given us": p. 347.

250 "a contempt for traditional views": Max Nordau, *Degeneration* (New York: Howard Fertig, 1968), p. 5. Page nos. from here to the end of the chap. refer to this work.

250 "false prophets arise": p. 6.

250 "their hands before pictures": p. 12.

250 "applause and wreaths are reserved for Tristan": ibid.

250 "A dissonant interval": pp. 12–13.

251 "of which the minor stages are designated as neurasthenia": p. 15.

251 "the predilection for inane revery": p. 21.

251 "for the most part to the multitude": p. 25.

251 "When he sees a picture": p. 26.

252 "he takes part . . . in the thousand events": p. 39.

252 "hinting at mysteries": p. 45.

252 "like floating fog in the morning wind": p. 57.

252 "a model of egotism": p. 252.

252 "The 'I' retires": ibid.

253 "the molecular movement takes place": pp. 353–354.

253 He extruded an especially strong venom toward Wagner: pp. 171–243.

254 "be blushing crimson": p. 181.

254 "In my belief . . . it cannot be doubted that every great war": pp. 207–208.

254 "Teutonomaniacal chauvinism": p. 209.

255 Nordau also launched an attack on Verlaine: pp. 119–128.

255 "we find, in astonishing completeness": p. 119.

256 "completely disconnected nouns": p. 126.

256 "completely delirious": p. 127.

Chapter 11. Christ the Neurotic

262 According to Beard: George Beard, *The Salem Witch Excitement* (New York: Putnam's, 1882), pp. 1–51.

262 Two hundred years later: J.-M. Charcot, *Diseases of the Nervous System* (London: New Sydenham, 1889), Vol. 3, pp. 169–206.

263 Many, especially in France: Theodore Zeldin, *Anxiety and Hypocrisy, France 1848–1945* (New York: Oxford Univ. Press, 1981), pp. 45–52. Also see Fritz Stern, *The Politics of Cultural Despair* (New York: Anchor Books, 1965), pp. 160–227.

264 Charcot and his followers: see especially Paul Richer, *Etudes Cliniques sur la Grande Hystérie* (Paris: Delahaye & Lecrosnier, 1885), with its numerous sketches.

264 The Salpêtrists depicted celebrated religious figures: J.-M. Charcot and Paul Richer, *Les Démoniaques dans l'Art* (Paris: Delahaye & Lecrosnier, 1887).

266 The facts of her life: see Augustus Rohling, *Louise Lateau: Her Stigmas and Ecstasy* (New York: Hickey & Co., 1879), and Désiré Bourneville, *Louise Lateau ou la Stigmatisée Belge* (Paris: Progrès Médical, 1875).

267 "Then came a period of sickness": Rohling, *Louise Lateau*, p. 6.

267 "suffered from intense headaches": ibid., p. 7.

268 "she instantly recovered consciousness": ibid., p. 9.

270 "Hemorrhages are frequent among hysterics": Bourneville, *Louise Lateau*, p. 28.

270 "sweat of blood": ibid., p. 32.

270 "Louise remained seated in her chair": Rohling, pp. 26–27.

271 "When she sees him kneel or fall": ibid., p. 28.

271 "Our Lord . . . with long, curly chestnut-colored hair": Bourneville, p. 45.

272 Bernadette was born in 1844: see René Laurentin, *Bernadette of Lourdes* (London: Darton, Longman & Todd, 1979).

275 No one was surprised when the novelist Emile Zola: Ernest Vizetelly, *Emile Zola, Novelist and Reformer* (London: John Lane, 1904), p. 318.

275 "At last the neckerchief fell aside": see F. De Grandmaisson, *Twenty Miracles at Lourdes* (St. Louis: B. Herder Book Co., n.d.), pp. 29–30.

275 "I'm cured! I'm cured!": ibid., p. 30.

276 In his article: see J.-M. Charcot, "The Faith Cure," *The New Review* (6:1893), pp. 18–31, and "La Foi Qui Guérit," *Archives de Neurologie* (25:1893), pp. 72–87.

276 "a natural phenomenon . . . at all times": Charcot, "The Faith Cure," p. 19.

278 Early in life James faced a painful dilemma: see Gay W. Allen, *William James: A Biography* (New York: Viking, 1967).

279 In 1870 he seems to have undergone a kind of religious experience: see ibid., pp. 165–167; S. P. Fullinwider, "William James' 'Spiritual Crisis,'" *The Historian* (38:1975), pp. 39–57; and Cushing Strout, "William James and the Twice-Born Sick Soul," *Daedalus* (Summer 1968), pp. 1062–82.

280 However, James remained a nervous sufferer: see Eugene Taylor, "William James on Psychopathology: The 1896 Lowell Lectures on 'Exceptional Mental States,'" *Harvard Library Bulletin* (30:1982), p. 463.

281 "Often . . . they have led a discordant inner life": William James, *The Varieties of Religious Experience* (New York: Modern Library, 1936), p. 8. Page nos. from here to the end of the chap. refer to this work.

281 "We are surely familiar": pp. 13–14.

282 "judge the religious life": p. 22.

282 "old hell fire theology": p. 89.

282 "coarse-meated": p. 90.

282 "*Question*: What does religion mean to you?": pp. 90–91.

283 "the world's meaning most comes home to us": p. 128.

283 "sanguine, healthy-minded . . . in darkness and apprehension": p. 133.

283 "a bottle or two of champagne": ibid.

283 "animal toughness . . . little irritable weakness": p. 38.

283 "Behold me then": p. 150.

284 "Whilst in this state of philosophical pessimism": p. 157.

285 "Francis of Assisi kisses his lepers": p. 279.

285 "he should never smell a flower": p. 297.

285 "psychopathic": p. 301.

285 "secretly caused an undergarment": pp. 301–303.

286 "A strange moral transformation": p. 292.

Chapter 12. Private Lives

290 George Sand: André Maurois, *Lélia: The Life of George Sand* (New York: Penguin Books, 1953), and William Atwood, *The Lioness and the Little One* (New York: Columbia Univ. Press, 1980).

290 Elizabeth Barrett Browning: Rosalie Mander, *Mrs Browning* (London: Weidenfeld & Nicolson, 1980); George Pickering, *Creative Malady* (London: Allen & Unwin, 1974); and F. E. Halliday, *Robert Browning: His Life and Work* (London: Jupiter Books, 1975).

290 Elizabeth Siddal Rossetti: Violet Hunt, *The Wife of Rossetti* (New York: Dutton, 1932); David Sonstroem, *Rossetti and the Fair Lady* (Middletown, Conn.: Wesleyan Univ. Press, 1970); and Brian Dobbs and Judy Dobbs, *Dante Gabriel Rossetti, an Alien Victorian* (London: MacDonald & Jane's, 1977).

290 George Eliot: Gordon S. Haight, *George Eliot: A Biography* (New York: Oxford Univ. Press, 1968).

290 Alice James: Jean Strouse, *Alice James* (New York: Bantam Books, 1980).

Chapter 13. Private Pain

322 Sigmund Freud: see many sources, e.g., Ernest Jones, *The Life and Work of Sigmund Freud* (New York: Basic Books, 1965); Henri F. Ellenberger, *The Discovery of the Unconscious* (New York: Basic Books, 1970); F. J. Sulloway, *Freud, Biologist of the Mind* (New York: Basic Books, 1979); Kenneth Levin, *Freud's Early Psychology of the Neuroses* (Pittsburgh: Univ. of Pittsburgh Press, 1978).

323 "scientific fairy tale": Max Schur, *Freud: Living and Dying* (New York: International Universities Press, 1972), p. 104.

323 Though many authors have questioned: see especially Sulloway, *Freud, Biologist of the Mind*, and Ellenberger, *Discovery of the Unconscious*.

325 Anna O./Bertha Pappenheim: see Josef Breuer and Sigmund Freud, *Studies on Hysteria* (New York: Nervous and Mental Disease Publishing Co., 1936); Lucy Freedman, *The Story of Anna O.* (New York: Walker & Co., 1972); and Dora Edinger, *Bertha Pappenheim, Freud's Anna O.* (Highland Park, Ill. Congregation Solel, 1968).

325 "autohypnotized": Breuer and Freud, *Studies on Hysteria*, p. 4.

330 Mme. D.: see Pierre Janet, *Névroses et Idées Fixes* (Paris: Baillière, 1898).

331 "Madame, prepare a bed": ibid., p. 116.

331 "Here he is": ibid., p. 117.

332 "Where are we": ibid., p. 118.

333 "What is the name of your intern?": ibid., p. 131.

334 "In a word": ibid., p. 141.

334 "Madame, prepare a bed": ibid., p. 146.

336 Dora/Rosa: Sigmund Freud, *Dora: An Analysis of a Case of Hysteria* (New York: Collier Books, 1963). Page nos. from here to citation of another work refer to this book.

336 "Bring her to reason": p. 42.

336 "getting nothing": ibid.

336 "the attack was, I believe": pp. 38–39.

337 "More interesting cases": p. 39.

337 "housewife's psychosis": p. 34.

338 "A house was on fire": p. 81.

338 "Then a return present": p. 87.

339 "I was walking about in a town": p. 114.

340 Years later, she was treated: Felix Deutsch, "A Footnote to Freud's Fragment of an Analysis of a Case of Hysteria," *Psychoanalytic Quarterly* (26:1957).

340 "one of the most repulsive of hysterics": ibid., p. 167.

340 "normal, conscious man": Breuer and Freud, *Studies on Hysteria*, p. 148.

342 "false step": Freud, *Dora: An Analysis*, p. 124.

Chapter 14. Angels and Oedipus

344 "primary addiction": Max Schur, *Freud: Living and Dying* (New York: International Universities Press, 1972), p. 61.

346 Madeleine: Pierre Janet, *De l'Angoisse à l'Extase* (Paris: Alcan, 1926), Vol. 1, pp. 1–200. Page nos. from here to citation of another work refer to this volume.

348 "The sound of shoes": p. 11.

349 "singular adventure": p. 1.

350 "to lead the life of a worker": p. 14.

351 "Ask God if he will": p. 56.

351 "delicious drunkenness . . . falls asleep again": p. 47.

353 "My being is drunk": p. 77.

353 "Virginity is a treasure": p. 71.

353 "I seem to be careening": p. 87.

354 "state of equilibrium": pp. 175–200.

356 Sergei the Wolf-man: see Muriel Gardiner, ed. *The Wolf-man and Sigmund Freud* (New York: Basic Books, 1971). Page nos. from here to citation of another work refer to this book.

358 "after greeting me": pp. 44–45.

358 "now embraced life fully": p. 50.

361 "turned out the lights": p. 77.

361 "with his gold-rimmed spectacles": p. 79.

361 "Of course, I told Professor Freud": p. 83.

362 "role of maître de plaisir": p. 84.

362 "When I saw her": p. 86.

362 "From the History of an Infantile Neurosis": see Sigmund Freud, in Gardiner, ed. *The Wolf-man and Sigmund Freud*, pp. 153–262.

364 "I dreamt that it was night": ibid., p. 173.

366 "God-shit" and "God-swine": ibid., pp. 209 and 226.

366 "persons who serve others": ibid., p. 167.

BIBLIOGRAPHY

Ackerknecht, E. H. *A Short History of Psychiatry*. New York: Hafner, 1968.

Alexander, F., and S. Selesnick. *The History of Psychiatry*. New York: Harper & Row, 1969.

Allbutt, Sir Clifford. "Nervous Diseases and Modern Life." *Contemporary Review*, 67:217, 1895.

Allen, Gay W. *William James: A Biography*. New York: Viking, 1967.

Allport, Gordon. "William James and the Behavioral Sciences." *Journal of the History of Behavioral Science*, 2(2):145–147, 1966.

Althaus, Julius. *The Failure of Brain Power (Encephalasthenia)*. London: Longmans, Green, 1898.

———. *The Spas of Europe*. London: Trubner & Co., 1862.

Amacher, Peter. "Thomas Laycock, I. M. Sechenov and the Reflex Arc Concept." *Bulletin of the History of Medicine*, 38:168–83, 1964.

American Journal of Neurology and Psychiatry. Review of Herbert Page, *Injuries of the Spine and Spinal Cord*. 2:561–566, 1883.

———. Review of Richard von Krafft-Ebing, *Psychopathia Sexualis*. 1:323–325, 1882.

American Law Reports. "Sufficiency of Proof that Mental or Neurological Conditions Complained of Resulted from Accident or Incident in Suit Rather than from Pre-existing Condition." 3d ser., 2:487–532, 1965.

Angel, R. W. "Jackson, Freud, and Sherrington on the Relation of Brain and Mind." *American Journal of Psychiatry*, 118:193–197, 1961.

Ansbacher, Heinz. "The Significance of the Socio-Economic Status of the

Patients of Freud and Adler." *American Journal of Psychotherapy*, 13:376–382, 1959.

Appellate Court of Indiana. Kalen v. Terre Haute and Indianapolis Railroad Company, 18:202–213, 1897.

Arndt, Rudolf. *Die Neurasthenie*. Vienna and Leipzig: Urban & Schwarzenberg, 1885.

Atwood, William. *The Lioness and the Little One*. New York: Columbia Univ. Press, 1980.

Aubry, Paul. *La Contagion du Meurtre*. Paris: Alcan, 1894.

Austen, Jane. *Sense and Sensibility*. New York: Nelson Doubleday, n.d.

Ballet, Gilbert (trans. P. Campbell Smith). *Neurasthenia*. London: Henry Kimpton, 1911.

Barraud, Henri-Jean. *Freud et Janet*. Toulouse: Edouard Privat, 1971.

Bate, W. Jackson. *John Keats*. Cambridge, Mass.: Belknap Press, 1963.

Baudouin, A. "Quelques Souvenirs de la Salpêtrière." *Paris Médical*, 21: May 23, 1925, pp. 517–520.

Baumer, Franklin. *Modern European Thought*. New York: Macmillan, 1977.

Beard, George M. *American Nervousness*. New York: Putnam's, 1881.

———. "The Elements of Electrotherapeutics." *Archives of Electrology and Neurology*, Vol. 1, No. 1: 158–164; Vol. 1, No. 2: 17–23; 184–194, 1874.

———. "Experimental Research in the Physiology of the Brain." *Archives of Electrology and Neurology*, Vol. 1, No. 1: 89–98, 1874.

———. *Herbert Spencer on American Nervousness: A Scientific Coincidence*. New York: Putnam's, 1882.

———. "The Involuntary Life." *Archives of Electrology and Neurology*, Vol. 1, No. 2: 220–257, 1874.

———. "The Newly-Discovered Force." *Archives of Electrology and Neurology*, Vol. 1, No. 2: 257–282, 1874.

———. "Obstinate Case of Hysteria in a Male." *Archives of Electrology and Neurology*, Vol. 1, No. 2: 209–216, 1874.

———. "Physical Future of the American People." *Atlantic Monthly* (June 1878), pp. 718–728.

———. *A Practical Treatise on Nervous Exhaustion (Neurasthenia)*. New York: William Wood, 1880.

———. *The Salem Witch Excitement*. New York: Putnam's, 1882.

———. *Sexual Neurasthenia*. New York: E. B. Trent, 1884.

———. *The Study of Trance, Muscle-Reading, and Allied Nervous Phenomena in Europe and America*. New York (publisher unknown), 1882.

———, and A. D. Rockwell. *A Practical Treatise on the Medical and Surgical Uses of Electricity*. New York: William Wood, 1871.

Bellak, Leopold, ed. *Contemporary European Psychiatry*. New York: Grove Press, 1961.

Ben-Horin, Meir. *Max Nordau, Philosopher of Human Solidarity.* New York: Conference of Jewish Social Studies, 1956.

Bernfeld, Siegfried. "Freud's Earliest Theories and the School of Helmholtz." *Psychoanalytic Quarterly*, 13:341–362, 1944.

Bernheim, Hippolyte. *Hypnotisme, Suggestion, Psychothérapie, Nouvelles Etudes.* Paris: Doin, 1891.

———. "La Suggestion Criminelle." *Revue de Hypnotisme*, 4:243–301, 1890.

———. *Suggestive Therapeutics.* New York: Putnam's, 1889.

Bettany, G. T. "Robert Cullen." *Dictionary of National Biography*, 5: 279–282. London: Oxford Univ. Press, 1917.

Binet, Alfred, and Charles Féré. *Animal Magnetism.* Trans. from the French. New York: Appleton, 1889.

Blum, H. "The Borderline Childhood of the Wolfman." *Freud and His Patients.* Ed. M. Kanzer and J. Glenn. New York: Aronson, 1980.

———. "The Psychogenic Influence of the Primal Scene: A Reevaluation." *Freud and His Patients.* Ed. M. Kanzer and J. Glenn. New York: Aronson, 1980.

Bourneville, Désiré. *Louise Lateau ou la Stigmatisée Belge.* Paris: Progrès Médical, 1875.

———, and Paul Regnard. *Iconographie Photographique de la Salpêtrière.* 3 vols. Paris: Progrès Médical, 1877–80.

Braceland, F. J. "Kraepelin: His System and His Influence." *American Journal of Psychiatry*, 113:871–876, 1957.

Bram, F. M. "The Gift of Anna O." *British Journal of Medical Psychology*, 38:53–58, 1965.

Bramwell, John Milne. "James Braid: His Works and Writings." *Proceedings of the Society of Psychical Research*, 12:127–166, 1896.

Brazier, Mary. "Rise of Neurophysiology in the 19th Century." *Journal of Neurophysiology*, 20:212–226, 1957.

Breuer, Josef. "Autobiography of Josef Breuer." Trans. C. P. Oberndorf. *International Journal of Psychoanalysis*, 34:64–67, 1953.

———, and Sigmund Freud. *Studies on Hysteria.* Trans. A. A. Brill. New York: Nervous and Mental Disease Publishing Co., 1936.

Brinton, Crane. *A History of Western Morals.* New York: Harcourt, Brace, 1936.

British Medical Journal. Review of R. von Krafft-Ebing, *Psychopathia Sexualis.* June 24, 1893, pp. 1325–26.

Browning, Don. "William James' Philosophy of the Person: The Concept of the Strenuous Life." *Zygon*, 10:162–174, 1975.

Browning, Elizabeth Barrett. *Aurora Leigh.* Chicago: Academy Chicago Ltd., 1979.

———, and Robert Browning. *Best Known Poems.* New York: London League of America, 1942.

Buchanan, G. "Healing by Faith." *Lancet*, Nov. 7, 1885, pp. 843–844.

Bullough, Vern, and Martha Voght. "Homosexuality and Its Confusion with the 'Secret Sin' in Pre-Freudian America." *Journal of the History of Medicine and Allied Sciences*, 28:143–144, 1973.

Burr, Anna Robeson. *Silas Weir Mitchell*. New York: Duffield & Co., 1929.

Buzzard, E. Farquhar. "Hughlings Jackson and His Influence on Neurology." *Lancet*, 2:909–913, 1934.

Bynum, W. F. "Rationales for Therapy in British Psychiatry, 1780–1835." *Medical History*, 18:317–334, 1974.

Carlson, Eric. Essay-review of Robert Fuller, *Mesmerism and the American Cure of Souls*. In *Transactions and Studies of the College of Physicians of Philadelphia*, 5(5):145–155, 1983.

———. "George M. Beard and Neurasthenia." *Essays in the History of Psychiatry*. Ed. E. R. Wallace and L. Presley. New York: William S. Hall Psychiatric Institute, 1980.

———. "The Nerve Weakness of the Nineteenth Century." *International Journal of Psychiatry*, 9:50–54, 1970.

———, and N. Pain. "The Psychotherapy That Was Moral Treatment." *American Journal of Psychiatry*, 117:519–524, 1960.

———, and Meribeth Simpson. "Models of the Nervous System in the Eighteenth Century." *Bulletin of the History of Medicine*, 63(2):101–105, 1969.

Carter, A. E. *The Idea of Decadence in French Literature*. Toronto: Univ. of Toronto Press, 1958.

Cassaguard, J. M. *Carrel et Lola devant le Miracle à Lourdes*. Lourdes: Imprimerie de la Grotte, 1958.

Charcot, J.-M. "Accidents Nerveux Provoqués par la Foudre." *Paris Médical*, May 23, 1925, pp. 475–478.

———. *Clinique des Maladies du Système Nerveux*. 2 vols. Paris: Progrès Médical, 1892–93.

———. *Diseases of the Nervous System*. Trans. Thomas Saville. 3 vols. London: New Sydenham, 1889.

———. "The Faith Cure." *The New Review*, 6:18–31, 1893.

———. "La Foi Qui Guérit." *Archives de Neurologie*, 25:72–87, 1893.

———. *Leçons du Mardi à la Salpêtrière*. 2 vols. Paris: Progrès Médical, 1889–92.

———. *Lectures on the Diseases of the Nervous System*. Trans. George Sigerson. Philadelphia: Henry C. Lea, 1879.

———. *Oeuvres Complètes*, Vols. 1, 2, 3, 9. Paris: Progrès Médical, 1886–90.

———. "Sur un Cas d'Amnésie Rétro-Antérograde, Probablement d'Origine Hystérique." *Revue de Médecine*, 12:80–96, 1892.

———, and Georges Gilles de la Tourette. "Hypnotism in the Hysterical." *Dictionary of Psychological Medicine*. Ed. Hack Tuke. 1:606–610. Philadelphia: Blakiston, 1892.

———, and Paul Richer. *Les Démoniaques dans l'Art*. Paris: Delahaye & Lecrosnier, 1887.

———, and Pierre Marie. "Hysteria." *Dictionary of Psychological Medicine*. Ed. Hack Tuke. 1:618–641. Philadelphia: Blakiston, 1892.

Chatel, John, and Roger Peele. "A Centennial Review of Neurasthenia." *American Journal of Psychiatry*, 126:10, 1404–13, 1970.

———. "The Concept of Neurasthenia." *International Journal of Psychiatry*, 9:36–49, 1970.

Chertok, L. "Freud in Paris: A Crucial Stage." *International Journal of Psychoanalysis*, 51:511–520, 1970.

———. "From Liébeault to Freud." *American Journal of Psychotherapy*, 22:96–101, 1968.

———. "A propos de la découverte de la méthode cathartique." *Bulletin de Psychologie* (Nov. 1960), pp. 33–36.

Cheyne, George. *The English Malady*. London: Strahan & Leake, 1733.

———. *An Essay on Regimen*. London: C. Rivington, 1740.

Chrzanowski, Gerard. "An Obsolete Diagnosis." *International Journal of Psychiatry*, 9:54–56, 1970.

Colin, N. "Charcot." *Annales Médico-Psychologiques* (May 1925), pp. 385–392.

Courbon, Paul. "Charcot et la Psychiatrie." *Annales Médico-Psychologiques* (May 1925), pp. 393–431.

Courchet, J. L. "Janet à la Salpêtrière." *L'Evolution Psychiatrique* (Jan.–Mar. 1950), pp. 357–364.

Cranefield, Paul. "Josef Breuer." *Dictionary of Scientific Biography*. Ed. Charles C. Gillespie. 2:445–450, 1972.

———. "Josef Breuer's Evaluation of His Contribution to Psychoanalysis." *International Journal of Psycho-Analysis*, 39:319–322, 1958.

Critchley, M. "The Contribution of John Hughlings Jackson to Neurology." *Cerebral Palsy Bulletin*, 2:7–9, 1960.

———. "Early Days of the National Hospital, Queen Square." *Cerebral Palsy Bulletin*, 2:5–6, 1960.

———. "Hughlings Jackson: The Man and the Early Days of the National Hospital." *Proceedings of the Royal Society of Medicine*, 53:613–618, 1960.

Cullen, William. *A Synopsis of Nosology*. Philadelphia: Dobson, 1816.

Cushing, Harvey. *Life of William Osler*. Oxford: Clarendon Press, 1925.

Dana, Charles. "Dr. George M. Beard." *Archives of Neurology and Psychiatry*, 10:428–435, 1923.

———. *Textbook of Nervous Diseases*. New York: William Wood, 1892.

Darnton, Robert. *Mesmerism and the End of the Enlightenment*. Cambridge: Harvard Univ. Press, 1968.

Darwin, Charles. *Autobiography*. New York: Norton, 1958.

———. *The Expression of the Emotions in Man and Animals*. New York: Appleton, 1873.

Davis, J. O. *Phrenology: Fad and Science*. New Haven: Yale Univ. Press, 1955.

Debove, G. M. "Eloge de J.-M. Charcot." *La Presse Médicale*, Dec. 19, 1900, pp. 200–204.

De Grandmaison, F. *Twenty Miracles at Lourdes*. St. Louis: B. Herder Book Co., n.d.

Dejerine, J. "L'Oeuvre Scientifique de Charcot." *Paris Médical*, May 23, 1925, pp. 509–511.

Delboeuf, Joseph. *Le Magnétisme Animal*. Paris: Alcan, 1889.

Deleuze, Gilles. *Sacher-Masoch*. London: Faber & Faber, 1971.

DeMonzie, M. A. "Eloge de Charcot." *Revue Neurologique* 41(1):1159–62, 1925.

Dercum, F. X., ed. *Nervous Diseases by American Authors*. Philadelphia: Henry C. Lea, 1895.

Dessoir, Max. *Bibliographie des Modernen Hypnotismus*. Berlin: Duncken, 1888.

————. *Erster Nachtrag zur Bibliographie des Modernen Hypnotismus*. Berlin: Duncken, 1890.

Deutsch, Felix. "A Footnote to Freud's Fragment of an Analysis of a Case of Hysteria." *Psychoanalytic Quarterly*, 26:159–167, 1957.

Diethelm, O. "An Historical View of Somatic Treatment in Psychiatry." *American Journal of Psychiatry*, 95:1165–79, 1939.

District of Columbia Appellate. The Washington and Georgetown Railroad Company v. Dashiell, 7:507–516, 1895.

Dobbs, Brian, and Judy Dobbs. *Dante Gabriel Rossetti, An Alien Victorian*. London: MacDonald & Jane's, 1977.

Dostoevski, Fyodor. *The Idiot*. Trans. Henry and Olga Carlisle. New York: a Signet Classic, 1969.

Dubos, René. *Louis Pasteur, Freelance of Science*. New York: Scribners, 1950.

Duchenne, Guillaume. *Mécanisme de la Physionomie humaine ou analyse électro-physiologique de l'expression des passions*. Paris: Baillière, 1876.

Dumas, Alexandre, fils. *Camille (la Dame aux Camélias)*. New York: New American Library, 1972.

Earnest, Ernest. *Silas Weir Mitchell, Novelist and Physician*. Philadelphia: Univ. of Pennsylvania Press, 1950.

Edinburgh Review. Review of John Thomsen, M.D., *An Account of the Life, Lectures and Writings of William Cullen, M.D.*, 50:461–479, 1832.

Edinger, Dora. *Bertha Pappenheim: Freud's Anna O*. Highland Park, Ill.: Congregation Solel, 1968.

Eisley, Loren. *Darwin's Century*. Garden City, N.Y.: Anchor Books, 1961.

Eliot, George. *The Works of George Eliot*. 3 vols. New York: P. F. Collier, n.d.

Ellenberger, Henri F. Review of D. Edinger, *Bertha Pappenheim: Leben und Schriften. Journal of the History of the Behavioral Sciences*, 2:94–96, 1966.

————. "Charcot and the Salpêtrière School." *American Journal of Psychotherapy*, 19:253–267, 1965.

————. *The Discovery of the Unconscious*. New York: Basic Books, 1970.

————. "The Pathogenic Secret and Its Therapeutics." *Journal of the History of the Behavioral Sciences*, 2:29–42, 1966.

———. "La Psychothérapie de Janet." *L'Evolution Psychiatrique* (Jan.–Mar. 1950), pp. 465–484.

Engelhardt, H. T. "The Disease of Masturbation: Values on the Concept of Disease." *Bulletin of the History of Medicine*, 48:234–248, 1974.

———. "John Hughlings Jackson and the Mind-Body Relation." *Bulletin of the History of Medicine*, 49(2):137–151, 1975.

Erb, Wilhelm. *Handbook of Electro-Therapeutics.* New York: William Wood, 1883.

Erikson, Erik. "Reality and Actuality." *Journal of the American Psychoanalytic Association*, 10:451–474, 1962.

Ey, H. "Force et Faiblesses des concepts génétiques et énergétiques de la psychopathologie de Pierre Janet." *Bulletin de Psychologie* (Nov. 1960), pp. 52–54.

———. "Hughlings Jackson's Principles of the Organo-dynamic concept of psychiatry." *American Journal of Psychiatry*, 118:673–682, 1962.

Ferrero, Gina Lombroso. *Criminal Man According to the Classification of Cesare Lombroso.* Intro. by Cesare Lombroso. New York: Putnam's, 1911.

———. *Cesare Lombroso: Storia della vita e delle opere.* Turin: Fratelli Bocca, 1915.

Fischer-Homberger, Esther. "Die Buchse der Pandora: Der Mythische Hintergrund der Eisenbahnkrankheiten des 19 Jahrhunderts." *Sudhoff's Archive* (1972), pp. 297–317.

———. "Charcot und die Atiologie der Neurosen." *Gesnerus*, 28:35–46, 1971.

———. "Hypochondriasis of the 18th Century, Neurosis of the Present Century." *Bulletin of the History of Medicine*, 46:391–401, 1972.

———. "Railway Spine und Traumatische Neurose—Seele und Rückenmark." *Gesnerus*, 27:96–111, 1970.

———. *Die Traumatische Neurose: Von Somatische zum Socialen Leiden.* Stuttgart: Hans Huber, 1975.

Fontane, Theodor. *Effi Briest.* Trans. Douglas Parmee. Baltimore: Penguin Books, 1967.

Foucault, Michel. *Madness and Civilization.* New York: Vintage Books, 1973.

Freedman, Lucy. *The Story of Anna O.* New York: Walker & Co., 1972.

Freud, Sigmund. *Dora: An Analysis of a Case of Hysteria.* New York: Collier Books, 1963.

———. *The Standard Edition of the Complete Psychological Works of Sigmund Freud,* Vols. 1–3. London: Hogarth Press, 1955.

Fullinwider, S. P. "William James' 'Spiritual Crisis.'" *The Historian*, 38: 39–57, 1975.

Furnas, T. C. *The Americans: A Social History of the United States.* New York: Putnam's, 1969.

Galdston, Iago, ed. *Freud and Contemporary Culture.* New York: Inter University Press, 1957.

Gardeil, Bruno de Jesus-Marie. "A propos de la 'Madeleine' de Pierre Janet." *Etudes Carmelitaines,* 16(1):21–61; (2):65–125, 1931.

Gardiner, Muriel, ed. *The Wolfman and Sigmund Freud.* New York: Basic Books, 1971.

Garrison, Fielding. *History of Neurology.* Rev. and enl. by Lawrence McHenry. Springfield, Ill.: Charles Thomas, 1969.

Gay, Peter. *Freud, Jews and Other Germans.* New York: Oxford Univ. Press, 1978.

Gedo, J., et al. " 'Studies on Hysteria.' A Methodological Evaluation." *Journal of the American Psychoanalytic Association,* 12:734–751, 1964.

Gerlach, Walter. "Herman von Helmholtz." *Neue Deutsche Biographie,* 8:498–501. Berlin: Duncken & Humblot, 1953.

Germain, J. "Pierre Janet." *Bulletin de Psychologie,* Nov. 2–4, 1960.

Gilles de la Tourette, Georges. *Leçons de Clinique Thérapeutique sur les Maladies du Système Nerveux.* Paris: Plon, 1898.

———. *Traité Clinique et Thérapeutique de l'Hystérique Normal.* Paris: Plon, 1891.

Goldstein, Jan. "The Hysteria Diagnosis and the Politics and Anticlericalism in Late Nineteenth-Century France." *Journal of Modern History.* 54:209–239, 1982.

Goncharov, Ivan. *Oblomov.* Trans. David Magarshack. New York: Penguin Books, 1954.

Goodhart, James. *The Common Neuroses.* London: H. K. Lewis, 1894.

Gorman, Warren. "Whiplash: Fictive or Factual?" *Journal of the American Association of Psychiatry and the Law,* 7(3):245–248, 1980.

Gover, Geoffrey. *The Life and Ideas of the Marquis de Sade.* London: Peter Owen, 1953.

Gowers, William. *A Manual of Diseases of the Nervous System,* Vol. 2. Philadelphia: Blakiston, 1893.

Grana, Cesar. *Bohemian versus Bourgeois: French Society and the French Man of Letters in the Nineteenth Century.* New York: Basic Books, 1964.

Greenblatt, Samuel. "The Major Influences on the Early Life and Work of John Hughlings Jackson." *Bulletin of the History of Medicine,* 39: 346–376, 1965.

Griswald, Wesley. *Train Wreck.* Brattleboro, Vt.: Stephen Greene Press, 1969.

Grob, Gerald. *Mental Institutions in America.* New York: Free Press, 1973.

———. *The State and the Mentally Ill.* Chapel Hill: Univ. of North Carolina Press, 1966.

Guillain, Georges. *J.-M. Charcot: His Life—His Work.* Trans. Pearce Bailey. New York: Paul Hoeber, 1959.

Guinon, Georges. "Charcot Intime." *Paris Médical,* May 23, 1925, pp. 511–516.

Gutman, Robert. *Richard Wagner: The Man, His Mind and His Music.* New York: Harcourt Brace Jovanovich, 1974.

Haeckel, Ernst. *The Riddle of the Universe.* Trans. Joseph McCabe. New York: Hargen Bros., 1900.

Haight, Gordon S. *George Eliot: A Biography.* New York: Oxford Univ. Press, 1968.

Hale, Nathan. "From Berggasse XIX to Central Park West: The Americanization of Psychoanalysis, 1919–1940." *Journal of the History of the Behavioral Sciences,* 14:299–315, 1978.

———. *Freud and the Americans.* New York: Oxford Univ. Press, 1971.

Hale-White, Sir William. *Great Doctors of the Nineteenth Century.* London: Edward Arnold, 1935.

Hall, Marshall. *Memoirs on the Nervous System.* London: Sherwood, Gilbert & Piper, 1837.

Haller, John. "Neurasthenia." *New York State Journal of Medicine,* Feb. 15, 1971, pp. 473–482.

Halliday, F. E. *Robert Browning: His Life and Work.* London: Jupiter Books, 1975.

Halport, E. "Lermontov and the Wolfman." *Freud and His Patients.* Ed. M. Kanzer and J. Glenn. New York: Aronson, 1980.

Hamilton, Nigel. *The Brothers Mann.* New Haven: Yale Univ. Press, 1978.

Hare, E. H. "Masturbatory Insanity: A History of an Idea." *Journal of Mental Science,* 108:1–25, 1962.

Hare, Hobart Amory. *The Medical Complications, Accidents, and Sequelae of Typhoid or Enteric Fever.* Philadelphia: Henry C. Lea, 1879.

Hauser, Arnold. *The Social History of Art,* Vols. 3 and 4. New York: Vintage Books, n.d.

Havens, L. "Charcot and Hysteria." *Journal of Nervous and Mental Diseases,* 141:505–516, 1965.

———. "Emil Kraepelin." *Journal of Nervous and Mental Diseases,* 141: 16–28, 1965.

———. "Pierre Janet." *Journal of Nervous and Mental Diseases,* 143: 383–398, 1966.

Hesnard, A. "La Conception de la Psychasthénie de P. Janet." *L'Evolution Psychiatrique* (Jan.–Mar. 1950), pp. 391–400.

———. "Un parallèle Janet-Freud." *Bulletin de Psychologie* (Nov. 1960), pp. 69–73.

Hillman, Robert G. "A Scientific Study of Mystery: The Role of the Medical and Popular Press in the Nancy-Salpêtrière Controversy on Hypnotism." *Bulletin of the History of Medicine,* 39:163–182, 1965.

Hoff, Hans, and Franz Seitelberger. "The History of the Neurological School of Vienna." *Journal of Nervous and Mental Diseases,* 116: 495–505, 1952.

Hofstadter, Richard. *Social Darwinism in American Thought.* Boston: Beacon Press, 1944.

Houghton, Walter E. *The Victorian Frame of Mind.* New Haven: Yale Univ. Press, 1957.

Hunt, Violet. *The Wife of Rossetti.* New York: Dutton, 1932.

Hutchinson, Jonathan. "The Late Dr. Hughlings Jackson: Recollections of a Life-Long Friendship." *British Medical Journal*, 2:1551–54, 1911.

Huxley, T. H. "Mr. Darwin's Critics." *Contemporary Review* (1871), pp. 443–476.

Hyman, Stanley. *The Tangled Bank: Darwin, Marx, Frazer and Freud as Imaginative Writers.* New York: Atheneum, 1962.

Jackson, J. Hughlings. *On Post-Epileptic States.* London: H. Wolff, 1888.

———. *Remarks on Evolution and Dissolution of the Nervous System.* London: H. Wolff, 1883.

———. *Selected Writings of John Hughlings Jackson.* 2 vols. Ed. James Taylor. London: Hodder & Stoughton, 1931–32.

Jackson, Stanley. "Galen on Mental Disorders." *Journal of the History of the Behavioral Sciences*, 5:365–384, 1969.

———. "The History of Freud's Concepts of Regression." *Journal of the American Psycho-Analytic Association*, 17:743–784, 1969.

James, Henry. *The Ambassadors.* New York: Penguin Books, 1979.

———. *The Americans.* New York: Penguin Books, 1979.

———. *The Wings of the Dove.* New York: Penguin Classics, 1978.

James, William. "Degeneration and Genius." *Psychological Review*, 2: 287–294, 1895.

———. "Great Men, Great Thoughts and the Environment." *Atlantic Monthly*, 46(274):440–459, 1880.

———. "The Importance of Individuals." *The Open Court*, 4: 2437–40, 1890.

———. "Notes on Automatic Writing." *Proceedings of the American Society on Psychical Research*, 1:548–564, 1886.

———. "Report of the Committee on Mediumistic Phenomena." *Proceedings of the American Society on Psychical Research*, 1:103–106, 1886.

———. *The Varieties of Religious Experience.* New York: Modern Library, 1936.

Janet, Jules. "Le Hystérie et l'hypnotisme, d'après la théorie de la double personnalité." *Revue Scientifique*, 41:616–623, 1888.

Janet, Pierre. *L'Automatisme Psychologique.* Paris: Alcan, 1889.

———. *De l'Angoisse à l'Extase.* 2 vols. Paris: Alcan, 1926.

———. *The Major Symptoms of Hysteria.* New York: Macmillan, 1920.

———. *The Mental State of Hystericals.* New York: Putnam's, 1901.

———. *Névroses et Idées Fixes.* 2 vols. Paris: Alcan, 1898.

———. "Psychoanalysis." *Journal of Abnormal Psychology*, 9:1–35, 153–187, 1914–15.

———. Trans. Dorothy Olson. In Carl Murchinson, ed. *History of Psy-*

chology in Autobiography, 1:123–133. Worcester: Clark Univ., 1930.

Janik, Allan, and Stephen Toulmin. *Wittgenstein's Vienna*. New York: Simon & Schuster, 1972.

Joffroy, M. "Jean-Martin Charcot." *Archives de Médecine et d'Anatomie Pathologique*, 5:577–606, 1893.

Johnston, William. *The Austrian Mind: An Intellectual and Social History, 1848–1938*. Berkeley: Univ. of California Press, 1972.

Jones, Ernest. *The Life and Work of Sigmund Freud*. 3 vols. New York: Basic Books, 1965.

———. "Professor Janet on Psychoanalysis: A Rejoinder." *Journal of Abnormal Psychology*, 9:400–410, 1914–15.

de Jonge, Alex. *Baudelaire, Prince of Clouds*. New York: Paddington Press, 1976.

Josephson, Matthew. *Edison*. New York: McGraw-Hill, 1959.

Kanzer, M. "Dora's Imagery: The Flight from a Burning House." *Freud and His Patients*. Ed. M. Kanzer and J. Glenn. New York: Aronson, 1980.

———. "Further Comments on the Wolfman: The Search for a Primal Scene." *Freud and His Patients*. Ed. M. Kanzer and J. Glenn. New York: Aronson, 1980.

Kennedy, F. "John Hughlings Jackson." *Bulletin of the New York Academy of Medicine*, 11:479–480, 1935.

Kentucky Reports. Louisville Southern Railroad Company v. Minogue. 90:369–377, 1890.

Kindt, Hildburg. "Freiherr Richard von Krafft-Ebing." *Neue Deutsche Biographie*, 12:649–650. Berlin: Duncker & Humblot, 1953.

Kippis, Andrew, ed. "Cheyne." *Biographia Britannica*, Vol. 3. London: C. Rivington, 1778–93.

Knight, David. *Robert Koch, Father of Bacteriology*. New York: F. Watts, 1961.

Krafft-Ebing, Richard von. *Nervosität und Neurasthenische Zustände*. Vienna: Alfred Hölder, 1900.

———. *Psychopathia Sexualis, mit Besonderer Berücksichtigung der Contraren Sexualempfindung*. 2d ed. Stuttgart: Ferdinand Enke, 1887.

———. *Psychopathia Sexualis, with Especial Reference to Contrary Sexual Instinct*. Trans. Charles Gilbert Chaddock. 7th ed. Philadelphia: F. A. Davis, 1894.

———. *Psychopathia Sexualis*. Trans. Victor Robinson. 12th ed. New York: Pioneer Publications, 1939.

———. *Textbook of Insanity*. Trans. C. G. Chaddock. Philadelphia: F. A. Davis, 1905.

Kris, Ernst. "The Significance of Freud's Earliest Discoveries." *International Journal of Psychoanalysis*, 31:108–116, 1950.

Kroll, J. "A Reappraisal of Psychiatry in the Middle Ages." *Archives of General Psychiatry*, 29:276–283, 1973.

Kurella, Hans. *Cesare Lombroso: A Modern Man of Science*. Trans. M. Eden Paul. New York: Robinson Co., 1910.

Lagache, D. "Janet au Collège de France." *L'Evolution Psychiatrique* (Jan.–Mar., 1950), pp. 411–417.

Langs, Robert. "The Misalliance Dimension in the Case of Dora." *Freud and His Patients.* Ed. M. Kanzer and J. Glenn. New York: Aronson, 1980.

———. "The Misalliance Dimension in the Case of the Wolfman." *Freud and His Patients.* Ed. M. Kanzer and J. Glenn. New York: Aronson, 1980.

Langworthy, O. R. "Hughlings Jackson—His Opinions Concerning Epilepsy." *Journal of Nervous and Mental Diseases,* 76:574–585, 1932.

Lassek, Arthur. *The Unique Legacy of Dr. Hughlings Jackson.* Springfield, Ill.: Charles Thomas, 1970.

Lattes, L. "Retour à Lombroso." *Revue Médicale de Liège,* 12:41–56, 1957.

Laughton, J. K. "Thomas Trotter." *Dictionary of National Biography,* 19:1181–82. London: Oxford Univ. Press, 1917.

Laurentin, René. *Bernadette of Lourdes.* Trans. John Drury. London: Darton, Longman & Todd, 1979.

Lazare, Aaron. "Conversion Symptoms." *New England Journal of Medicine,* Vol. 305, No. 13: 745–748, 1981.

Legiardi, Laura. "Lombroso and Freud." *Medical Life,* 39:109–121, 1932.

LeGrand, André. "A propos de la 'Madeleine' de Pierre Janet." *Etudes Carmelitaines,* 16(2):43–64, 1931.

LeMasle, Robert. *Le Professeur Adrien Proust.* Paris: Lipschutz, 1936.

Levillain, Fernand. *La Neurasthénie: Maladie de Beard.* Paris: A. Maloine, 1891.

Levin, Kenneth. *Freud's Early Psychology of the Neuroses.* Pittsburgh: Univ. of Pittsburgh Press, 1978.

———. "Freud's Paper 'On Male Hysteria' and the Conflict Between Anatomical and Physiological Models." *Bulletin of the History of Medicine,* 48:377–397, 1974.

Lewin, Bertram. "The Train Ride: A Study of One of Freud's Figures of Speech." *Psychoanalytic Quarterly,* 39:71–89, 1970.

Lhermite, Jean. "L'Ecole de la Salpêtrière, J.-M. Charcot, psychophysiologiste." *Encéphale,* 4:297–310, 1950.

Liébeault, Auguste Ambroise, "Confession d'un Médecin Hypnotiseur." *Revue de l'Hypnotisme,* 1:105–110, 143–148, 1886.

Liégeois, Jules, "L'Ecole de Paris et Ecole de Nancy." *Revue de L'Hypnotisme,* 1:33–41, 1886.

Lindesmith, Alfred, and Yale Levin. "The Lombrosian Myth in Criminology." *American Journal of Sociology,* 42:653–671, 1937.

Lombroso, Cesare. *Crime: Its Causes and Remedies.* Trans. Henry P. Horton. Boston: Little, Brown, 1911.

———. Intro. to Gina Lombroso Ferrero, *Criminal Man According to the Classification of Cesare Lombroso.* New York: Putnam's, 1911.

———. *L'Homme Criminel.* 2 vols. Paris: Alcan, 1895.

————. *L'Uomo Delinquente.* First pub., 1876; Rome: Napoleone, 1971.

————. *Man of Genius.* Trans. from the Italian. London: Walter Scott, 1891.

————, and William Ferrero. *The Female Offender.* New York: Appleton, 1895.

————. *La Femme Criminelle et la Prostituée.* Paris: Alcan, 1896.

Löwenfeld, L. *Die Moderne Behandlung den Nervenschwäche.* Wiesbaden: J. F. Bergmann, 1895.

Luton, Alfred. "Névrose." *Nouveau Dictionnaire de Médecine et de Chirurgie,* 23:803–859. Paris: J. B. Baillière, 1877.

MacDonald, Robert H. "The Frightful Consequences of Onanism: Notes on the History of a Delusion." *Journal of the History of Ideas,* 28: 423–431, 1967.

MacMillan, M. B. "Beard's Concept of Neurasthenia and Freud's Concept of the Actual Neuroses." *Journal of the History of the Behavioral Sciences,* 12:376–390, 1976.

————. "Delboeuf and Janet as Influences in Freud's Treatment of Emmy Von N." *Journal of the History of the Behavioral Sciences,* 15(4): 299–309, 1979.

Male, Pierre. "L'Automatisme Psychologique." *L'Evolution Psychiatrique* (Jan.–Mar. 1950), pp. 366–375.

Mander, Rosalie. *Mrs. Browning.* London: Weidenfeld & Nicolson, 1980.

Mann, Thomas. *Buddenbrooks.* Frankfurt: Fischer, 1975.

————. *Die Erzählungen.* 2 vols. Frankfurt: Fischer, 1975.

Marcus, Steven. *The Other Victorians.* New York: Basic Books, 1966.

————. *Representation: Essays on Literature and Society.* New York: Random House, 1976.

Marie, Pierre. "Eloge à J.-M. Charcot." *Revue Neurologique,* Vol. 1, No. (Jan.–Mar. 1950), pp. 366–375.

Marshall, J. H. "Insanity Cured by Castration." *Medical and Surgical Reporter,* 13:363–364, 1865.

Marx, Otto. "American Psychiatry Without William James." *Bulletin of the History of Medicine,* 42:52–61, 1968.

————. "Nineteenth-Century Medical Psychology." *Isis,* 61:33, 355–370, 1970.

————. "A Reevaluation of the Mentalists in Early 19th-Century German Psychiatry." *American Journal of Psychiatry,* 121:752–760, 1965.

Massachusetts Reports. Frank H. Warren v. Boston and Maine Railroad and Others, 163:484–490, 1845.

Massachusetts Reports. Laura M. Homans v. Boston Elevated Railway Company, 180:456–458, 1901.

Massachusetts Reports. Margaret C. Spade v. Lynn and Boston Elevated Railroad Company, 168:285–290, 1897.

Matthiessen, F. O. *The James Family.* New York: Knopf, 1947.

Maudsley, Henry. *Body and Mind.* London: Macmillan, 1870.

Maurois, André. *Lélia: The Life of George Sand.* Trans. Gerard Hopkins. New York: Penguin Books, 1953.

May, Arthur. *Vienna in the Age of Franz Josef.* Norman, Okla.: Univ. of Oklahoma Press, 1966.

McGillicuddy, T. J. *Functional Disorders of the Nervous System in Women.* New York: William Wood, 1896.

Mercier, C. "The Late Hughlings Jackson." *British Medical Journal,* 1: 85–86, 1912.

Merz, John. *A History of European Thought in the 19th Century,* Vols. 1 and 2. London: Blackwell, 1896–1914.

Mettler, Cecilia. *History of Medicine.* Philadelphia: Blakiston, 1947.

Michaud, L. G., ed. "Philippe Pinel." *Biographie Universelle,* 33:356–359. Paris: Delagrane, 1811–28.

Minkowski, E. "A propos des derniers publications de Pierre Janet." *Bulletin de Psychologie* (Nov. 1960), pp. 121–127.

Mitchell, S. Weir. "The Evolution of the Rest Cure." *Journal of Nervous and Mental Diseases,* 368–373, 1904.

———. *Fat and Blood: And How to Make Them.* Philadelphia: Lippincott, 1878.

———. *Lectures on Diseases of the Nervous System, Especially in Women.* Philadelphia: Henry C. Lea, 1881.

———. *Roland Blake.* New York: Century Co., 1913.

———. *Wear and Tear, or Hints for the Overworked.* Philadelphia: Lippincott, 1897.

Mochulsky, Konstantin. *Dostoevsky: His Life and Work.* Trans. Michael A. Minihan. Princeton, N.J.: Princeton Univ. Press, 1967.

Modlin, Herbert. "The Trauma in 'Traumatic Neurosis.'" *Readings in Law and Psychiatry.* Ed. Richard Allen, E. Z. Ferster, and Jesse G. Rubin. Baltimore: Johns Hopkins Press, 1968.

Moebius, Paul Julius. *Neurologische Beiträge.* Leipzig: Abel, 1894.

Mora, George. "Antecedent to Neurosis." *International Journal of Psychiatry,* 9:57–60, 1970.

———. "One Hundred Years from Lombroso's First Essay, 'Genius and Insanity.'" *American Journal of Psychiatry,* 121:562–571, 1964.

Moreau (de Tours), J. J. *La Psychologie Morbide.* Paris: Victor Masson, 1859.

Moreau (de Tours), Paul. *De la Folie Chez les Enfants.* Paris: Baillière, 1888.

Morel, B. A. *Traité des Dégénérescences.* Paris: Baillière, 1857.

———. *Traité des Maladies Mentales.* Paris: Victor Masson, 1860.

Morris, James. *Heaven's Command.* New York: Harvest/Harcourt Brace Jovanovich, 1980.

———. *Pax Britannica.* New York: Harvest/Harcourt Brace Jovanovich, 1980.

Morrison, W. Douglas. Introd. to C. Lombroso and M. Ferrero, *Female Offender.* New York: Appleton, 1895.

Mosse, George. Introd. to Max Nordau, *Degeneration.* New York: Howard Fertig, 1968.

Müller, Franz Carl, ed. *Das Handbuch der Neurasthenie.* Leipzig: F. C. W. Vogel, 1893.

Müller, Johannes. *Elements of Physiology.* Trans. John Bell. Philadelphia: Henry C. Lea, 1843.

Munk, Hermann. "Johannes Müller." *Allegemeine Deutsche Biographie,* 22:625–628. Berlin: Duncken & Humblot, 1967.

Munthe, Axel. *The Story of San Michele.* London: John Murray, 1929.

Murphy, Gardiner. "William James on the Will." *Journal of the History of the Behavioral Sciences,* 7(3):249–260, 1971.

Muslin, Hyman, and Merlin Gill. "Transference in the Dora Case." *Journal of the American Psycho-Analytic Association,* 26:311–328, 1978.

Neame, Alan. *The Happening at Lourdes.* London: Hodder & Stoughton, 1968.

New York Reports. Annie Mitchell, Respondent, v. Rochester Railway Company, Appellant, 151:107–111, 1896.

New York Supplement. Becker v. Albany Railway, 54:395–398, 1848.

Nicoll, John. *Dante Gabriel Rossetti.* New York: Macmillan, 1975.

Nordau, Anna, and Maxa Nordau. *Max Nordau: A Biography.* New York: Nordau Committee, 1943.

Nordau, Max. *Degeneration.* Trans. from the German. New York: Appleton, 1895.

———. *Degeneration.* Trans. from the German. New York: Howard Fertig, 1968.

———. *Paradoxes.* Trans. from the German. Chicago: L. Schick, 1886.

———. *The Shackles of Fate.* New York: F. Tennyson Neely, 1897.

Occasional Correspondent. "Hypnotism in Paris." *Lancet,* 1882: (May), pp. 842–843; (June), pp. 1057–58; (July), pp. 163–165; (Nov.), pp. 786–787; (Dec.), pp. 1057–58.

Oppenheim, Hermann. *Diseases of the Nervous System.* Philadelphia: Lippincott, 1900.

———. *Die Traumatische Neurosen.* Berlin: August Hirschwald, 1889.

———. "Wie sind diejenigen Fälle von Neurastheine aufzufassen, welche sich nach Erschütterungen das Rückenmarkes inbesondere nach Eisenbahnunfällen entwickeln?" *Deutsche Medizinische Wochenschrift,* 14:194–196, 1888.

Osler, William. *Principles and Practice of Medicine.* New York: Appleton, 1892.

Owen, Alan. *Hysteria, Hypnosis and Healing: The Work of J.-M. Charcot.* New York: Garrett, 1971.

Page, Herbert. *Injuries of the Spine and Spinal Cord and Nervous Shock.* Philadelphia: Blakiston, 1885.

Painter, George. *Marcel Proust.* 2 vols. New York: Vintage Books, 1978.

Parcheminery, G. "La Conception de l'Hystérie." *L'Evolution Psychiatrique* (Jan.–Mar. 1950), pp. 377–390.

Parker, Gail Thain. *Mind Cure in New England.* Hanover, N.H.: Univ. Press of New England, 1973.

Parmelee, Maurice. Introd. to C. Lombroso, *Crime: Its Causes and Remedies.* Trans. H. P. Hortan. Boston: Little, Brown, 1911.

Pastore, Nicholas. "William James: A Contradiction," *Journal of the History of the Behavioral Sciences,* 13(2):126–130, 1977.

Payne, J. F. "George Cheyne." *Dictionary of National Biography,* 4: 217–219. London: Oxford Univ. Press, 1917.

Pearsall, Ronald. *The Worm in the Bud: The World of Victorian Sexuality.* New York: Penguin Books, 1983.

Pelner, Louis. "The Other Max Nordau." *New York State Journal of Medicine,* 69:973–977, 1969.

Pennsylvania Reports. Ewing et ux., Appellants, v. Pittsburgh, Cincinnati and St. Louis Railway Company, 147:40–45, 1892.

Peterson, Frederick. Introd. to R. von Krafft-Ebing, *Textbook of Insanity.* Philadelphia: F. A. Davis, 1964.

Petitfils, Pierre. *Verlaine.* Paris: Julliard, 1981.

Pickering, George. *Creative Malady.* London: Allen & Unwin, 1974.

Pieron, H. "Conscience et conduite chez Pierre Janet." *Bulletin de Psychologie* (Nov. 1960), pp. 149–153.

Pinel, Philippe, and Isidore Brichetau. "Névrose." *Dictionnaire des Sciences Médicales,* 35:557–581. Paris: Panckoucke, 1819.

———. *A Treatise on Insanity.* New York: Hafner, 1962.

Playfair, William S. *The Systematic Treatment of Nervous Prostration and Hysteria.* Philadelphia: Henry C. Lea, 1883.

Podolsky, Edward. "Cesare Lombroso and Criminal Man." *Indian Journal of the History of Medicine,* 6(1):11–20, 1961.

Pollock, G. "The Possible Significance of Childhood Object Loss in the Josef Breuer-Bertha Pappenheim-Sigmund Freud Relationship." *Journal of the American Psycho-Analytic Association,* 16:711–739, 1968.

Proceedings of the Royal Society of London. "Hermann von Helmholtz." 59:17–30, 1896.

Proceedings of the Royal Society of London. "Johannes Müller." 9:556–563, 1859.

Proust, Adrien, and Gilbert Ballet. *Hygiène du Neurasthénique.* Paris: Victor Masson, 1897.

———. *The Treatment of Neurasthenia.* London: Henry Kimpton, 1902.

Proust, Marcel. *A la Recherche du Temps Perdu.* 3 vols. Paris: Gallimard, 1954.

Putnam, J. J. "Recent Investigations into the Pathology of So-Called Concussion of the Spine." *Boston Medical and Surgical Journal,* 109(10):217–223, 1883.

Rambo, Lewis. "Ethics, Evolution and the Psychology of William James." *Journal of the History of the Behavioral Sciences,* 16(1):50–57, 1980.

Reichart, S. "A Re-examination of 'Studies in Hysteria.'" *Psychoanalytic Quarterly,* 25:155–177, 1956.

Renan, Ernest. *Vie de Jesus.* Paris: Michel, 1870.

Renterghem, A. W. van. "Liébeault et son Ecole." *Zeitschrift für Hypnotismus,* 4:333–375, 1896; 5:95–127, 46–55, 1897; 6:11–44, 1897.

Reynolds, J. R. "Remarks on Paralysis and Other Disorders of Motion and Sensation, Dependent on Idea." *British Medical Journal,* Nov. 6, 1869, pp. 483–485.

Richards, Lawrence. "Head Trauma, Traumatic Neurosis, and the Forensic Report." *Journal of the American Association of Psychiatry and the Law,* 7(3):232–238, 1980.

Richardson, Joanna. *Verlaine.* London: Weidenfeld & Nicolson, 1971.

Richer, Paul. *Etudes Cliniques sur la Grande Hystérie.* Paris: Delahaye & Lecrosnier, 1885.

Rieff, Philip. *Freud: The Mind of the Moralist.* London: Victor Gollancz, 1960.

———. Introd. to S. Freud, *Dora: An Analysis of a Case of Hysteria.* New York: Collin Books, 1963.

Riese, Walther. "The Pre-Freudian Origin of Psychoanalysis." *Science and Psychoanalysis, Volume I.* Ed. Jules Masserman. New York: Grune & Stratton, 1958.

———, and W. Gooddy. "An Original Clinical Record of Hughlings Jackson, with an Interpretation." *Bulletin of the History of Medicine,* 29:230–238, 1955.

Risse, Guenter. "The Quest for Certainty in Medicine: John Brown's System of Medicine in France." *Bulletin of the History of Medicine,* 45:1–12, 1971.

Rivane, Georges. *Influence de l'Asthme sur L'Oeuvre de Marcel Proust.* Paris: Nouvelle Edition, 1945.

Robertson, G. M. "Hypnotism at Paris and Nancy." *Journal of Mental Science,* 38:494–531, 1892.

Robinson, Victor. Introd. to R. von Krafft-Ebing, *Psychopathia Sexualis.* 12th ed. New York: Pioneer Publications, 1939.

Rockwell, Alphonso. *Rambling Recollections: An Autobiography.* New York: Paul B. Holbin, 1920.

Rogow, A. "A Further Footnote to Freud's 'Fragment of an Analysis of a Case of Hysteria.'" *Journal of the American Psycho-Analytic Association,* 26:331–356, 1978.

Rohling, Augustus. *Louise Lateau: Her Stigmas and Ecstasy.* Trans. W. J. Walsh. New York: Hickey & Co., 1879.

Romanell, P. "Medicine and Pragmatism in William James." *Connecticut Medicine,* 39(9):577–580, 1975.

Romberg, Moritz Heinrich. *A Manual of the Nervous Diseases of Man.* Trans. E. H. Sieveking. London: Sydenham Society, 1853.

Rosenberg, Charles. "The Place of George Beard in Nineteenth-Century Psychiatry." *Bulletin of the History of Medicine,* 36:245–259, 1962.

———. *The Trial of the Assassin Guiteau.* Chicago: Univ. of Chicago Press, 1968.

Rouart, Julien. "Janet et Jackson." *L'Evolution Psychiatrique* (Jan.-Mar. 1950), pp. 485–496.

Rousseau, Jean-Jacques. *The Confessions.* New York: Random House, n.d.

———. *Discours sur l'Origine de l'Inégalité (Extraits).* Paris: Larousse, n.d.

———. *The Social Contract and Other Essays.* New York: Carlton House, n.d.

Sacher-Masoch, Leopold von. *Venus in Furs.* In Gilles Deleuze, *Sacher-Masoch.* London: Faber & Faber, 1971.

de Sade, Marquis. *Justine, or the Misfortunes of Virtue.* Trans. Helen Wearn. New York: Putnam's, 1966.

Salomon, M. I. "Doctors Afield: Max Nordau." *New England Journal of Medicine,* 274:1258–59, 1966.

Sand, George. *La Mare au Diable* and *François le Champi.* Paris: Garnier, n.d.

Scharfman, M. A. "Further Reflections on Dora." *Freud and His Patients.* Ed. M. Kanzler and J. Glenn. New York: Aronson, 1980.

Schivelbusch, Wolfgang. *The Railway Journey.* New York: Urizen Books, 1979.

Schlesinger, Arthur M. *The Rise of the City, 1878–1898.* New York: Macmillan, 1938.

Schlesinger, Nathan, et al. "The Scientific Style of Breuer and Freud in the Origins of Psychoanalysis." *Journal of the American Psycho-Analytic Association,* 15:404–422, 1967.

Schmid, Magnus. "Ruodlf Arndt." *Neue Deutsche Biographie,* 1:362. Berlin: Duncken & Humblot, 1953.

Schneck, Jerome. "Jean-Martin Charcot and the History of Experimental Hypnosis." *Essays in the History of Psychiatry.* Ed. E. R. Wallace and Elsie Pressley. Columbia, S.C.: William S. Hall Psychiatric Institute, 1980.

Schoenwald, Richard. "Recent Studies of the Younger Freud." *Bulletin of the History of Medicine,* 29:261–268, 1955.

Schonbauer, Leopold. "Josef Breuer." *Neue Deutsche Biographie,* 2:606–607. Berlin: Duncken & Humblot, 1953.

Schorske, Carl E. *Fin-de-Siècle Vienna.* New York: Vintage Books, 1981.

Schule, H. "Neurolog Richard von Krafft-Ebing." *Allgemeine Zeitschrift für Psychiatrie,* 60(3):305–329, 1903.

Schur, Max. *Freud: Living and Dying.* New York: International University Press, 1972.

Sellers, William. "Memoir of the Life and Writings of Robert Whytt, M.D." *Transactions of the Royal Society of Edinburgh,* 23:99–131, 1861.

Shaw, George Bernard. *The Perfect Wagnerite.* New York: Dover Publications, 1967.

Sickerman, Barbara. "The Uses of a Diagnosis: Doctors, Patients and

Neurasthenia." *Journal of the History of Medicine* (1977), pp. 33–54.

Simon, Robert. "Great Paths Cross: Freud and James at Clark University, 1909." *American Journal of Psychiatry*, 124:831–834, 1967.

Skelton, Geoffrey. *Richard and Cosima Wagner: Biography of a Marriage.* Boston: Houghton Mifflin, 1982.

Smith, Hubert Winston. "Problems of Proof in Psychic Injury Cases." *Syracuse Law Review*, 14:586–633, 1962–63.

———, and Harry Solomon. "Traumatic Neurosis in Court." *Virginia Law Review*, 30:87–165, 1943.

Smith-Rosenberg, Carroll. "The Female World of Love and Ritual: Relations Between Women in 19th-Century America." *Signs* (Autumn 1975), pp. 1–29.

———. "The Hysterical Woman: Sex Roles and Role Conflict in 19th-Century America." *Social Research*, 29:652–678, 1972.

Sonstroem, David. *Rossetti and the Fair Lady.* Middletown, Conn.: Wesleyan Univ. Press, 1970.

Sontag, Susan. *Illness as Metaphor.* New York: Farrar, Straus & Giroux, 1977.

Soupault, Robert. *Marcel Proust de Côté de la Médecine.* Paris: Plon, 1967.

Souques, A. "Charcot Intime." *La Presse Médicale*, May 27, 1925, pp. 693–698.

———. "Essai sur l'Amnésie Rétro-Antérograde." *Revue de Médecine*, 12:367–401, 867–881, 1892.

South Carolina Reports. S. S. Mack v. South Bound Railroad Company, 52:323–344, 1897.

Southern Reporter. Lapleine v. Morgan's L&T R&SS Company, 4:875–878, 1888.

Southwestern Reporter. Gulf, Colorado and Santa Fe Railway Company v. Hayter, 55:128, 1899.

Spanos, N. P. "Witchcraft in Histories of Psychiatry: A Critical Analysis and an Alternative Conceptualization." *Psychological Bulletin*, 85:417–439, 1978.

Spencer, Herbert. "The Gospel of Relaxation." *Popular Sciences Monthly* (Jan. 1803), pp. 354–359.

Spitz, René. "Authority and Masturbation." *Psychoanalytic Quarterly*, 21:490–527, 1952.

Spitzka, Edward. *Insanity.* New York: Bermingham & Co., 1883.

Stafford, Ann. *Bernadette and Lourdes.* London: Hodder & Stoughton, 1967.

Starkie, Enid. *Arthur Rimbaud.* New York: New Directions, 1961.

Steiner, Andreas. *Das Nervöse Zeitalter.* Zurich: Neue Reihe, 1964.

Stengel, Erwin. "Hughlings Jackson's Influence on Psychiatry." *British Journal of Psychiatry*, 109:348–355, 1963.

Stephen, J. "Thomas Trotter, M.D." *Gentlemen's Magazine* (1832), p. 476.

Stern, Fritz. *The Politics of Cultural Despair.* New York: Anchor Books, 1965.

Stookey, Bryon. "A Lost Neurological Society with Great Expectations." *Journal of the History of Medicine,* 16:280–291, 1961.

Stronach, G. "Robert Whytt." *Dictionary of National Biography,* 21:174–175. London: Oxford Univ. Press, 1917.

Strouse, Jean. *Alice James.* New York: Bantam Books, 1980.

Strout, Cushing. "William James and the Twice-Born Sick Soul." *Daedalus* (Summer 1968), pp. 1062–82.

Sulloway, F. J. *Freud, Biologist of the Mind.* New York: Basic Books, 1979.

Sutter, Jean. "Les Attitudes directives chez Pierre Janet, leur portée et leur limites." *Phychotherapy and Psychosomatics,* 29:358–360, 1978.

Taine, Hippolyte Adolphe. *The Modern Regime.* New York: Henry Holt, 1980.

Taylor, Eugene. "William James on Psychopathology: The 1896 Lowell Lectures on 'Exceptional Mental States.'" *Harvard Library Bulletin,* 30(4):455–479, 1982.

———. *William James on Exceptional Mental States.* New York: Scribners, 1983.

Taylor, G. R. *The Angel Makers.* London: Heinemann, 1958.

Taylor, W. S. "Pierre Janet." *American Journal of Psychology,* 60:637–645, 1947.

Temkin, Owsei. *The Falling Sickness.* Baltimore: Johns Hopkins Press, 1945.

Texas Reports. Gulf, Colorado and Santa Fe Railway Company v. J. O. Hayter, 93:239–243, 1900.

———. J. H. Hill et al. v. H. H. Kimball, 76:210–217, 1890.

Thomsen, Robert, and H. Oppenheim. "Uber das Vorkommen und die Bedeutung der Sensorischen Anasthesie bei Erkrankungen des Zentral Nervensystems." *Archiv für Psychiatrie,* 15:559–583, 633–680, 1884.

Thornton, E. M. *Hypnotism, Hysteria and Epilepsy: An Historical Synthesis.* London: Heinemann Medical Books, 1976.

Tibbits, Flora Woodward. "Neurasthenia: The Result of Nervous Shock as a Groound for Damages." *Central Law Journal,* 59:83–89, 1904.

Tomlinson, J. C., and W. Haymaker. "Jean-Martin Charcot." *Archives of Neurology and Psychiatry,* 77:44–48, 1957.

Toulouse, Edouard. *Emile Zola: Enquête Médico-Psychologue.* Paris: Société d'Editions Scientifiques, 1896.

Trotter, Thomas. *A View of the Nervous Temperment.* Newcastle: Edward Walker, 1807.

Veith, Ilza. "English Melancholy and American Nervousness." *Bulletin of the Menninger Clinic,* 32:301–317, 1967.

———. *Hysteria: The History of a Disease.* Chicago: Univ. of Chicago Press, 1965.

————. "On Hysterical and Hypochondriacal Afflictions." *Bulletin of the History of Medicine*, 30:233–240, 1956.

Vigouroux, A., and P. Juquelier. *La Contagion Mentale*. Paris: Doin, 1905.

Vizetelly, Ernest. *Emile Zola, Novelist and Reformer*. London: John Lane, 1904.

Wagner von Jauregg, J. "Richard von Krafft-Ebing." *Wiener Medizinische Wochenschrift*, 42:2305–11, 1908.

Walker, Edwin. "An Unusual Hysterical Symptom Group." *Archives of Medicine*, 10:85–88, 1883.

Wallon, H. "Pierre Janet, psychologue réaliste." *Bulletin de Psychologie* (Nov. 1960), pp. 154–156.

Walton, G. L. "Two Cases of Hysteria." *Archives of Medicine*, 10:88–95, 1883.

Walton, Richard. "What Became of the Degenerate?" *Journal of the History of Medicine and Allied Sciences*, 11:422–429, 1956.

Weber, Marianne. *J. J. Moreau de Tours 1804–1884, und die experimentalle und therapeutische Verwendung in Haschisch in der Psychiatrie*. Zurich: Juris Verlag, 1971.

Weiner, Dora [D. B.]. "The Apprenticeship of Philippe Pinel." *American Journal of Psychiatry*, 136:1128–34, 1979.

————. "Health and Mental Health in the Thought of Philippe Pinel: The Emergence of Psychiatry During the French Revolution." *Healing and History: Essays for George Rosen*. Ed. C. E. Rosenberg. New York: Science History Publications, 1979.

Weitzenhoffer, André. "What Did He (Bernheim) Say?" Postscript and addendum, in *Journal of Clinical and Experimental Hypnosis*, 28:252–260, 1980.

Westernhagen, Curt von. *Wagner: A Biography*. Cambridge: Cambridge Univ. Press, 1977.

Wettley, Annemarie. "Zur Problemgeschichte der 'Degenerescence.'" *Suffhoff's Archiv*, 43(3):193–212, 1959.

Whytt, Robert. *Works*. Edinburgh: Balfour, Auld, & Smellie, 1768.

Wiener, Philip. "G. M. Beard and Freud in 'American Nervousness.'" *Journal of the History of Ideas*, 117:269–274, 1956.

Winslow, Forbes. *On the Obscure Diseases of the Brain and Disorders of the Mind*. London: John Churchill, 1868.

Wolfgang, M. E. "Pioneers in Criminology: Cesare Lombroso." *Journal of Criminal Law and Criminology*, 52:361–391, 1961.

Wyckoff, James. *Franz Anton Mesmer: Between God and Devil*. Englewood Cliffs, N.J.: Prentice Hall, 1975.

Young, Robert. *Mind, Brain and Adaptation in the Nineteenth Century*. Oxford: Clarendon Press, 1970.

Zeldin, Theodore. *Ambition and Love, France 1848–1945*. New York: Oxford Univ. Press, 1979.

————. *Anxiety and Hypocrisy, France 1848–1945*. New York: Oxford Univ. Press, 1981.

————. *Politics and Anger, France 1848–1945*. New York: Oxford Univ. Press, 1979.

————. *Taste and Corruption, France 1848–1945*. New York: Oxford Univ. Press, 1980.

Zilboorg, Gregory, and George Henry. *A History of Medical Psychology*. New York: Norton, 1953.

Zola, Emile. *Le Docteur Pascal*. Paris: Livre de Poche, 1978.

————. *La Fortune des Rougon*. Paris: Livre de Poche, 1978.

————. *Germinal*. Paris: Livre de Poche, 1978.

————. *Nana*. Paris: Livre de Poche, 1978.

INDEX

PERMISSIONS (continued)

Thanks are due to the following authors, museums, galleries, archives, and publishing houses for permission to use materials included:

American Medical Association
Chicago, Ill.
Photograph of George Beard in *Archives of Neurology and Psychiatry*, p. 427, vol. 10 (1923). Copyright 1923, the American Medical Association.

Basic Books
New York, N.Y.
Photographs of the Wolf-man, Therese and the Primal Scene in *The Wolf-man: The Double Story of Freud's Most Famous Case* by the Wolf-man, ed. by Muriel Gardiner (1971). Copyright 1971 by Basic Books, Inc., Publishers. Reprinted by permission of the publishers.

Courtesy of the Francis A. Countway Library of Medicine
Harvard University
Boston, Mass.
Prints of *Pinel Freeing the Madwomen at the Salpêtrière* by Antoine Fleury, *A Clinical Lesson of Dr. Charcot at the Salpêtrière* by André Pierre Brouillet, and *Docteur Charcot* by Dr. Renouard

Bibliothèque Nationale
Paris, France
Intérieur d'un Omnibus and *Magnétisme Animal* by Honoré Daumier

Art Museum of Chicago
Chicago, Ill.
Saint Martin and the Beggar by El Greco

University of Chicago Press
Chicago, Ill.
Man with electrodes attached to his head in Charles Darwin, *Expression of the Emotions in Man and Animals* (1965), reprinted from Guillaume Duchenne, *Mécanisme de la Physionomie Humaine* (1862).

Credo-Verlag
Würzburg, West Germany
Photograph of Louise Lateau in Johannes Maria Höcht, *Träger der Wundmale Christi*.

Courtesy of the Fogg Art Museum, Harvard University
Cambridge, Mass.
Bequest—Collection of Maurice Wertheim, class of 1906
La Gare St-Lazare by Claude Monet

Mary Evans Picture Library of London
London, England
Photograph of Sigmund Freud

Grenada Publishing, Ltd.
St. Albans, Hertfordshire, England
Photograph of hydrotherapy in Harry Keen (ed.), *Triumphs of Medicine* (1976).

Hamburger Kunsthalle
Hamburg, West Germany
Wanderer in a Sea of Mist by Caspar David Friedrich

Studios Janet-Le Caisne
Paris, France
Photograph of Pierre Janet

Courtesy of the Alan Chesney Medical Archives
The Johns Hopkins Medical Institutions
School of Medicine
Baltimore, Md.
The Four Doctors by John Singer Sargent

Kunsthistorisches Museum
Vienna, Austria
Saint Katherine of Siena by Giovanni Battista Tiepolo

The Makins Collection
Washington, D.C.
Mariana by John Everett Millais

Medizinhistorisches Institut
Universität Zurich
Zurich, Switzerland
Photographs of Auguste Ambroise Lièbeault and Hippolyte Bernheim

Collection of the Mutual Assurance Company
Philadelphia, Penn.
John Singer Sargent portrait of S. Weir Mitchell, M.D.
Photography by Will Brown

Casa Editrice Roberto Napoleone
Rome, Italy
Tattoos in Cesare Lombroso, *L'Uomo Delinquente* (1971).

Ny Carlsberg Glypotek
Copenhagen, Denmark
The Absinthe Drinker by Edouard Manet

Philosophical Library
New York, N.Y.
The phrenological brain in A. A. Roback and T. Kiernan, *Pictorial History of Psychology and Psychiatry* (1969).

Oxford University Press
Oxford, England
Photograph of John Hughlings Jackson in *Neurological Biographies and Addresses* (1956).

Alfred A. Knopf
Random House
New York, N.Y.
Sketch of William James by himself in F. O. Matthiessen, *The James Family* (1947).

Stiftung Oskar Reinhart
Winterthur, Switzerland
The Chalk Cliffs of Rügen by Caspar David Friedrich

Benno Schwabe and Company
Basel, Switzerland
Portrait of Paul Verlaine in Gerhart Haug, *Verlaine: Die Geschichte des Armen Lelian* (1944).

The Tate Gallery
London, England
Beata Beatrix by Dante Gabriel Rossetti and *King Cophetua and the Beggar-Maid* by Edward Burne-Jones

Studio Noël Viron
Lourdes, France
Photograph of St. Bernadette of Lourdes

Richard-Wagner-Museum
Bayreuth, West Germany
Photograph of Richard Wagner

The Walker Art Gallery
Liverpool, England
The Murder by Paul Cézanne

Wallraf-Richartz-Museum
Cologne, West Germany
The Stigmatization of Saint Francis by Peter Paul Rubens